Cases in Paediatric Critical Care Transfer and Retrieval Medicine

T0201406

Cases in Paediatric Critical Care Transfer and Retrieval Medicine

Edited by
Shelley Riphagen
Evelina London Children's Hospital

Sam Fosker
Evelina London Children's Hospital

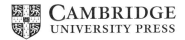

CAMBRIDGE
UNIVERSITY PRESS

University Printing House, Cambridge CB2 8BS, United Kingdom

One Liberty Plaza, 20th Floor, New York, NY 10006, USA

477 Williamstown Road, Port Melbourne, VIC 3207, Australia

314–321, 3rd Floor, Plot 3, Splendor Forum, Jasola District Centre, New Delhi – 110025, India

103 Penang Road, #05–06/07, Visioncrest Commercial, Singapore 238467

Cambridge University Press is part of the University of Cambridge.

It furthers the University's mission by disseminating knowledge in the pursuit of education, learning, and research at the highest international levels of excellence.

www.cambridge.org
Information on this title: www.cambridge.org/9781108931113
DOI: 10.1017/9781108946438

© Cambridge University Press 2022

First published 2022

Printed in the United Kingdom by TJ Books Limited, Padstow Cornwall

A catalogue record for this publication is available from the British Library.

ISBN 978-1-108-93111-3 Paperback

Contents

List of Contributors viii
Preface xv
List of Abbreviations xvi

1 **Models of Care** 1
Shelley Riphagen

2 **Logistics and Organisation** 3
Shelley Riphagen and Karen Starkie

3 **Air Retrieval** 7
Karen Starkie

4 **Improving Team Performance** 13
Shelley Riphagen and
Karen Starkie

5 **I Like Children, but I Don't Fancy Intubating One …** 19
Rumiko King and Joanne Perkins

6 **Upper Airway Obstruction** 29
Gareth Waters and Andrew Nyman

7 **Just Bronchiolitis?** 35
Sam Fosker and Shelley Riphagen

8 **Foreign Body Aspiration** 41
Alexander Hall and Andrew Nyman

9 **A Child with Facial Swelling** 48
Michael Carter and
Shelley Riphagen

10 **Pneumonia and Empyema** 53
Elizabeth Daisy Dunn and
Marilyn McDougall

11 **The Child with a Cough and Concerning White Cell Count** 59
Jo Dyer and Maja Pavcnik

12 **Worsening Stridor, to Intubate … or Not to Intubate** 65
Joanna Davies and Shelley Riphagen

13 **Difficult Asthma** 70
Christopher Hands and
Andrew Nyman

14 **Transfer of Child with Pulmonary Hypertension** 74
Kenneth MacGruer and
Alison Pienaar

15 **A Blue Baby** 79
Joanna Davies and Shelley Riphagen

16 **A Shocked Blue Baby Who Won't Improve** 84
Jenny Budd and Shelley Riphagen

17 **Under a Spell** 89
Catia Pinto and Miriam
Fine-Goulden

18 **A Decline in Function** 94
Shelley Riphagen

19 **Rash, Tachycardia and Irritability** 99
Shelley Riphagen

20 **Is the Baby's Heart Rate Supposed to Be Slower than Mine?** 105
Olga Van Der Woude and
Shelley Riphagen

21 **A Pale Lethargic Girl** 109
Maria Gual Sanchez and
Shelley Riphagen

22 **Too Fast for Comfort** 116
Sarah Hardwick and
Miriam Fine-Goulden

23 **Chickenpox and Other Bugs** 122
Michelle Alisio and Marilyn
McDougall

24 **When Amoxicillin Just Doesn't
Cover It** 127
Michael Carter and Marilyn
McDougall

25 **Tumour Lysis** 135
Jo Dyer and Shelley Riphagen

26 **Respiratory Insufficiency on
Maximal Support: Is That It?** 141
Federico Minen and Jon Lillie

27 **Cardiac Arrest** 148
Abi Whitehouse and Jon Lillie

28 **A Neurosurgical Emergency** 154
Livia Procopiuc and Alison Pienaar

29 **A Fall from Height** 159
Caroline Smith, Sam Fosker and
Shelley Riphagen

30 **Brain against the Clock** 165
Tanmay Toteja and Sam Fosker

31 **When Vomit Turns to Blood** 171
Anna Canet Tarres and
Shelley Riphagen

32 **Bilious Vomiting and Distended
Abdomen? Let's Find
a Surgeon** 178
Xabier Freire-Gomez and
Alison Pienaar

33 **What Can't Go Down, Must
Come Up** 185
Emily Cadman and
Alison Pienaar

34 **Not All Burns Can Be Seen** 191
Alex Williams and Ariane Annicq

35 **Drowning and Organ Donation** 197
Emma Prower and Joanne Perkins

36 **The Cold Shocked Child** 202
Sam Fosker and Shelley Riphagen

37 **Encephalopathy** 207
Fiona Bickell and Shelley Riphagen

38 **Adolescent Psychosis and Seizures:
Infection, Ingestion or
Encephalitis?** 210
Sasha Herring and Marilyn McDougall

39 **The Collapsed Neonate** 216
Ain Satar and Shelley Riphagen

40 **A Floppy Breathless Child** 221
Sam Fosker and Shelley Riphagen

41 **Fever in the Time of COVID-19
(SARS-CoV2)** 227
Marilyn McDougall

42 **A Palliative Care
Transfer Home** 231
Miriam Fine-Goulden and Jo Laddie

43 **A Story that Just Doesn't
Add Up** 237
Emma Smith and Shelley Riphagen

44 **Multidrug Overdose: A Practical
Guide to Stabilisation
and Transfer** 243
Nav Somasinghe and
Joanne Perkins

45 **Death Is a Possible Outcome** 248
Dawn Knight and Shelley Riphagen

46 **A Cold, Unconscious 12-Year-
Old Girl** 253
Louisa Brock and
Marilyn McDougall

47 **Another Collapsed Neonate** 259
Hannah Hayden and
Maja Pavcnik

48 **The Challenges
of Chemotherapy** 263
Heather Burnett and Maja Pavcnik

49 **Diarrhoea and Vomiting** 267
Georgina Humble and
Shelley Riphagen

50 **A Life-Threatening Sickle Cell Crisis** 272
Juan Ramon Valle Ortiz and
Shelley Riphagen

51 **A Baby with Acute Liver Failure** 277
Marilyn McDougall

52 **Air Transport of a Critically Ill Baby** 281
Joanna Davies and
Shelley Riphagen

53 **Crew Resource Management** 288
Sam Fosker

54 **Chest Drain Insertion** 293
Marilyn McDougall

55 **Paediatric Airway Clearance for Acute Management on Retrieval** 299
Rosalie Summers

56 **Use of Ultrasound for Paediatric Retrieval** 303
Ariane Annicq

57 **Vasoactive Drugs on Retrieval** 306
Benedict Griffiths

Index 311

Colour plates can be found between pages 142 and 143.

Contributors

Editors

Sam Fosker is an anaesthetic trainee with an interest in pre-hospital and retrieval medicine and is currently undertaking a clinical fellow role at the Evelina London Children's Hospital and South Thames Retrieval Service. He is a Fellow of the Academy of Wilderness Medicine and has worked on projects in multiple different countries.

Shelley Riphagen is a South-African and Canadian-trained paediatric intensivist and clinical lead for the South Thames Retrieval Service, integrated within the Evelina London Children's Hospital PICU. She has a keen interest in retrieval medicine and triage and the electronic technology to support this. She continues to jointly deliver a successful paediatric critical care advanced practitioner training programme for senior nurses and allied health professionals that started in 2003.

Contributors

Michelle Alisio is a South-African trained paediatrician working at the Royal London Hospital as a Senior Clinical Fellow in Paediatric Emergency Medicine (PEM). She is currently assisting in creating an online PEM teaching programme with Don't Forget the Bubbles. Outside of work, she enjoys being in nature, travelling and music. She draws inspiration from Nelson Mandela's quote 'There can be no keener revelation of a society's soul than the way in which it treats its children.'

Ariane Annicq is a paediatrician from Belgium who has specialised in paediatric intensive care and retrieval medicine since 2014, having worked in a number of international models of care. She became a consultant at the Evelina London Children's Hospital in 2019. She is continuing to develop the Paediatric Critical Care Advanced Practitioners Masters' program with Riphagen. Ariane has a special interest in point-of-care ultrasound (POCUS) and is a POCUS trainer.

Fiona Bickell is currently the Lead Nurse for PICU and the South Thames Retrieval Service at the Evelina London Children's Hospital. She has been a paediatric intensive care nurse for over 25 years and has a passion for retrieval and transport medicine. Her appointment as Lead Nurse will enable her to enhance the experience of families in PICU and ensure the development of PICU nurses of the future.

Louisa Brock is an Adult and Paediatric Emergency Medicine Consultant working in South West London. She completed a year-long post Certificate of Completion Training secondment with South Thames Retrieval Service to gain more experience in retrieval medicine and stabilisation of the critically unwell child. Prior to settling in London, she worked in Emergency Departments in Wales, Manchester and South Africa and is grateful for the varied and valuable experience these places have offered her. Away from work she enjoys horse riding, triathlons and supporting Welsh rugby.

Jenny Budd is a paediatric intensive care nurse with 20 years of experience within this speciality. Budd is a qualified Advanced Nurse Practitioner (ANP) and is the nursing lead for ECMO at the Evelina London Children's Hospital. She is proud to be part of an outstanding team at Evelina and South Thames Retrieval Service. She hopes that this book provides useful information for those undertaking paediatric retrieval.

Heather Burnett is an ANP working on PICU at the Evelina London Children's Hospital, and for the South Thames Retrieval Service. She previously worked on the PICU at St Mary's Hospital.

Emily Cadman is a final year paediatric emergency medicine trainee from London. She studied in Bristol and started training in the south west. Early experiences in training gave her a taste for retrieval and transport medicine and her younger self wishes this book existed back then. As well as acute and emergency medicine, she interested in medical education, ethics and law and is Vice-Chair of a London research ethics committee.

Anna Canet Tarres is a paediatrician from Spain who has been training in paediatric intensive care since 2017. Since September 2019, she has been a PICU fellow at the Evelina London Children's Hospital and part of the South Thames Retrieval Service.

Michael Carter is an NIHR Academic Clinical Lecturer in Paediatrics at King's College London, and Sub-speciality Registrar in Paediatric Intensive Care and Retrieval Medicine at Evelina London Children's Hospital. He works in the Schools of Life Course Sciences, and in Dr Shankar-Hari's group (Immunology and Microbial Sciences) to investigate the pathophysiology of severe inflammation following cardiac surgery and in sepsis. He aims to take a 'life course' view of our patients in intensive care, acknowledging that the consequences of each admission to an intensive care unit will have profound importance for a patient's long-term health.

Joanna Davies trained at the Nightingale School of Nursing. She has worked in PICU for 27 years and has been a Retrieval Nurse Practitioner (RNP) for South Thames Retrieval Service for the last 14 years. She is co-author for *Children in Intensive Care: a Survival Guide*, now on its third edition.

Elizabeth Daisy Dunn is a senior paediatric trainee, with a particular interest in high dependency care in unwell children, simulation training and medical education. Having been part of the team at the Evelina London Children's Hospital Paediatric Intensive Care Unit, she is now currently undertaking a Medical Education Fellowship in Paediatrics at St George's Hospital, and is also an honorary senior lecturer at St. George's University of London Medical School. She is heavily involved in both undergraduate and postgraduate medical education and is herself undertaking a Postgraduate Certificate in Healthcare and Biomedical Education. Having trained both within London and the surrounding area, Dunn hopes this book will help to educate and inform all those involved in the care of unwell children, thus helping to provide better care to the patients they treat.

Jo Dyer has been a paediatric intensive care nurse since 2000, training in Southampton before joining the Evelina London Children's Hospital PICU team in 2006. She qualified as a RNP in 2014 and now works both as an RNP for South Thames Retrieval Service and a Band 7 nurse on the PICU.

Miriam Fine-Goulden is a paediatric intensive care consultant at the Evelina London Children's Hospital, Guy's & St. Thomas' NHS Foundation Trust and South Thames Retrieval Service for Children. She is an honorary clinical senior lecturer at King's

College London. She trained in the UK at Cambridge University and at University College London. She has written for *The Science of Paediatrics: MRCPCH Mastercourse* (Elsevier) and co-edited *Challenging Concepts in Paediatric Critical Care* (OUP). Her specialist interests include: ECMO, education, child mortality, healthcare policy and strategy and medical communications. She tweets @finegoulden.

Xabier Freire-Gomez is a qualified paediatrician trained in Spain, pursuing a career in paediatric intensive care. He has worked at the Evelina London Children's Hospital PICU as a senior fellow (ECMO and Airway Fellow) with a special interest in congenital heart disease and mechanical ventilation, including non-invasive ventilation. He's currently working as a critical care retrieval consultant in Barcelona and is very excited about his future job at RCHM PICU (Melbourne).

Benedict Griffiths is an intensive care and retrieval medicine consultant at the Evelina London Children's Hospital with South Thames Retrieval Service. He started his medical career as a physiotherapist. He has an interest in fluid shifts in critical illness and paediatric difficult airways.

Alexander Hall is a senior anaesthetic registrar with an interest in paediatric anaesthesia and difficult airway management. He is currently undertaking his advanced paediatric anaesthetic fellowship at the Evelina London Children's Hospital. Hall has an interest in peri-operative care and is completing a postgraduate diploma in anaesthesia and perioperative medicine.

Christopher Hands trained in paediatrics and paediatric intensive care in London. He is a clinical fellow in paediatric intensive care at Evelina London Children's Hospital, and an honorary lecturer in child health at the Liverpool School of Tropical Medicine.

Sara Hanna is a paediatric intensive care consultant at the Evelina London Children's Hospital. She is a Cambridge graduate and completed paediatric intensive care training at Guy's and St Thomas' and Royal Melbourne Children's Hospital. She is also Medical Director of the Evelina London.

Sarah Hardwick works as an ANP in PICU at the Evelina London Children's Hospital and for South Thames Retrieval Service. She joined Evelina in 2000 and qualified as an ANP in 2009. Prior to this she worked in children's and adult nursing in various settings after qualifying in 1991.

Hannah Hayden is a UK-trained paediatric intensivist with an interest in organ donation, retrieval medicine, global health and education. She has worked in many countries overseas including teaching on ETAT+ Courses as well as Masters of Health Professions Education in Somaliland with King's Somaliland Partnership.

Sasha Herring began her nursing career in Australia and worked in PICU at the Royal Children's Hospital Brisbane. Since 1998 she has been at the Evelina London Children's Hospital, beginning her training as an RNP in 2003. Her area of special interest is the continuing professional development of non-medical prescribers who are prescribing for children.

Georgina Humble qualified as a paediatric nurse at Kingston University. Post qualifying she started working in PICU at St George's Hospital and after 7 years relocated to PICU at the Evelina London Children's Hospital to undertake ANP training. She currently works as a paediatric critical care ANP for South Thames Retrieval Service and in the PICU.

Paul James is South-African and British-trained doctor who has specialised in paediatric anaesthesia and intensive care. His main areas of interest are paediatric airway management, paediatric cardiac anaesthesia and ECMO. He also enjoys taking these skills outside the UK and works for a number of charities including Healing Little Hearts, Chain of Hope and Medical Education for Kenya. Outside work he is never off his bike or running up a hill and enjoys long distance ultra-triathlons.

Rumiko King is an anaesthetic registrar at St. George's Hospital in London with interest in paediatric anaesthesia.

Dawn Knight. After nearly 11 years practicing as a corporate lawyer Knight qualified as a children's nurse in 2002 from Southbank University London. On qualification she joined Evelina London Children's Hospital and after a 1-year rotation, joined PICU where she remains. She qualified as an RNP in 2013 and shortly after as a non-medical prescriber. Since then she has consolidated this RNP role and developed as an ANP on PICU.

Jon Lillie is a paediatric intensivist and ECMO lead at the Evelina London Children's Hospital. Having worked across six PICUs and three ECMO centres, he has realised that there are different valid approaches to the same problem and dogma prevents improvement within paediatric critical care. The right answer is not always offered by those that shout the loudest and there may not even be a 'right' answer. Through research and teamwork, he hopes to enjoy the next 20 years, improving care and knowledge within the speciality. He tweets @DrJonLillie.

Kenneth MacGruer is a final year paediatric intensive care medicine (PICM) trainee. After studying in Edinburgh, he trained in paediatrics in Manchester and Melbourne before starting PICM in Evelina London Children's Hospital.

Marilyn McDougall completed her paediatric training in Cape Town, South Africa and now works as a full-time paediatric intensive care consultant at the Evelina London Children's Hospital and South Thames Retrieval Service. She is the Clinical Director of the South Thames Paediatric Network and an honorary senior lecturer at Kings College London. She enjoys teaching and has developed a particular interest in simulation education. She co-authored *Children in Intensive Care: A Survival Guide*, now in its third edition and published by Elsevier in 2018.

Federico Minen is an Italian-trained paediatrician who moved to the UK to specialise in paediatric intensive care. Currently a senior fellow in the Evelina London Children's Hospital paediatric intensive care, he has a special interest in cardiac diseases, airway management and procedural sedation.

Andrew Nyman is a paediatric intensive care consultant at the Evelina London Children's Hospital, Guy's & St. Thomas' NHS Foundation Trust and South Thames Retrieval Service for Children. He is an honorary clinical senior lecturer at King's College London. He obtained his medical training in South Africa and completed paediatric specialisation in the UK, with further subspecialty training in Australia. His specialist interests include: bronchoscopy and airway pathology, ECMO, clinical research and health informatics.

Juan Ramon **Valle Ortiz** completed paediatric training in Spain and is currently working in paediatric intensive care and anaesthesia.

Maja Pavcnik is a paediatric intensive care consultant at the Evelina London Children's Hospital, Guy's & St. Thomas' NHS Foundation Trust, and South Thames Retrieval Service for children. She is from Slovenia and has worked in a number of international models of care. Her specialist interests include: education, retrieval medicine and child mortality.

Joanne Perkins is a consultant in paediatric intensive care and in paediatric anaesthesia at the Evelina London Children's Hospital. She completed medical training in Ireland and came to London to complete post-Certificate of Completion Training fellowship in paediatric intensive care. Her areas of interest include audit, education and medicine safety.

Alison Pienaar has worked as a consultant in paediatric intensive care at the Evelina London Children's Hospital Guy's and St Thomas' Foundation Trust and South Thames Retrieval Service from 2013. She is an Honorary Clinical Senior Lecturer at King's College London. She completed her training in South Africa and her areas of clinical interest include transport medicine, extracorporeal life support and patient safety.

Catia Pinto is currently training to become an ANP at the Evelina London Children's Hospital. She started her intensive care training in an adult cardiac intensive care unit where she developed an interest in congenital heart disease. She later specialised in a PICU at Great Ormond Street Hospital before moving to Evelina in 2019 to start her ANP training.

Livia Procopiuc is a German trainee in anaesthesia and adult intensive care currently pursuing an out of programme Fellowship in Paediatric Intensive Care at the Evelina London Children's Hospital and the South Thames Retrieval Service.

Emma Prower is a senior registrar in Intensive Care Medicine based at Kings College Hospital. She has a particular interest in intensive care outreach and the deteriorating patient.

Maria Gual Sanchez studied medicine in Barcelona and then moved to Madrid (Hospital Universitario La Paz) for her paediatric training. The last part of her training was focused on the critically ill child. Since September 2019 she has been a PICU fellow in Evelina Children's Hospital and part of the South Thames Retrieval Service.

Ain Satar is a trainee paediatrician working in the Evelina PICU. As part of her training she is developing a particular interest in allergy, simulation and high dependency care. Satar is a passionate educationalist currently completing a Postgraduate Certificate in Medical Education, and is active in both undergraduate and postgraduate education in London.

Caroline Smith is a maxillofacial clinical fellow at the Royal London Hospital having worked previously in other maxillofacial teams and dental practice. She is a Dental Officer in the British Army and has a Masters in Humanitarianism and Conflict Response.

Emma Smith is a senior paediatric registrar who has trained at a number of central London hospitals including Evelina Children's Hospital, where she spent a year working on PICU and as part of the South Thames Retrieval Team. She has a special interest in paediatric high dependency care as well as simulation.

Nav Somasinghe is an adult nephrology and intensive care medicine trainee with an interest in retrieval medicine and pre-hospital care.

Karen Starkie is a paediatric, intensive care nursing sister based at the Evelina London Children's Hospital. She has been retrieving for over 17 years and is currently the South Thames Retrieval Service Co-ordinator.

Rosalie Summers is a Highly Specialist Paediatric Respiratory Physiotherapist who has worked within Evelina London Children's Hospital and its PICU since 2005. Physiotherapists are an integral part of the PICU team within Evelina and Rosalie feels confident this improves patient care. She has a keen interest in using her knowledge of ventilation and physiotherapy techniques to treat critically unwell children often at the point of admission. She has led work developing an online learning package to assist in training her physiotherapy colleagues and the wider multidisciplinary team, ensuring effective quality care for all.

Tanmay Toteja is a paediatric intensive care trainee presently at the Royal Brompton Hospital, London. He trained as a paediatrician in New Delhi, India and then in London at the Imperial College NHS trust and the Evelina London Children's Hospital. Initially trained in neonatal intensive care, he is currently pursuing PICM training. He has a keen interest in medical education, simulation learning (part of the London School of Paediatrics simulation programme), cardiac intensive care and retrieval of sick children.

Olga Van Der Woude is an anaesthetist from the Netherlands who moved to the UK after completing her specialist training in Utrecht, the Netherlands. She specialised in paediatric anaesthesia at Royal Manchester Children's Hospital and currently is a Senior Clinical Fellow in Paediatric Cardiac Anaesthesia and Intensive Care at the Evelina London Children's Hospital.

Gareth Waters is a UK PICM Grid trainee, currently working on PICU at the Evelina London Children's Hospital. His background is in anaesthesia, and he trained in the Oxford Deanery, after having studied medicine at the University of Oxford.

Abi Whitehouse is a general paediatric registrar with special interests in both respiratory and HDU medicine. She enjoys cycling, walking and sewing alongside completing her paediatric training. Whitehouse also has a keen research background, with a PhD in paediatric respiratory medicine and ongoing research projects looking at interventions to prevent the health effects associated with air pollution exposure.

Alex Williams is an ANP. He works at Evelina London Children's hospital on Paediatric Intensive Care and South Thames Retrieval Service. He has worked in PICU since 2010.

Preface

The Service

The South Thames Retrieval Service (STRS) is a paediatric emergency inter-hospital transfer service for critically ill children. Integrated within the Paediatric Intensive Care Unit (PICU) at the Evelina London Children's Hospital (ELCH), it operates two retrieval teams 24/7 all year round.

STRS is the hub of a Paediatric Critical Care Network for South London and the South East of England, serving 20 district general hospitals in the region and three network PICU's in South London at the Evelina, St George's Hospital and Kings College Hospital.

STRS supports the care of children presenting critically ill to their local hospitals from the first referral call until resolution of the case. This support is facilitated through a dedicated phone line. The calls are taken by doctors (PICU fellows) or paediatric critical care retrieval advanced nurse practitioners, who are able to take details of the referral and provide immediate advice to referrers. Calls are then triaged by the responsible retrieval consultant, with additional resuscitation and stabilisation advice to the local team. The STRS team is dispatched to undertake the transfer, as soon as it is ascertained that the child will need ongoing critical care and it is necessary to transfer the child.

Over the past 20 years, STRS has transferred between 500 and 1000 children per annum, rapidly rising from lower levels in the year 2000 to current numbers. This has provided a huge number of interesting and challenging cases of very sick children, many of which are expanded in this book.

The Book

Learning from personal and from other's experience is a fundamental learning tool in medicine.

The aim of this book is to use challenging cases in the management of critically ill children, from presentation to transfer and admission to PICU to identify key learning from others' experience. It provides an opportunity to participate in the resuscitation, stabilisation and transfer virtually, without the stress associated with having the critically ill child and distressed family in front of you. It provides an opportunity to consider how you would have done things, perhaps differently, and review what was done. It has the benefit of seeing the case through from start to finish, so that personal management strategies applied can be reviewed without impact to the child. It also gives opportunity to learn from the good practice or insight of others and to take this learning forward, to ensure that the next child with similar presentation has the best outcome.

Abbreviations

(D+) HUS	Diarrhoea positive haemolytic uraemic syndrome
AKI	Acute kidney injury
ALL	Acute lymphoblastic leukaemia
ALT	Alanine aminotransferase
AML	Acute myeloid leukaemia
APLS	Advanced Paediatric Life Support
APTT	Activated partial thromboplastin time
APTTR	Activated partial thromboplastin time ratio
ARDS	Acute respiratory distress syndrome
ASD	Atrial septal defect
AV	Atrioventricular
AVNRT	Atrioventricular node re-entry tachycardia
AVPU	Alert, verbal, pain, unresponsive
AVRT	AV re-entry tachycardia
BE	Base excess
BNP	Brain natriuretic peptide
BP	Blood pressure
BPD	Bronchopulmonary dysplasia
Bpm	Beat per minutes
BSPED	British Society of Paediatric Endocrinology and Diabetes
BTS	British Thoracic Society
BVM	Bag valve mask ventilation
CATS	Children's Acute Transport Service
CDH	Congenital diaphragmatic hernia
CHD	Congenital heart disease
CNS	Central nervous system
CO	Cardiac output
CPAP	Continuous *positive airway pressure*
CPAP/BiPAP	Continuous/bilevel positive airway pressure
CPR	Cardiopulmonary resuscitation
CRP	C-reactive protein
CrUSS	Cranial ultrasound
CSF	Cerebrospinal fluid
CT	Computed tomography
CVVH	Continuous veno-venous haeomofiltration
CXR	Chest X-ray/radiograph
DBD	Donation after brain death
DCD	Donation following circulatory death
DGH	District general hospital
DKA	Diabetic ketoacidosis
DNAR	Do not attempt cardiopulmonary resuscitation
DOPES	Displacement, obstruction, pneumothorax, equipment, stomach

ECG	Electrocardiogram
ECMO	Extracorporeal membrane oxygenation
ENT	Ear, nose, throat
ESR	Erythrocyte sedimentation rate
ETCO$_2$	End-Tidal Carbon Dioxide
ETT	Endotracheal tube
FiO$_2$	Fraction of inspired oxygen
GAS	Group A *Streptococcus*
GCS	Glasgow Coma Scale
HDU	High dependency unit
HFNC	High flow nasal cannula
HFOV	High frequency ventilation
HIE	Hypoxic ischaemic encephalopathy
HR	Heart rate
HUS	Haemolytic uraemic syndrome
ICP	Intracranial pressure
INR	International Normalized Ratio
IV	Intravenous
IVIG	Intravenous immunoglobulin
LMA	Laryngeal mask airway
MAP	Mean airway pressure
MAS	Meconium aspiration
MCCD	Medical Certificate of Certification of Death (usually referred to as 'death certificate')
MHI	Manual hyperinflation
MRI	Magnetic resonance imaging
MRSA	Multi-resistant *Staphylococcus aureus*
NBP	Non-invasive blood pressure
NDMA	N-methyl-D-aspartate receptor
NICE	National Clinical Institute of Excellence
NICU	Neonatal intensive care unit
NIV	Non-invasive ventilation
NPIS	National Poisons Information Service
NSAID	Non-steroidal anti-inflammatory drug
ODT	Organ donation team
OPA/NPA	Oropharyngeal/nasopharyngeal airways
OSI	Oxygen saturation index
OI	Oxygenation index
PALISI	Paediatric Acute Lung Injury and Sepsis Investigators
PaO$_2$	Partial pressure of oxygen
pCO$_2$	Partial pressure of carbon dioxide
PCR	Polymerase chain reaction
PCT	Procalcitonin
PDA	Patent ductus arteriosus
PEEP	Positive end-expiratory pressure
PEG	Percutaneous endoscopic gastrostomy
PFO	Patent foramen ovale

PICU	Paediatric intensive care unit
PIM-TS	Paediatric Multisystem Inflammatory Syndrome – Temporally Associated with SARS-CoV-2
POCUS	Point of care ultrasound
PT	Prothrombin time
PEA	Pulseless electrical activity
PVL	Panton-Valentine Leukocidin
RBC	Red blood cells
RCPCH	Royal College of Paediatrics and Child Health
RICP	Raised intracranial pressure
ROSC	Return of spontaneous circulation
RR	Respiratory rate
SA	Sinoatrial
SaO$_2$	Arterial oxygen saturation
SCIWORA	Spinal cord injury without radiological abnormality
SCUBU	Special Care Baby Unit
SIRS	Systemic inflammatory response syndrome
SMA	Spinal muscular atrophy
SNOD	Senior Nurses in Organ Donation
SOFA	Sequential (or sepsis-related) organ failure assessment
SORT	Southampton and Oxford Retrieval Service
SpO$_2$	Pulse oximetry
STRS	South Thames Retrieval Service
SV	Stroke volume
SVR	Systemic vascular resistance
SVT	Supraventricular tachycardia
TAPVD	Total anomalous pulmonary venous drainage
TGA	Transposition of the great arteries
TLS	Tumour lysis syndrome
TSS	Toxic shock syndrome
VBG	Venous blood gas
VILI	Ventilator-induced lung injury
VSD	Ventricular septal defect
VT	Ventricular tachycardia
WCC	White cell count

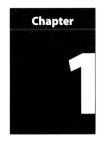

Chapter 1

Models of Care

Shelley Riphagen

Paediatric Critical Care Retrieval Services

Since 1995, Paediatric Critical Care Retrieval has been growing and developing in the UK. In the late 1990s, Paediatric Retrieval was delivered by almost every PICU in the United Kingdom with over 20 services of varying size, throughout the country.

In 1997, the South Thames Retrieval Service (STRS) was established to deliver paediatric critical care retrieval for the PICU at Evelina Children's hospital, based at Guys hospital at that time, and additionally for two smaller specialised PICU's at Kings College(hepatology, neurosurgery and trauma) and St George's hospitals (oncology, neurosurgery and trauma) in South London.

The number of children being admitted into these three intensive care units from South London and the South East of England, the most densely populated and rapidly growing area in the UK, meant that the retrieval activity quickly reached a critical mass. This justified the establishment of two teams, with availability 24/7 all year round. This remains the case today.

Integrated or Independent

While STRS amalgamated retrieval activity from three intensive care units very early on to achieve a cost-effective critical mass to deliver an excellent service, most other PICUs continued to deliver their own transfers. The exception, in the early 2000's was the establishment of the Children's Acute Transport Service (CATS), serving north London and North Thames. This service amalgamated the transfer activity from three PICU's in north London. The newly formed service moved out of its base at Great Ormond Street Hospital to develop the first stand-alone retrieval service, not integrated within any PICU.

Many retrieval services across the UK followed suit, with all except two of the ten present in 2020, regarded as 'stand-alone' services, and the service in South England – Southampton and Oxford Retrieval Service (SORT), based in the Southampton PICU – representing the only other integrated service.

Choosing the Best Model

There is no straightforward answer to the question of 'what is the best model of retrieval service?' The model chosen for regional retrieval needs to be a balance of activity, staffing, funding, accommodation for the service and many other factors.

There are advantages and disadvantages to both, as evidenced by the fact that throughout the rest of the world, including North America, Europe and Australia, good examples of both types of service, operating well, continue to exist.

The most important factors that keep STRS integrated in the Evelina PICU are:

- Significant national and international recruitment factor for nurses and doctors for the PICU/STRS.
- Ability to train doctors and nurses to solo competence/independent retrieval practice in a short time in the relative safety and with direct consultant supervision in the PICU or the Evelina operating theatres with the combined volume of work in PICU and STRS providing ample clinical experience.
- Flexibility of doctors and nurses to work between services as the need arises on a specific day, with the immediate availability of staff to step into a retrieval position if a team member calls in ill.
- Doctors and nurses can work clinically in the PICU, supporting colleagues, while awaiting tasking of the retrieval team, without risk of losing clinical skills or becoming bored in the quieter periods. Year-on-year for 23% of shift time, there is no retrieval activity, and this time can be spent supporting colleagues in PICU, for example undertaking in-hospital patient transfers to CT, MRI etc.
- Skill and knowledge levels of retrieval teams are maintained at high level due to ongoing clinical activity and exposure both on retrieval and in the PICU.
- Parents commend the fact that their child may be retrieved by a doctor or nurse the day before and then looked after by the same clinical team the following day or week. This provides huge comfort and continuity for the child and family, and some closure to the team regarding the outcome of care after transfer.
- Lastly drugs and equipment can be rotated from the retrieval service into the PICU to ensure that equipment used infrequently on retrieval but more commonly in PICU does not become out of date.

However, a significant compromise is that:

- The STRS working day is always clinically busy with little 'downtime' to recharge and reflect. Professional support with prevention of burnout and stress-related problems has become an increasing focus in medicine in general, with paediatrics and PICU considered high-risk areas. Time for case-based reflection needs to be part of the normal working day to mitigate this.
- Due to the clinically busy nature of the job, there is little time for publishing research or audit. Anything of this nature is generally undertaken in team personal time, above and beyond their clinical commitment
- Conflict of need can arise if the retrieval teams are not supernumerary to the PICU numbers. STRS does not work in this manner, and retrieval teams are rostered separately, above the clinical numbers required to undertake care in the PICU.

Logistics and Organisation

Shelley Riphagen and Karen Starkie

Organisation

The success of an organisation is dependent on some fundamental requirements being met. This is true for a retrieval service.

- There must be a clear and compelling **philosophy or mission** with a **shared sense of purpose** supported by all involved.
  - ○ The best critical care outcome for the child and family, delivered by expert teams working collaboratively, from presentation to discharge.
- A **culture of trust and respect** must exist within the organization.
  - ○ Every team member, involved in all aspects of care of child and family, is supported to deliver the highest quality of care.
- User friendly **systems** are in place that **augment service delivery.**
  - ○ Guidelines, drug calculator, referral algorithms, checklists improve speed and quality of care.
- There is a strong **focus** on the **end user.**
  - ○ The child and family's care must be optimised and the district general hospital and retrieval teams must feel valued and supported.
- The workforce must be **empowered** to deliver an **ever improving service** based on creative ideas and problem-solving identified at the front line.
  - ○ Good ideas, creative thinking and problem solving from the point of delivery of care must be encouraged. New ways of working should challenge old dogma and be positively supported to drive improvement.

Logistics

The logistics of the retrieval process must be clearly articulated, documented and practiced so that the complex task of retrieval becomes simple and automatic.

- The referral call is received via a single paediatric critical care network referral number.
- The telephone call and all the clinical information must be recorded digitally for record, legal and audit purposes.
- The call is taken by a clinically capable individual who can document and prioritise relevant clinical information quickly.
- After or while the call is taken, it must receive immediate paediatric critical care retrieval consultant attention for triage, further advice and outcome decision.
- If and when retrieval has been agreed, all members of the team must be activated swiftly.

- Pre-checking of equipment, drugs and travel routes must complete within the shortest time possible. Preferably some checks should be completed at shift start.
- Once activated, and en route to the child's bedside, the team must make contact with the referrers for update status of the child.

Checklists

Checklists of repeated processes and tasks ensure that these can be undertaken at speed, under pressure without important aspects being omitted, independent of the team experience.

STRS has a number of checklists seen below in Table 2.1 to ensure standardisation and speed, independent of clinical teams.

Table 2.1. STRS Checklists

STRS checklists	Details
Ambulance start shift	Complete vehicle checks: fuel, tyres, brakes, check vehicle clean. All electrical equipment is on charge and in good working order. Oxygen cylinders three-quarters full or above and operational.
Retrieval team start shift	Check and prepare equipment; ventilators, emergency grab bag restocked and sealed, to ensure team can launch quickly.
Retrieval team call activation	Prepare patient/weight-specific equipment; ventilator, airway adjuncts, drugs, including controlled/fridge drugs and fluids. Print drug and equipment calculator.
Pre-departure at base	Paperwork; medical, nursing, parent information, emergency drug calculation sheet. Destination hospital and receiving PICU details and phone numbers. Mobile phone with base consultant contact numbers.
Pre-departure in ambulance	All kit present: cardiac monitor, suction, defibrillator, infusion pumps fully charged and working. Oxygen cylinders checked and turned on, spare identified, oxygen splitter present for use in theatres. Weight-appropriate ambulance securing harness or baby pod available for use. Stretcher secured safely in floor bracket, ambulance inverter activated. Team introduce themselves, confirm fit to travel, confirm hospital destination.
Pre-departure after stabilisation	Ensure patient has identification band and parents aware of transfer. Airway patent, secure and suctioned, spare airway equipment to hand, ventilation adequate and oxygen cylinders full plus an extra cylinder. Patent IV access ×2, with an extension set 'rescue line' attached, emergency drugs sedation, paralysis and fluid boluses prepared and available. Monitor physiological alarms set, pupils checked and lubrication applied if intubated, blood gas and glucose checked. Urinary catheter inserted if required or clean nappy. Referring hospital notes, X-rays copied for transfer, STRS consultant and receiving PICU updated on interventions, infusions, condition and ETA.

Table 2.1. (cont.)

STRS checklists	Details
Pre-departure, child in ambulance	Patient secured safely on stretcher and stretcher secured in vehicle. All equipment secured in place, accessible and charging. Ambulance power supply activated (inverter), ventilator switched from oxygen cylinder to ambulance wall supply. Parent shown where to sit and informed of need to remain seated and secured (seatbelt) at all times, even in an emergency.
Child delivered to PICU, pre team departure	Full patient handover given by the medical and nursing team. All patient's notes, results and paperwork handed over to the receiving team. Drug infusion doses checked and confirmed, social issues, safeguarding concerns or incidents are handed over to the receiving team. Parents are introduced and shown where to wait.
Kit restocking	On arrival back at base team complete 'hot debrief' to identify areas of good practice and what could have worked better, and to ensure all are physically and psychologically well. The team then take the used kit and drugs to retrieval base, clean and restock ambulance and kit, and take a short break.

Air retrieval adds an additional layer of complexity to retrieval.

- Weather adds a degree of unpredictability. Temperature control of patient and team must be added to checklist.
- Where there is no helipad on site, a road transfer is required on either side of the team either arriving at the child or at the PICU, and the logistics and communication of this must be added to checklist.
- Air-retrieval-specific checklists should be in place.

Data Quality and Audit

- All members of the service are responsible for data accuracy.
- All data relating to the referral and the retrieval must be recorded on a written or electronic form.
- Data quality and accuracy should be reviewed in a time-sensitive manner so that where there are questions regarding information recorded, this can be validated by the team members involved, with direct memory that is fresh enough to be accurate.
- Retrieval data must be captured electronically at some point in the process of retrieval, so that activity can be audited daily, weekly, monthly and annually.
- The reporting and recording of clinical and other incidents must be encouraged and made easy, so that patterns can be detected and learning instituted.

- Where there is learning that may pertain to other retrieval services, there should be a mechanism to share information in an anonymous but timely manner with other retrieval services.
- Activity data covering quantity and quality of service delivery must be published and available to the network clinical teams so that performance can be evaluated and acted upon.
- Service activity should be benchmarked against other similar services to ensure performance is optimised.

Air Retrieval

Karen Starkie

Logistics

Tasking an Air Retrieval

Ambulance road transfers are the easiest and most economic means of transferring an intensive care patient over relatively shorter travel distances. They account for 97% of all STRS patient transfers but represent a smaller proportion for other teams internationally, where air retrieval can represent up to 15% of the transfer activity, dependent on a combination of geography, aircraft and landing site availability and patient acuity.

When distance, speed of retrieval or urgency of team attendance are critical, aeromedical transfer should be considered.

This may be in the form of rotary (helicopter) or fixed wing (aeroplane) aircraft.

Rotary Transfer

The aircraft used in the inter-hospital transfer helicopter service provided for children in the UK are bespoke, purpose-designed vehicles equipped for children's intensive care support in the air and funded entirely charitably through the Children's Air Ambulance (Figure 3.1). The significant advantages of rotary transfer are avoidance of airport delays, with significantly reduced travel times, the ability to transfer hospital to hospital and to avoid the effects of altitude and acceleration, experienced with fixed wing air transfers. These have to be weighed against the disadvantages of confined space, noisy environment, increased communication challenges, lack of access to mains electricity, limited number of providers and the flight restrictions imposed by weather.

Fixed Wing

Aeromedical fixed wing transfers have the added advantage of being almost unrestricted by weather, along with more room to treat the patient. There is less noise, communication is easier and it is also easier for the team to undertake medical and nursing interventions.

Fixed wing aircraft have the advantage of speed and over-water flight; however, access to airports, travel time to and from airport to hospital, and set landing time are significant limitations. There are additional clinical considerations relating to the effects of altitude on hypoxia and gas expansion, and the acceleration/deceleration effects on cardiovascularly or neurologically unstable children.

Due to the fact that fixed wing transfers are commonly used for longer distance transfers, and staff are undertaking prolonged, high concentration work in a hypoxic

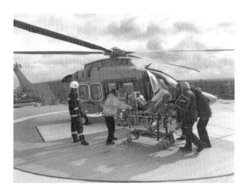

Figure 3.1 The Children's Air Ambulance preparing for a retrieval. (A black and white version of this figure will appear in some formats. For the colour version, please refer to the plate section.)

environment, greater planning is required to ensure the team are able to take rest and sleep breaks to maintain patient safety.

As a retrieval service, it is important to be ready for any eventuality.

Forward planning saves time and lives. Easy accessibility to contact details of reputable air providers is essential. Staff and patient safety is paramount. STRS will only undertake aeromedical transfers, rotary or fixed wing, if the aircraft has two pilots available during transfer.

Other Considerations

- Space available on board.
- Facilities on board: oxygen piped or cylinders only. Check cylinders have both a flow meter and Schraeder valve outlet and patient ventilator is compatible with the valve.
- All equipment and kit must be safely secured at all times in the aircraft.
- Cost of the aircraft transfer and whether medical personnel from the air provider have to accompany the team. This provides the benefit of the team being able to remain as medical passengers but may reduce the opportunity for one or both parents to accompany their child on flight transfer.
- Ambulance transfer from airport to patient bedside and back to aircraft.
- Requirement to refuel during transfer.
- Commercial flights are often more difficult to organise as the times and dates are less flexible, securing equipment and oxygen more challenging. and there is limited room to operate in the cabin, usually in full public view.
- Large airports usually have a medical centre available for the team prior to boarding.

Landing Sites

- Hospital helipad or helideck makes inter-hospital transfers smoother and faster by reducing patient bed to bed transfer time. Not all helipads are lit, restricting 24-hour use.
- If there is no helipad on site, a secondary road transfer will be required. Arranging the ambulance in advance is essential. Check compatibility of ambulance trolley with air stretcher, ability to secure equipment safely in vehicle, and confirmed expected time of arrival to prevent patient and team waiting in a field. Clear instructions regarding pick

up point are essential. Using the 'what3words' app will help ambulance crews find the team's exact location.

- A second ambulance transfer may also be required from the airfield to the receiving PICU or hospital. The more land transfers required, the longer the journey and potential increase in delays, incidents and patient instability. Adding all these time points may negate the usual time saving afforded by air transfer.

Team

- Team composition is dependent on staff availability and experience, number of seats and weight of personnel for rotary wing aircraft transfers. One team member must be flight trained.
- A parent is usually taken in preference to a third team member.
- All members of the team, including the parent, must declare themselves 'fit to fly'.
- International medical flights require the same identification and visa approvals as non-medical flights. The patient and parent also require valid travel documents.

Parents

STRS always tries to accommodate at least one parent to accompany their child during retrieval. For flight transfers the parent must be able to speak good English, to understand emergency instructions from the pilot.

Flight Equipment

- Establish how the patient can be secured in the aircraft: vacuum mattress, stretcher compatible with aircraft, baby pod, or incubator. Patient-securing harnesses and straps must be flight certified and compatible for both road and air if a secondary road transfer is required.
- Medical equipment must be flight certified and able to be secured safely in the aircraft (Figure 3.2).
- Flight bags size and contents (Table 3.1) should be minimised to essentials only (Figure 3.3).

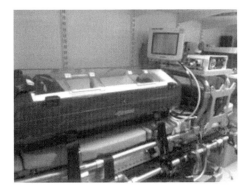

Figure 3.2 Baby pod secured to air stretcher. (A black and white version of this figure will appear in some formats. For the colour version, please refer to the plate section.)

Table 3.1. Flight bags

Cabin Bag	Intervention Bag
Patient-specific airway bag	Cannulation pack
Controlled drugs and cardiac arrest drugs"	Intubation kit
Grab pouch	Nasogastric and catheter pack
Intra-osseous vascular access kit (e.g. EZ IO)	Chest drain kit
Paperwork	Arterial kit
Pneumothorax kit	Central line kit
Oxygen equipment	IV fluids pack
IV equipment	Cricothyroidotomy kit
IV fluids in flight	

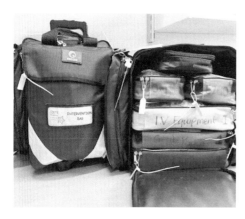
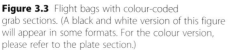

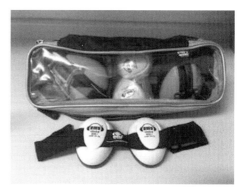

Figure 3.4 A selection of in-flight patient ear defenders. (A black and white version of this figure will appear in some formats. For the colour version, please refer to the plate section.)

Figure 3.3 Flight bags with colour-coded grab sections. (A black and white version of this figure will appear in some formats. For the colour version, please refer to the plate section.)

- Essential equipment includes: portable suction with yankaur and suction catheters; portable manual suction unit; cardiac monitor with ECG, pulse oximetry, non-invasive blood pressure with age appropriate cuff and temperature probe. Capnography is standard of care if the patient is ventilated. Invasive pressure monitoring is ideal if the patient is requiring inotropic support; however, these infusions must be run through syringe drives not via pressure bags.
- A back up monitor, defibrillator or pulse oximeter and extra leads should also be available. Take extra straps to ensure all equipment can be secured.
- Portable syringe infusion pumps should be used in preference to fluid bags where air within the bag will expand during fixed wing flights and potentially infuse the incorrect amount.
- To ensure patient comfort, ear defenders (Figure 3.4) should be worn during rotary flights. Temperature must be actively managed using a suitable patient warming device:

for example, Transwarmer, Cositherm, incubator, blankets, as the cabin temperature decreases with altitude.

- Intubation and emergency drugs should be drawn up if the patient is intubated, along with fluid boluses and inotropic infusions. Ensure all essential drugs and equipment remain in the cabin with the patient.
- Spare batteries for the monitor and infusion pumps should be packed and stored in a suitable, certified container in case of battery content leakage.

Extra Considerations
- Medical and flight paperwork
- Passport for international flights
- Food and drink if a long flight, tissues and vomit bags
- Warm clothes, jacket, gloves, umbrella if raining and head torches for evening transfers
- Mobile phone and contact numbers of air desk, base, receiving hospital and team, ambulance provider if secondary transfer required
- Confirm flight details with base team before departure.

Pre-departure Checks
Prior to departure it is essential to complete safety checks (Table 3.2) to ensure everyone is well and all equipment or patient specific kit is packed.

Table 3.2. Pre-departure flight checks

Pre-departure checks	Details
Medical team & parent	Name, weight, flight trained, helmet size, all team fit and well to fly? Parent checklist completed, fit to fly, able to understand English and instructions during the flight. Maximum luggage – 5 kg bag.
Patient	Name, weight, condition, patient securing harness/baby pod, ear defenders, flight restrictions, i.e. fly at sea level, one way transfer.
Equipment & weight	Air stretcher with securing device to hold all equipment; cardiac monitor, ventilator, drug infusion pumps, suction. Medical kit required for stabilisation, usually one for use in cabin and medical intervention bag in the hold, along with the clip deck required for stretcher transfer. All equipment weighed and air desk informed during tasking process.
Medical gases	Calculate oxygen requirement for flight, then double the volume (see STRS oxygen calculator). Check oxygen cylinders available with flow meter and Schrader valve, compatible with ventilator.
Pick up/drop off points/times	Paperwork – nursing/medical, tasking form, parent information booklet. Clear plan of destination, landing site/airport and receiving hospital, 'contact numbers at destination and base contact if any issues arise. Confirm with flight provider and have contact details in case of any issues.
Land ambulance	Will an ambulance transfer be required to take team from helipad to hospital and back and to the receiving destination. Confirm arrangements pre departure quoting HELIMED call sign. Identify location with 'what3words' and have contact numbers in case of any issues.

Patient Safety during Flight

Rotary wing transfers are less challenging to the medical team as the helicopter flies at lower altitude. This reduces complications caused by gas expansion, reduction in temperature and hypoxia associated with increase in altitude.

Further Reading

Oxygen Calculator, STRS Aeromedical Guidance. www.evelinalondon.nhs.uk/resources/our-services/hospital/south-thames-retrieval-service/Aeromedical-transfer-2017.pdf

Improving Team Performance

Shelley Riphagen and Karen Starkie

The Retrieval Team

There are a number of components of retrieval where improvements can be achieved through either organisational elements or through team training.

Team members must know who they are working with for the shift, and as a team they should have pre-checked a number of elements at the start of the shift. This ensures that when a call comes in and is accepted for transfer, there is minimal delay and fewer items to check.

Where possible, equipment should be stored in the ambulance and checked by the team in situ at the start of each shift (Figures 4.1a and 4.1b). An ambulance checklist is completed and signed at the commencement of each shift to ensure this is undertaken and auditable. A second ambulance checklist, regarding the vehicle itself, must be completed by the ambulance technician.

For STRS, the patient monitor with all the requisite leads and monitoring devices, defibrillator, suction device, infusion pumps, glucometer, baby pod and stretcher all remain in the ambulance.

STRS has a standard kit bag which is restocked after every retrieval, checked for completeness, and returned to the ambulance, pending the next retrieval. Inside the box,

(a)

(b)

Equipment wall with electrical appliances safely secured and charging.

    A   Cardiac monitor
    B   Defibrillator
    C   Non invasive ventilators
    D   Ventilator
    E   Intravenous infusion pumps
    F   Suction
    G   Nitric oxide bracket
    H   Stretcher with leads
    I   Equipment bridge

Figure 4.1 (a) STRS bespoke ambulance interior; (b) Ambulance equipment wall checklist. (A black and white version of this figure will appear in some formats. For the colour version, please refer to the plate section.)

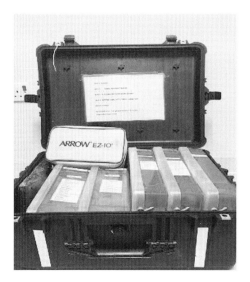

Figure 4.2 Ambulance kit box. (A black and white version of this figure will appear in some formats. For the colour version, please refer to the plate section.)

(a)

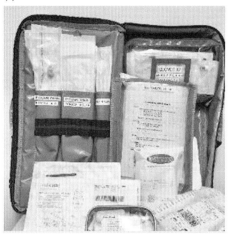

(b)

Pleural catheters, straight soft radio-opaque
10Fr x 200mm, 12Fr x 250mm, 16Fr x 450mm
Portex seldinger chest drain 12Fr x 300mm; 18Fr
Heimlich drainage valve
Triple lumen CVP catheter set: 5Fr x 5cm, x 8cm, x 15cm
General procedure pack
Sterile gloves Size 6-8 x 2 each
Y connectors, straight connectors, luer lock connector
Straight mosquito forceps x 2
Surgical blade size 10, size 15
Sterile scissors, suture needle holder
Lignocaine
Biopatches
Silk sutures 2.0 x 2

Figure 4.3 (a) Central venous access and chest drain kit. (b) Central venous access and chest drain box contents. (A black and white version of this figure will appear in some formats. For the colour version, please refer to the plate section.)

all elements are arranged in a systematic order in subsection boxes with a checklist on each box lid. This means when the team are looking for disposables, they are easy to locate and when restocking, only the opened boxes need to be restocked. Once restocked, boxes are sealed and signed to identify they are complete and checked. This saves an enormous amount of time at the bedside, but also when restocking (Figure 4.2).

Over the past 17 years, STRS has systematically reduced the kit in the bag. Only the essentials are taken, on the assumption that most district general hospitals (DGH) use similar equipment, and it will be available. For tasks that are rarely undertaken, such as chest drain insertion and tracheostomy, the equipment required is stored in the ambulance in separate boxes (Figures 4.3a and 4.3b). This is only brought to the bedside when required. The equipment in these boxes is checked monthly to ensure it remains within expiry date and circulated into the PICU stock within three months of expiry.

Medications Used on Transfer

Drug commonly used on retrieval are prepacked by the pharmacy into small labelled boxes, and stored in the main pharmacy retrieval box (Figure 4.4). STRS has undertaken three audits over the past 15 years looking at commonly used drugs on retrieval and the drug bag contains only these to avoid drug wastage (Table 4.1).

Table 4.1. STRS pharmacy supplies

Pharmacy pack with individual boxes

Box A	Adrenaline 10 mg/10 ml
Box B	Propofol 200 mg/20 ml; sodium bicarbonate (8.4%)10 ml
Box C	Adrenaline 1 mg/10 ml (1in 10,000); hydrocortisone 100 mg; calcium gluconate 2.2 mmol in 10 ml
Box D	Milrinone 10 mg/10 ml; noradrenaline 4 mg/4 ml (1 in 1000)
Box E	Adenosine 6 mg/2 ml; flumazenil 500 mcg/5 ml; phenytoin sodium 250 mg/5 ml; salbutamol 5 mg/5 ml
Box F	Atrophine sulphate 600 mcg/1 ml; chlorphenamine maleate 10 mg/1 ml; frusemide 20 mg/2 ml; magnesium sulphate 4 mmol/2 ml
Box G	Thiopental sodium 500 mg
Box H	Dopamine HCl 200 mg/5 ml
Box I	Potassium chloride 20 mmol/10 ml (15%). Controlled drugs. Sodium chloride polyfuser 2.7% in 500 ml (referred to as 3% hypertonic saline)

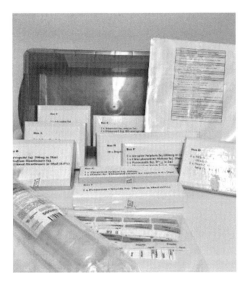

Figure 4.4 Nurse drug fridge pack and controlled drug box. (A black and white version of this figure will appear in some formats. For the colour version, please refer to the plate section.)

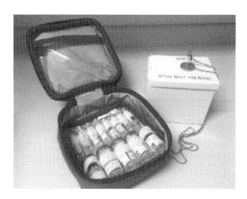

Figure 4.5 Nurse drug fridge pack and controlled drug box. (A black and white version of this figure will appear in some formats. For the colour version, please refer to the plate section.)

Rarely, when children need unusual drugs, the specific drug is taken from the intensive care stock. The exception to this is for metabolic drugs, where a prepacked STRS metabolic drug box and calculator are kept in the PICU drug room, for the occasions when these are required. Children needing these drugs are usually clearly identified prior to retrieval being activated.

The retrieval nurse also packs controlled drugs (CD), including ketamine, fentanyl, morphine and midazolam, used during and after intubation. The CDs are kept in a locked cabinet in the main PICU drug store room and need to be checked out by two retrieval nurses for every retrieval (Figure 4.5).

Fridge drugs such as rocuronium, suxamethonium, prostaglandin and lorazepam are stored in a fridge pack, kept refrigerated in the PICU drug room and only removed for each specific retrieval. Portable ice packs keep them cold during retrieval

Team Training

Retrieval Team

The efficiency of the team with respect to the timed element of retrieval can be monitored and reported.

The team attempt to mobilise retrieval within 20 minutes of the call being accepted. The national standard for mobilisation is 30 minutes.

In this 20-minute period the team must:

- call the DGH regarding decision to transfer
- check controlled and fridge drugs
- print off a patient specific drug calculator and
- ensure that the any drugs and fluids that are anticipated to be used on the retrieval and are not standard are added to the kit.

A patient-specific airway bag is packed by the retrieval lead including ambubag, anaesthetic circuit, appropriate sized masks, guedel airways, laryngeal mask airway and endotracheal tube (ETT) with laryngoscopes.

The retrieval lead ensures the correct ventilator and tubing for size of child, and correct sized end tidal CO_2 monitoring is packed and ready to take.

Twenty minutes passes quickly if the team do not work collaboratively.

Local Referring Team

En route to the child, much time can be saved by phoning ahead from the ambulance, for a clinical update from the team taking care of the child.

This allows time to be saved upon arrival, as there is often minimal additional information that needs to be relayed to the retrieval team after arrival if this catch-up call has been made.

On arrival at the DGH, any additional information that has not been relayed can be handed over. The retrieval team need to:

- Check the ETT is the correct size, in good position, patent, with good ventilation and no evidence of respiratory complications. The risk of the ETT becoming dislodged during transit must be actively minimised. For this reason, tube taping/strapping must be ultra-secure. The DGH anaesthetic team involved in the child's care can competently perform all these tasks and should be asked to do so.

- Good secure vascular access is essential. Depending on the clinical condition of the child, a number of appropriate sized, well placed and secured peripheral lines may suffice. Where the child has required resuscitation or is supported on inotropes, a central venous line is usually recommended. This is often challenging in critically ill children. The anaesthetic team can be tasked with central line insertion, under ultrasound guidance. If unsuccessful, the retrieval team should attempt vascular access with a strict time limit on attempts, and with a secure back-up plan to use external jugular or intra-osseous access if a central venous line cannot be secured in the crisis situation.

- If the blood pressure can be reliably read by non-invasive cuff measurements, an arterial line is not essential for transfer, or even ongoing intensive care in many situations. The insertion of an arterial line can wait until the child is admitted to PICU, if it is deemed necessary for ongoing care. This is not a life-saving, or life-changing procedure and time should not be wasted on undertaking this procedure if it proves difficult in an unstable child, provided a reliable cuff pressure can be obtained. Where children have had significant resuscitation and are on inotropes, or require targeted blood pressure, for example for neurosurgical emergency transfers, an arterial line is preferable but not essential.

- A nasogastric tube and urinary catheter is essential in a sedated, muscle-relaxed, ventilated child. A nappy may suffice for a baby. These are all tasks that can be undertaken by the local team nurses.

If the local team works well with the retrieval team, directing tasks required to undertake safe transfer (both from a medical and nursing point of view), the team can be ready to leave with the child fully prepared and made safe for transfer within 60 minutes of arrival at the bedside. This requires good directive leadership from the retrieval team and collaborative team working.

For every procedure that the retrieval team need to undertake, an additional 10 minutes are added to the stabilisation time.

Factors that commonly delay retrieval are:

- The child has been taken for CT scan or is awaiting a portable X-ray.
- Blood products, where necessary, have not been ordered.

- The child is profoundly unstable, and it is difficult to find the 'window' to leave safely with the child. In some instances, stabilisation may never be achieved but still has to be attempted. In this case the parents should be fully informed and the team need to take all the necessary precautions to deal with potential cardiac arrest en route.
- The responsible retrieval consultant should be updated regularly in the case of very unstable children and be made aware if the child is profoundly unstable, and likely to deteriorate significantly or arrest en route.
- The parents are not with the child and need to be recalled.
- A referral letter has not been written.

Team Training

One way we have found useful over the years to evaluate team training is to undertake simulated retrievals together.

- STRS team attendance at annual simulation training is compulsory for every team member. This demonstrates good practice, communication and leadership, and exposes practices that compromise team performance

The same training is offered to every one of the 20 DGH teams in the region, so that local anaesthetic, paediatric and emergency medicine doctors and nurses working locally can practice resuscitation and stabilisation of a critically ill child, in the form of a manikin.

- STRS uses real life cases from the region to identify learning and good practice to be shared with all teams.
- Although this training is not compulsory for staff not in the STRS team, it is generally well attended and very well evaluated, and those teams that train together in this manner, generally perform at a higher level and work better together, even though managing a critically ill child is a rare event.

Chapter

5

I Like Children, but I Don't Fancy Intubating One …

Rumiko King and Joanne Perkins

Introduction

When children become critically ill or suffer trauma, they are usually brought to their local hospital, where local teams are responsible for assessment, initial management and stabilisation of the sick child. Tracheal intubation is carried out, in the majority of cases, by local teams, rarely comprising paediatric specialist anaesthetists.

This chapter is aimed to help those anaesthetising children in these emergency situations.

Once the decision is made to intubate a child, it is important to prepare the equipment, drugs, patient, team and run through the likely course of events with plans for deterioration prior to undertaking this task.

Table 5.1. Indications for intubation

Indications for intubating a child may be anticipated, impending or already present:
- Maintain airway patency, e.g. upper airway obstruction, burns
- Protect the airway against aspiration, e.g. neurological dysfunction
- Support oxygenation or ventilation
- Reduce work of breathing and oxygen consumption and support failing haemodynamics
- Facilitate neuroprotection.

Prepare Equipment

The equipment below is required for all intubations and will allow management of difficult ventilation and intubation. If difficulty is anticipated, more advanced equipment in the correct paediatric sizes should be immediately available as well as a detailed escalation plan.

Table 5.2. Intubation equipment

Emergency intubation equipment:
Oxygenation:
- Face masks
- Oropharyngeal/nasopharyngeal airways
- Breathing systems (e.g. Ayres T piece for <25 kg, Mapleson C >25 kg)
- Nasal prong
- Suction (airway secretions and gastric contents)
- Nasogastric tube.

Table 5.2. (cont.)

Primary intubation:
- Laryngoscopes with blades × 2
- Endotracheal tube (ETT) (plus size above and below)
- Stylet
- Bougie
- Magill's forceps
- Lubrication gel
- Syringe (for cuffed tubes)
- Tapes to secure ETT.

Rescue oxygenation:
- Laryngeal mask airway.

Alternative strategies (if needed):
- Videolaryngoscopes
- Fibre-optic approaches
- Emergency surgical airway kit.

Oxygenation

A modified rapid sequence induction is advised. This involves:

- Pre-oxygenating the child via a manual ventilation circuit with positive end-expiratory pressure (PEEP).
- Gastric distention will rapidly impede ventilation. A nasogastric tube must be placed and aspirated continuously during mask ventilation to prevent this.
- Small children have limited respiratory reserve and will desaturate quickly with apnoea. This is exaggerated in the critically ill child with increased metabolic requirements. Gentle facemask ventilation is required after induction.
- Optiflow for apnoeic oxygenation may be of use to maintain saturation during laryngoscopy.
- Evidence for cricoid pressure to prevent aspiration is weak. It distorts the upper airway anatomy and should not be used routinely.
- If difficulties with oxygenation arise during induction, a two-handed, two-person technique should be used for mask ventilation with adjuncts (oropharyngeal/nasopharyngeal airways). Attention to finger placement is needed to avoid soft tissue compression.
- A supraglottic airway device (e.g. laryngeal mask airway) must be available for rescue ventilation.

Maintaining acceptable oxygenation is the primary goal of all airway management. Remember the saturation targets in some neonates with congenital heart disease may differ.

Intubation

Age and weight-based calculators for equipment size are readily available online or on paediatric emergency apps. These tools can help in preparing the correct size equipment.

Tracheal tubes are sized according to age, rather than weight. Equipment calculators for tube size are only useful over 1 year of age.

The following is a guide to size a tracheal tube in under 1's

- Neonates 2.5–3.5mm inner diameter
- Infants 3.5–4.0mm inner diameter.

Length of the tube can be determined either by the black depth markers on the tube being placed at the vocal cords or by using standard length calculation methods, which only apply over 1 year of age.

- Oral length (cm) = (Age/2) + 12
- Nasal length (cm) = (Age/2) + 15.

These length calculations should be confirmed appropriate by noting:

- Depth marking on the tube (thick black line) at the vocal cords
- Position at the lips or nose
- A consistent end tidal CO_2 trace
- Bilateral air entry
- Tube in the correct position on CXR. (Tip between thoracic inlet at T1 and carina at T4. Ideal tube placement is T2–3 neutral neck position.)

Do not cut endotracheal tubes (ETT's) until you have confirmed appropriate tube position on CXR.

Head movement in infants can easily displace the tube. ('Head up tube up.')

Endobronchial intubation in children is common and can quickly lead to contralateral lung collapse with subsequent hypoxia and hypercarbia.

The tube must be carefully securely to prevent migration or accidental extubation, which should never occur during the acute stabilisation or transfer phase.

Traditionally, uncuffed tubes have been used for children below 8 years of age. Newly designed cuffed tubes (e.g. Microcuff) allow for a better seal with less cuff pressure and have become popular in younger patients with difficult oxygenation or ventilation.

Cuffed tubes have some advantages over uncuffed tubes. These include:

- Avoidance of repeated laryngoscopy due to incorrect initial tube size
- Ability to deliver higher ventilatory pressures and PEEP.

Cuffed tubes, especially in critically ill neonates, should be used with caution due to the risk of subglottic stenosis in a child with borderline tracheal mucosal perfusion (e.g. in shock).

Blades

Laryngoscope blades comes in different shapes and sizes. Straight blades are traditionally used for neonates to lift up their long, floppy and U-shaped epiglottis but these can obscure the view of the glottis as the tube passes through the cords.

Those competent in the use of curved blades can continue to use the more familiar equipment. Common reasons for obtaining a poor view at laryngoscopy are using a blade that is too small and placing the child's head in the incorrect position.

Suction

A Yankaur suction should be placed near the patient's head,with an endobronchial suction catheter available to deal with any secretions in the chest or tube immediately after intubation. As a general rule, the size of the suction catheter is double that of the ETT inner diameter.

Preparing for Difficulty

When there is difficulty intubating, a stylet and bougie can be useful. A stylet can be particularly useful when using smaller ETT's which can kink easily, or when there is airway narrowing, such as in croup. The tip must not protrude beyond the ETT as this can cause airway trauma.

Videolaryngoscopes (e.g. AirTraq, Glideoscope or C-MAC) or fibre-optic broncho-scopes (e.g. 2.8 mm bronchoscope) can be prepared for anticipated difficult intubation.

Monitoring

Full cardiorespiratory monitoring is required when anaesthetising a critically ill child. Continuous capnography will confirm tube placement as well as giving information on adequacy of ventilation and cardiac output. If a capnography trace is completely flat or non-continuous, oesophageal intubation should be assumed until proven otherwise (**No trace = Wrong place**), and the situation corrected immediately.

Table 5.3. Intubation monitoring

Monitoring:
• Capnography
• Pulse oximeter (audible beeps)
• ECG
• Blood pressure (on 2-minute cycles)
• Stethoscope.

Prepare Drugs

Intubation Drugs

It is important to appreciate that most anaesthetic drugs, gases, analgesia and sedatives are myocardial depressants and blunt the sympathetic drive, causing vasodilatation. Safe induction can be challenging and haemodynamic decompensation is common.

The choice and dose of drugs used for induction and maintenance will depend on the cardiovascular and neurological status of the child. Most critically ill children require reduced doses to achieve adequate anaesthesia. Paediatric drug doses may be unfamiliar and so it is important to double check the drugs and doses prior to administration. Online drug calculators are helpful.

Table 5.4. Intubation drugs

Standard intubation drugs often used in paediatric critical illness are:
• Fentanyl 1–2 mcg/kg
• Ketamine 1–2 mg/kg
• Rocuronium 1 mg/kg.

Ketamine

This is the preferred induction agent in shock or haemodynamic compromise. It offers the most cardiovascular stability over other induction agents. Previous concerns about ketamine raising intracranial pressures are unfounded and hypotension caused by other agents is far more detrimental to patients with a traumatic brain injury. Increased secretions induced by ketamine may make intubation conditions less favourable.

Propofol

This is a less suitable agent in a critically ill child due to its hypotensive effects but would be the preferred agent in status epilepticus. Prior administration of anti-epileptic drugs can cause profound hypotension on induction. Dose reduction is necessary.

Fentanyl

Fentanyl is a synthetic opioid and exhibits some cardiovascular stability. It must still be carefully titrated as it is a sympatholytic and can cause hypotension by suppressing the stress-induced catecholamine response. High doses are associated with chest wall rigidity.

Rocuronium

This is the muscle relaxant of choice and produces ideal intubating conditions in 60 seconds. It has largely replaced suxamethonium with its many side effects (muscle pain, arrhythmias, hyperkalaemia, rise in intra-ocular and intracranial pressure, anaphylaxis and malignant hyperthermia).

Emergency Drugs

During induction of anaesthesia in critically ill children, instability should be anticipated and preparation for this eventuality put in place prior to induction.

- For bradycardias not related to hypoxia: atropine 20 mcg/kg
- For hypotension: 10–20 ml/kg fluid bolus (0.9% NaCl or Hartman's), phenylephrine 1–2 mcg/kg boluses, adrenaline 1 mcg/kg boluses
- For cardiac arrest: adrenaline 10 mcg/kg
- If the patient is haemodynamically unstable following adequate fluid resuscitation and requires inotropes, a peripheral inotrope infusion can be started prior to inserting a central line.

Post intubation Sedation

- Morphine 10–40 mcg/kg/hr
- Midazolam 1–4 mcg/kg/hr.

Overt awareness must be avoided in the paralysed child post intubation, but it must be remembered that high doses or multiple sedative agents are likely to cause cardiovascular instability. Awareness during transfer is psychologically traumatic, and in school-age children, low dose midazolam infusion can provide retrograde and antegrade amnesia, avoiding this situation. Short-term propofol infusions, at the recommended dose, can be used in older children (1–4 mg/kg/hr).

Prepare the Patient

Assess

A quick history and examination of the patient is required. It is important to find out about any allergies or drugs that should be avoided. An airway assessment will predict any difficulties that may be encountered.

Table 5.5. Predictors of a difficult airway

Anatomical predictors of difficult intubation:
- Previous difficult intubation
- Stridor and symptoms of upper airway obstruction
- Significant facial dysmorphism
- Small receding jaw
- Prominent overbite
- Syndromes with known difficult airways, e.g. Treacher Collins, mucopolysaccharidosis.

Anatomically difficult airways are rare in children. More commonly, difficult intubations are a result of:

- Incorrect choice of equipment, e.g. too small laryngoscope blade
- Incorrect positioning of head in extended position especially in younger children
- Underlying precarious physiology, leading to limited time and reserve.

IV Access

Check that IV access is secure and working before induction. Induction via an intra-osseous line may be required if venous cannulation is difficult and causing delays. IV access may be very difficult in critically ill children due to peripheral vasoconstriction. Scalp and long saphenous veins are useful places to look in neonates, with external jugular vein useful in older children in emergencies.

Optimisation

Failure to optimise the patient prior to and during intubation may increase the risk of life-threatening adverse events. General anaesthesia and the administration of positive pressure ventilation can worsen venous return and cause profound hypotension. Fluid boluses and the use of vasoactive drugs may be required to mitigate physiological derangements prior to intubation.

Position

A poor view at laryngoscopy is commonly due to poor patient positioning. The patient's head should be at the top of the bed at the correct height for the intubator. Neonates may require a neck/shoulder roll to achieve a neutral position due to their large head and prominent occiput.

Prepare the Team

Location

Where to intubate the child will depend on the clinical scenario, but it is usually done in A&E or in operating theatres. If the patient is too unstable for transport then the specialised equipment must be brought to the patient.

Assign Roles

These emergencies can be very stressful to everyone concerned and good teamwork and communication are key to a successful outcome. Intubation in an environment that is not your usual place of work with team members you may not have met before is challenging on its own. In order to minimise the situational risks, it is important to introduce team members, assign roles and plan ahead to allow for clear decision making.

Table 5.6. Roles during intubation

Assign roles:
- Team leader
- Primary intubator
- Secondary intubator
- Airway assistant
- Monitoring/drugs.

The team leader should not be the intubator. The intubator must work within their competencies and in a high-risk intubation, the primary intubator needs to be the most experienced person. The airway assistant's role is to hand over airway equipment to the intubator and provide external laryngeal manipulation if required. There should also be a dedicated person to administer drugs and someone to continuously monitor the patient's vital signs. Audio cues from the cardiac monitor should be optimised.

Team Briefing

If difficulties are anticipated, these should be discussed and management strategies verbalised to the team. The Difficult Airway Society' (DAS) has provided guidelines on management of difficult airways in children and this plan should be followed. Plan A to D of the intubation strategies must be stated and a clear upper limit for the number of attempts at each plan set. Fixation errors are common in these situations, and observers need to be empowered to raise concern if there is deviation from the set plans.

Checklist

The pre-procedural checklist improves safety and it is important to go through the emergency intubation checklist before induction (Figures 5.1 and 5.2).

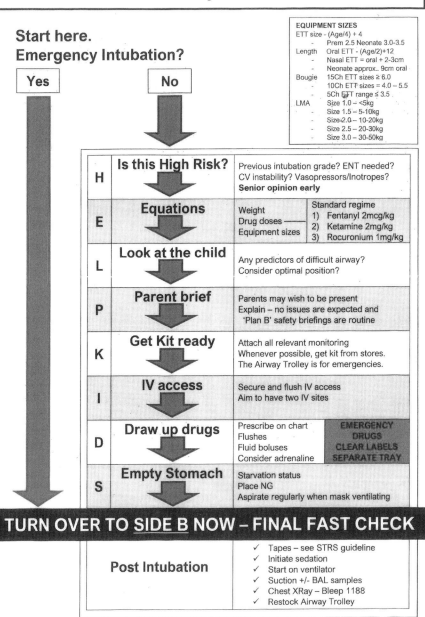

Figure 5.1 Example of intubation checklists – Intubation Pathway.

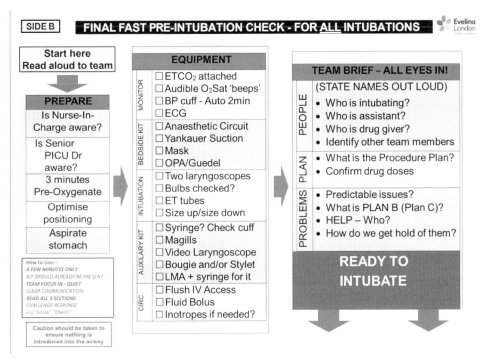

Figure 5.2 Example of intubation checklists – Final Fast Pre-Intubation Check.

Parental Presence

It is up to the team to decide whether to have parents present for induction and or intubation or not. Either way, a dedicated staff member should be present to support and manage parents at all times.

Post Intubation

It is important to prepare for instability after intubation and continue with resuscitation. Patients may become hypotensive once the stimulus of intubation has receded. Ventilation may be difficult.

Before Transfer

Table 5.7. Check before transfer

Check before transfer:
- CXR to confirm ETT position
- ETT properly secured with tapes
- Two IV access
- Ongoing sedation +/- muscle relaxation
- Pre-prepared drugs and fluids
- Establish ventilation on transfer ventilator
- Maintain euglycaemia
- Maintain normothermia
- Update parents
- Prepare transfer documentation.

Debrief

Treating critically ill and injured children can be distressing. After the event debriefing of the team should be conducted if possible. This will allow the team to express concerns and reflect on clinical practice in a supportive environment.

Improving Safety

Intubation of children in emergencies is rare and challenging. System-based measures can improve safety and these include standardisation of approach, dedicated paediatric and neonatal emergency equipment, use of checklists and multi-disciplinary team training in technical and non-technical aspects of emergency intubations. Regular simulation sessions are useful in keeping skills up to date. Regular audit of performance and review of cases in each department can also support staff to improve knowledge, reflect on how cases are managed and to identify areas for improvement.

Further Reading

The acutely or critically sick or injured child in District General Hospital: A team response. Department of Health, 2006. www.networks.nhs.uk/nhs-networks/north-west-north-wales-paediatric-critical-care/resources-1/Critically%20Sick%20Child%20in%20the%20DGH%20-DoH%20publication.pdf.

Cook TM, Woodall N, Frerk C. Major complications of airway management in the UK; results of the Fourth National Audit Project of the RCOA and DAS. *Br J Anaesthes* 2011;106(5):617–31.

Long E, Barrett MJ, Peters C, et al. Emergency intubation of children outside the operating room. *Paediatr Anaesthes* 2019; 30 (3):319–330. doi: 10.1111/pan.13784.

Paediatric Difficult Airway Guidelines 2015. http://www.das.uk/com/guidelines/downloads.html

South Thames Retrieval Service (STRS). http://www.strs.nhs.uk

Zeiler FA, Teitelbaum J, West M, Gillman LM. The ketamine effect on ICP in traumatic brain injury. *Neurocritical Care.* 2014;21 (1):163–73.

Upper Airway Obstruction

Gareth Waters and Andrew Nyman

An ex-premature infant, now 2 months corrected gestational age, is referred to your retrieval service. The baby was born at 24 weeks' gestation at a birthweight of 538 g. She was intubated and ventilated for the first 6 weeks of her NICU stay and since then has remained continuous positive airway pressure (CPAP) dependent, with a diagnosis of chronic lung disease. She was transferred as a step down to the referring hospital special care baby unit (SCUBU) 2 weeks ago. She weighs 3.4 kg now.

Over the last 3 days, the SCUBU team have noticed that the baby's work of breathing has been increasing and she has not been tolerating her CPAP breaks. At the time of referral to you, she is tachypnoeic at 80 breaths per minute, with significant work of breathing. Over the last 2 hours, she has developed biphasic stridor, which is new for her. Saturations are 85% in FiO_2 of 0.5, CPAP 6. She is tachycardic at 190 bpm (sinus rhythm), with well-maintained BP of 86/40, normal perfusion but increasing irritability.

Management so far by the SCUBU team has been to increase CPAP from 5 to 6, increase FiO_2, and initiate management for upper airway obstruction – dexamethasone 0.15 mcg/kg, plus adrenaline and budesonide nebulisers. There has been no clinical improvement with these interventions, and the SCUBU consultant has asked the team to refer her as she is concerned about airway obstruction that may need ENT input.

This morning's blood results are shown in Table 6.1.

Questions

1. What is the most likely underlying pathology and why is it important to consider this?
2. How would you anaesthetise this patient in order to safely secure her airway prior to transport?
3. Following induction of anaesthesia, the infant becomes apnoeic. Direct laryngoscopy is attempted, but reveals no view of the glottis (Cormack and Lehane grade 4). Attempts at bag mask ventilation are unsuccessful. The infant begins to desaturate. How do you proceed?

1. What is the most likely underlying pathology and why is it important to consider this?

This infant has upper airway obstruction, and the most likely pathology in this case is acquired subglottic stenosis in view of the prolonged period of intubation and ventilation

Table 6.1. Blood tests

Blood tests		Capillary blood gas	
Hb	128 g/dL	pH	7.42
White cell count	5.4 (10^3/mm^3)	pO$_2$	7.3 kPa
Platelets	412 (10^3/mm^3)	pCO$_2$	6.4 kPa
Na	141 mmol/L	HCO$_3^-$	22 mmol/L
K	4.9 mmol/L	Base excess	−1.0 mEq/L
Creatinine	27 U/L	Lactate	0.9 mmol/L
Urea	1.2 mmol/L	Glucose	5.8 mmol/L

Table 6.2. Aetiology of upper airway obstruction

Causes of airway obstruction	Characteristics
Transient post-intubation oedema	• Onset shortly after extubation • Good response to nebulised adrenaline and/or systemic steroids
Subglottic stenosis	• Stridor may be biphasic • Dyspnoea • Recurrent infections • History of intubation trauma
Laryngomalacia	• Presents within first few weeks of life • Inspiratory stridor, exacerbated by feeding or lying supine
Subglottic cysts	• History of tracheal intubation at birth (may be short duration) • Biphasic stridor
Subglottic haemagioma	• Asymptomatic at birth • Biphasic stridor age 2–6 months
Tracheomalacia	• Coughing • Expiratory stridor • Frequent infections • Acute life threatening events
Laryngeal cleft	• Feeding difficulties • Stridor • Cyanotic spells • Recurrent infections

and the inability to wean off CPAP. Other potential causes of airway obstruction are given in Table 6.2, with subglottic haemangioma an important consideration.

Subglottic stenosis can be congenital or acquired. Acquired subglottic stenosis is related to intubation, either trauma or tube size. Patients present with stridor (which may be biphasic), breathlessness or recurrent infections.

Table 6.3. McCaffery staging system

McCaffrey classification	Site involved	Length of stenosis (cm)
Stage 1	Confined to the subglottis **or** trachea	<1
Stage II	Confined to the subglottis	>1
Stage III	Both subglottis **and** trachea	N/A
Stage IV	Extends to the glottis. Fixation/paralysis of at least one vocal cord	N/A

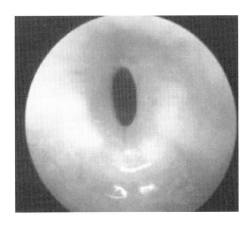

Figure 6.1 Tight grade 3 subglottic stenosis. (A black and white version of this figure will appear in some formats. For the colour version, please refer to the plate section.)

There are two classification systems for subglottic stenosis: the Myer-Cotton system is used for mature, firm, circumferential stenosis, confined to the subglottis. The four grades are based on the degree of reduction in the cross-sectional area of the subglottis, from grade 2 with 50–70% reduction, to grade 4 with no detectable lumen.

The McCaffrey classification system is based on the site and length of the stenosis. Four stages are described and specified in Table 6.3.

Diagnosis is established by diagnostic laryngoscopy, bronchoscopy (Figure 6.1), and oesophagoscopy, performed under general anaesthesia. Treatment choices for clinically significant subglottic stenosis are laser and/ or repeated balloon dilation with a success rate of approximately 73%.

In patients with severe narrowing, the treatment will initially be a tracheostomy to bypass the obstruction, and then at a later stage a laryngotracheal reconstruction. In this procedure, a wedge of cartilage taken from a costal cartilage is slotted anteriorly into a vertical incision made in the complete cricoid cartilage ring to increase the diameter of the airway lumen. Some stenotic lesions may also require a posterior cartilage wedge. After surgery, the airway is assessed and if the patency is adequate, the tracheostomy is decan-nulated after 3–6 months. Success rates are in the region of 80–90% for this surgery.

Postoperative ventilation for about a week after laryngotracheal reconstruction is common. Restenosis and long-term voice development remain major concerns.

2. How would you anaesthetise this patient in order to safely secure her airway prior to transport?

This child would classify as an airway emergency. She has symptoms and signs of severe airway obstruction and requires urgent attendance of the anaesthetic team as well as senior paediatric support.

Experience is important when deciding the need for tracheal intubation, and the urgency with which this should proceed. Immediate intubation should be considered in the case of increasing respiratory failure, indicated by:

- Rising $PaCO_2$
- Exhaustion
- Hypoxia (SpO_2 <92% despite high flow oxygen administered via mask)
- Decreasing level of consciousness.

This baby will need her airway definitively secured for transfer. This may be extremely challenging in a young infant with tight subglottic stenosis.

Planning for intubation should start at an early stage, particularly with regard to the personnel required. An early decision should be made regarding whether an ENT surgeon experienced in performing an emergency tracheostomy is required. This procedure in this age group will not have been performed by many surgeons and the level of anxiety in undertaking this will be high. It may take time to assemble an appropriately experienced and skilled team. Difficult intubation should be anticipated.

Ideally two experienced airway specialists should be present for intubation, with the most experienced one identified to lead the procedure. In paediatric retrieval medicine, this will often be the local anaesthetist and paediatric consultant experienced in neonatal intubation. A skilled anaesthetic assistant will help reduce stress levels. The ENT surgeon should be scrubbed and ready to perform a tracheostomy immediately if intubation is unsuccessful.

In the emergency situation, the airway and respiratory status override the requirement for a period of fasting before anaesthesia. In this situation, some precautions can be taken against the 'full' stomach, such as utilising a degree of head-up tilt and inserting a nasogastric tube to empty the stomach. The use of cricoid pressure and the rapid sequence induction has no place in this scenario. Pre-oxygenation is essential with standard anaesthetic monitoring.

It is important to consider that if the infant is still breathing and able to be transferred to theatre, the safest way to induce this patient will be using an inhalational induction with maintenance of spontaneous ventilation until airway is secure. Using sevoflurane in 100% oxygen provides maximal oxygenation, and the volatile agent also has useful bronchodilatory effects. Induction may be slow due to the compromised airway, and patience is required to achieve a deep enough plane of anaesthesia prior to attempting airway instrumentation.

If the child becomes apnoeic during induction, the upper airway should be kept patent using a chin lift, and a tight seal should be applied with the facemask, whilst waiting for the child to resume spontaneous ventilation. Airway obstruction may worsen due to loss of airway tone as anaesthesia deepens, but careful positioning, gentle application of jaw thrust and application of 5–10 cmH$_2$O of CPAP will generally maintain airway patency.

Once a suitable depth of anaesthesia (pupils small and central with no response to firm jaw thrust) has been achieved, IV access should be obtained if this was not already in place, before gentle laryngoscopy is attempted to allow assessment of the laryngeal inlet.

Intubation with an uncuffed endotracheal tube (ETT) that is considerably smaller than predicted must be anticipated. In older children a 'croup tube' (extra-long, standard diameter) may be useful. In extreme cases the subglottic narrowing may be so severe that it is necessary to 'intubate' the glottis with a bougie loaded with the smallest ETT that will take a suction catheter (2.5 mm internal diameter tube), and gently advance the well-lubricated ETT over the bougie.

Once the airway obstruction is bypassed, most infants will be easy to ventilate, except those who develop post-obstructive pulmonary oedema. Following intubation, the tracheal tube should be carefully secured at the correct depth to avoid any accidental dislodgement. The child should be sedated and paralysed to ensure the continued safety of the artificial airway. A CXR should be performed to confirm the tracheal tube position, and to exclude any other respiratory pathology.

The anaesthetist and other airway specialists should remain with the child until transfer to a suitable paediatric intensive care team has been completed. Detailed documentation of the difficulty and techniques used to access the airway successfully are important.

3. Following induction of anaesthesia, the infant becomes apnoeic. Direct laryngoscopy is attempted, but reveals no view of the glottis (Cormack and Lehane grade 4). Attempts at bag mask ventilation are unsuccessful. The infant begins to desaturate. How do you proceed?

This is a 'cannot intubate, cannot ventilate' (CICV) scenario, which is a life-threatening emergency. Continue to ventilate with two-person technique and apply 100% oxygen. All your help should already be around you. If the infant is not maintaining oxygen saturations above 80%, preparations should be made to proceed to tracheostomy immediately.

Standard airway opening manoeuvres and airway adjuncts should be used in a rapidly escalating manner. Gastric distention should be managed by passing a naso- or orogastric tube and allocating an individual to continuously empty the stomach using 50ml syringe aspiration of the tube.

The ENT surgeon should proceed to surgical tracheostomy. If adequate precautions have been taken and ENT called to attend in a timely manner, emergency cricothyroidotomy can be avoided. Most anaesthetists will never encounter this clinical situation in their career, especially in smaller children, and it should be avoided by preparation and anticipation. It is better to have called the ENT team to attend and not require their help, than to have to undertake this procedure in an emergency.

Further Reading

The Difficult Airway Society (DAS) and Association of Paediatric Anaesthetists (APA) Guidelines for difficult airway management in children. https://das.uk.com/guidelines/paediatric-difficult-airway-guidelines.

Ho AM-H, Mizubuti GB, Dion JM, et al. Paediatric postintubation subglottic stenosis. *Arch Dis Child* 2019;0:1. doi:10.1136/archdischild-2018-316517.

Maloney E, Meakin GH. Acute stridor in children. *Contin Educ Anaesthesia Crit Care Pain* 2007;7: 183–6. https://doi.org/10.1093/bjaceaccp/mkm041.

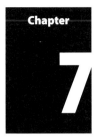

Just Bronchiolitis?

Sam Fosker and Shelley Riphagen

A 6-month old, 8-kg baby was brought into A&E by ambulance, after mother called 999 following a pale, blue, floppy episode at home.

The baby had been unwell for the previous 2 days with coryzal symptoms, poor feeding and was noted to be generally "not himself".

He had been born at 28 weeks gestation, remained in the special care baby unit on continuous positive airway pressure (CPAP) for the first 2 days of life, and then gradually improved, gaining weight and was well enough to be discharged home at 36 weeks and 2.3 kg. He had been thriving since discharge and was fully immunised.

On admission the following was noted:

- His temperature was unrecordable.
- During the first hour in A&E he had recurrent apnoeic episodes with associated bradycardia but was alert in between.
- Respiratory rate was 50 breaths per minute, saturations 98% in 3 L nasal cannula oxygenation.
- Baby had visible intercostal and subcostal recession and fine crackles on auscultation.
- Heart rate was 140 bpm with no heart murmur heard.
- His abdomen was soft with 3 cm liver palpable.
- He was moving and normally responsive to handling. Fontanelle was flat.

Initial blood gas and abnormal laboratory results are displayed in Table 7.1.

A referral call was made to the paediatric retrieval service because of the ongoing concern regarding recurrent apnoea and bradycardia, and the probable need for intubation and ventilation.

Questions

1. What management plan should you suggest to the referring team?
2. Before leaving to retrieve the child, you receive a call saying the child has been intubated but they are having difficulty with ventilation. How would you assess and manage this? What specific interventions should be carried out based on the X-rays sent to you?
3. When you arrive, the mother says she has two other children currently at nursery but needs to arrange care for them and can't the child be treated locally? What would you explain to the mother?

Table 7.1. Admission blood gas and key laboratory results

Bloods	Na 130 mmol/l
	Hb 129 g/L
	WCC 40.6
	(N 15, L 25)
Venous blood gas	pH 7.05
	pCO_2 11 kPa
	Base excess −8 Eq/L

Table 7.2. Criteria for severe respiratory disease

Saturations <92%
Respiratory rate >70 breaths per minute
Signs of severe respiratory distress
Apnoea
Decreased level of consciousness
A lower threshold for intervention should be used for high risk groups

1. What management plan should you suggest to the referring team?

The first question to ask before deciding on treatment strategy is whether this is an immediate or impending emergency. The answer is yes, this is an impending emergency requiring urgent treatment before it deteriorates further. The baby has respiratory failure with signs of decompensation. Emergency respiratory support is required, as oxygen is clearly insufficient support.

Despite the baby's reassuring oxygen saturations, the recurrent apnoea is likely to lead to the need for intubation and ventilation, unless non-invasive respiratory support proves to be adequate. This warrants a carefully monitored, short trial of CPAP of 5–6 cm H_2O or high flow nasal cannula at 2 L/kg/min. The stimulation and respiratory support this provides may reduce the work of breathing and stop the apnoeic episodes. A carefully monitored response to treatment is crucial. Assessment of adequacy of the intervention should demonstrate cessation of apnoea, improving heart rate and work of breathing in the next hour. The baby already has signs of severe respiratory disease (Table 7.2) and falls into the high-risk group (Table 7.3) due to its prematurity. If the apnoea and bradycardia continue in the hour following escalation of respiratory support, preparation for intubation and ventilation and referral to PICU should commence.

Prior to initiation of CPAP, ensure that the baby's nose and nasopharynx are clear of secretions, and that a nasopharyngeal aspirate is sent to virology. Other important considerations in babies with 'bronchiolitis', who require admission to hospital, is to exclude other

Table 7.3. High risk group characteristics

Prematurity and neonates
Pre-existing respiratory condition
Congenital heart disease
Neuromuscular conditions (**but beware these children may not
have signs of respiratory distress**)
Immune deficiency

serious underlying pathology, where bronchiolitis has only been the 'tipping' point. This should include a thorough cardiovascular and neurologic examination. Standard blood tests should include electrolytes and chemistry including CRP and full blood count. Pay specific attention to the presence of low sodium, as a sign of severity of respiratory illness, and elevated CRP suggestive of bacterial superinfection. Full blood count should be examined to exclude anaemia (associated with apnoea), and evaluate white cell count, especially in young babies who have not been fully immunised for pertussis. In this baby, you will have noticed that the white cell count is very elevated, with marked lymphocytosis, despite being fully immunised. As well as a pertussis swab, the full blood count should be repeated and a blood film requested. The presence or absence of hepatosplenomegaly and lymphadenopathy should be established. If the abnormality persists in the repeat sample, investigation will need to be escalated.

Bronchiolitis is a viral illness with respiratory syncytial virus (RSV), the commonest viral pathogen, but many other respiratory viruses (adenovirus, influenza, parainfluenza and human metapneumovirus) cause a similar clinical picture. In about 30% of those with bronchiolitis requiring PICU admission, secondary viral or bacterial co-infection will exist, often resulting in more severe disease. In severe bronchiolitis requiring intensive care admission, empiric antibiotic cover as per local guidelines is reasonable for the first 48 hours until bacterial cultures are available. Co-amoxiclav provides broad spectrum cover for older children, with ceftriaxone (cefotaxime <1 month) +/- acyclovir if there are significant CNS concerns (unless penicillin allergic). Once bacterial cultures are available and the 48-hour course of disease has been noted, decision can be made regarding antibiotic course.

You will also have noted that the sodium level in this baby is low. Hyponatraemia may predispose to seizures. Seizures in very young infants (<3 months) may present as apnoea. Other causes of hyponatraemia, including neurologic causes, should be considered. Although the baby has been feeding poorly for the past two days, babies with bronchiolitis are rarely dehydrated. On the contrary, many have evidence of excessive anti-diuretic hormone release, associated with change in intrathoracic pressure due to air trapping. The baby should remain fluid restricted, at 50% maintenance, until the sodium starts normalising over the next few days. It will need to be checked daily. Small volume frequent feeds via nasogastric tube are ideal but not until the course of respiratory failure has been established. For the next hour, the baby should remain nil enterally with normal saline/dextrose infusion at reduced volume. Although many studies have looked into their use, there is no role for nebulised salbutamol, ipratropium bromide, adrenaline, steroids, hypertonic saline or caffeine.

2. Before leaving to retrieve the child, you receive a call saying the child has been intubated but they are having difficulty with ventilation. How would you assess and manage this? What specific interventions should be carried out based on the X-rays sent to you?

Firstly, you must rapidly establish the current clinical condition of the child. Is this an emergency? You will need up to date clinical information relating to saturations, heart rate, blood pressure, current ventilation parameters and more details regarding the size and position of the endotracheal tube (ETT). You must understand fully what is meant by 'difficulty ventilating'.

The local team have intubated the baby with a 3.0 mm microcuff ETT which has been taped at the mouth at 12 cm. They performed a CXR, but the baby started desaturating shortly thereafter. The ETT was long on the CXR, so they pulled it back 1 cm. There is now very poor air entry bilaterally with no chest movement on the left. The saturations are 82% and falling in 100% oxygen with hand bagging. The chest feels non-compliant and high pressures are being used. Heart rate is 186 bpm and blood pressure 51/36. You can hear on the call that the local team is panicked.

This is an emergency: Respiratory failure, mainly worsening hypoxia, with impending shock. You need to work remotely with the team by telephone to establish the problem in a rapid and systematic manner, in order to determine the likely cause and thus, ideal treatment.

Where oxygenation or ventilation are identified as significant problems in ventilated children, the acronym **DOPES** can be used to identify possible causes rapidly:

- **D**isplaced ETT – check ETCO$_2$ trace and exact length of tube, remember 'no trace, wrong place'; 11 cm at the mouth may still be too long for an oral ETT in this baby.
- **O**bstruction – suction ETT and check suction catheter passes beyond the end. Check the heat and moisture exchanger (HME) filter is not full of secretions. Small increases in resistance in the very young can make a big difference. Check there is no obstruction to oxygen delivery to the patient in the bagging or ventilator circuit.
- **P**neumothorax/**p**leural collections – it may be difficult to exclude with clinical examination alone if the chest hyperinflated due to air trapping. Bedside ultrasound or CXR can help.
- **E**quipment – check ventilator settings including O$_2$ delivery. Using a second person to check with you. 'Fresh eyes' can ensure you aren't missing something.
- **S**tomach and **s**ecretions – ensure stomach is decompressed with nasogastric tube aspirated with 50 ml syringe. Ensure the ETT tube has been well suctioned for secretions, which may need thinning by saline lavage.

Assess DOPES first and then request a CXR if problem has not resolved.

As shown in the X-rays acquired by the local team (Figures 7.1 and 7.2), the initial ETT was too long and displaced into the right main bronchus resulting in collapse of the left lung. This would have made oxygenation difficult and the chest non-compliant. Before the CXR, the team would have increased ventilation pressures to compensate for the falling saturations. The tube needs to be withdrawn to an appropriate length between T1 and T4. Direct laryngoscopy can establish ETT ideal length marker ('black line') is at the vocal cords. Take care as high pressure ventilation could result in barotrauma to the ventilated

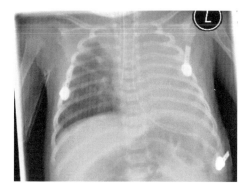

Figure 7.1 Initial chest radiograph post intubation.

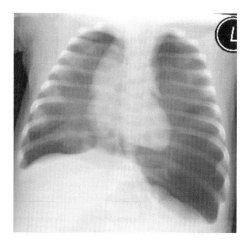

Figure 7.2 Repeat chest radiograph post withdrawal of endotracheal tube.

side and potential for pneumothorax. When the ETT is withdrawn the collapsed side will need gentle re-recruitment.

There are bilateral pneumothoraces with evidence of tension on the left (heart shadow is small and diaphragm inverted). There is clinical corroboration with cardiovascular impairment already noted. Worryingly the underlying lung has not fully collapsed, suggesting widespread consolidation. This should ring alarm bells in the setting of the very abnormal white cell count.

The presence of tension pneumothorax requires immediate decompression via a wide bore cannula without delay. Formal chest drain insertion (Chapter 54) should follow prior to transfer, because of the ongoing risk of re-accumulation on positive pressure ventilation.

This age group may present difficulties in finding a clinician willing to insert the chest drains due to the 'Goldilocks Phenomenon': the baby is 'too big' for the neonatal team but 'too small' for the anaesthetic team and the paediatric team may not have recent experience in chest drain insertion.

The most appropriate person must undertake the procedure, supported by the team. This cannot wait for the retrieval team.

It is always worth checking what chest drain equipment the local hospital has as this may need to be added to your retrieval kit, if possible with Heimlich (flutter) valves to help with ease of transfer.

3. When you arrive, the mother says she has two other children currently at nursery but needs to arrange care for them and can't the baby be treated locally? What would you explain to the mother?

Your primary concern is the safety of the child you are transferring. The question the mother has asked reveals a certain lack of insight into the gravity of the situation, possibly because there has been lack of time to update the mother on the course of the child, and the question may reveal a relatively unsupported mother.

Ongoing intensive care cannot be delivered locally, but you will need to ensure that the final destination PICU is as clinically appropriate and geographically sensible for the family as possible.

The local team and you have a duty of candour to fully update the mother, in a calm and empathetic manner, on the current situation and the course of events resulting in intubation and then bilateral chest drains. She needs to understand the gravity of the situation.

The local team and the retrieval team need to understand her social support available and establish the safety of the other children.

Outcome

This baby had bilateral chest drains inserted with the CXR seen below in Figure 7.3.

Ongoing concern of possible more significant underlying pathology remained, in view of the widespread consolidation. The baby recovered from RSV bronchiolitis with *Pneumocystis carinii* detected on bronchoalveolar lavage. During this admission he was diagnosed with Subacute Combined Immunodeficiency syndrome and subsequently underwent a successful bone marrow transplant.

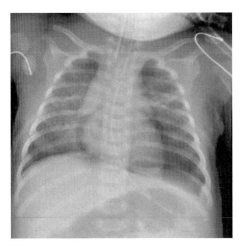

Figure 7.3 Chest radiograph post insertion of chest drains.

Foreign Body Aspiration

8

Alexander Hall and Andrew Nyman

A 13-month-old child presented from home, where he had begun choking and coughing. He had been eating pizza for dinner. When his mum turned around, she found he had opened her wallet that had been dropped on the floor. At home, he turned blue, went floppy and became unresponsive. His mum administered five back blows, which caused a cough and phlegm production, but nothing else.

On arrival to hospital, he had a runny nose and a cough with phlegm which was occasionally blood stained. He remained unsettled during the initial examination. Observations are noted in Table 8.1. The CXR is shown in Figure 8.1.

As the referring hospital did not have out-of-hours ENT cover, the local anaesthetist suggested that retrieval to a centre with this provision would be ideal. The child was referred to the paediatric retrieval service.

Questions

1. What are the common issues around ingested/aspirated foreign bodies?
2. Should the child be intubated prior to transfer, and, if so, how should the intubation be undertaken?
3. Are there any child safeguarding issues to consider?

1. What are the common issues around ingested/aspirated foreign bodies?

The main risks are obstruction, chemical burns or secondary infection. To ensure the correct management of the child, the exact nature of the foreign body must be established. The history is usually of sudden onset of coughing, choking or stridor without any preceding illness. A full history must be taken regarding the type of object ingested/aspirated, time elapsed since ingestion/aspiration, likely entry point (nose or mouth) and current location of the foreign body. Impending or anticipated medical emergencies must be considered.

Problems can arise when ingestion or aspiration has not been witnessed. For this reason, ingestion or aspiration should be considered in differential diagnosis of many presentations. Smaller children more commonly ingest/aspirate coins, batteries, safety pins, pen lids and hairpins, and these are usually visible on x-ray, whereas older children more commonly ingest or aspirate radiolucent food-based items. Absence of relevant history does not rule out foreign body aspiration.

Inspiratory and expiratory films can increase sensitivity for identification of radiolucent foreign bodies, when unilateral lung collapse or hyper-inflation may be present. Foreign

Table 8.1. Observations

Heart rate	145bpm
Respiratory rate	28 breaths per minute
SpO_2	95% on room air
Blood pressure	85/50 mmHg
AVPU	Alert, quiet
Temperature	36.2°C

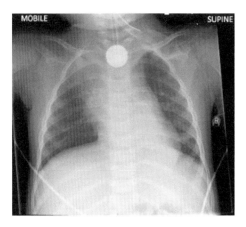

Figure 8.1 Admission chest radiograph.

body ingestion/aspiration is seen more commonly in children aged 6 months to 3 years but it is necessary to retain a low threshold for suspicion in children of all ages.

Obstruction: Obstruction of any lumen is likely to be an emergent issue.

- **Oesophageal** – swallowed foreign bodies usually pass through the bowel without incident. Impaction (becoming stuck) is most common at the level of cricopharyngeus (C5) at the thoracic inlet. Confirming the position of the foreign body can be difficult. For the safe transfer of these children to a tertiary centre, minimising intervention is the best approach.
- **Tracheal** – aspirated foreign bodies generate most anxiety for patient and clinician. Stridor is often a primary presenting complaint of extra-thoracic tracheal objects, with low pitched wheeze present when objects are intrathoracic. Some children are entirely asymptomatic. During stabilisation and transfer, attempt to keep the child self-ventilating to achieve less turbulent airflow, and reduce risk of migration of the object.
- It is also important to rule out other common differential diagnoses causing acute onset stridor or wheeze.
- Clinical diagnosis can be extremely difficult. The plain radiograph may be normal. If in doubt, definitive laryngo-bronchoscopy is recommended.
- The vast majority of deaths from foreign body airway obstruction (FBAO) occur in pre-schoolers. Blind 'finger sweeps' should not be attempted as these can further impact the foreign body. The Resuscitation Council (UK) algorithm (Figure 8.2) for a child with

Table 8.2. Radiographic findings

Radiograph findings	Management
Radiopaque foreign body	Button battery within the oesophagus is a surgical referral and should be removed as an emergency
Halo effect/double rim	If in the stomach and symptomatic should be referred as an emergency
Step off on lateral X-ray	If battery >15 mm and child <6 years, repeat X-ray in 4 days – if still in situ, should be removed surgically

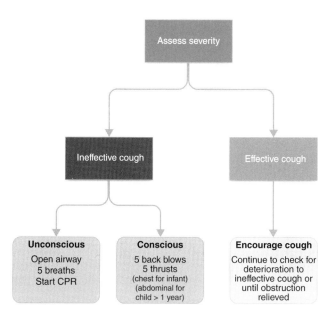

Figure 8.2 Resuscitation Council (UK) Paediatric Choking Algorithm.

suspected foreign body obstruction recommends evaluation based on presence or absence of an effective cough.

Chemical/Burn

By far the most common cause of chemical burn or char injury secondary to foreign body ingestion/aspiration is due to 'button' batteries, but other causes include ingestion or aspiration of caustic alkaline substances. The batteries contain metals such as lithium, silver or mercury with sodium or potassium hydroxide to create the chemical reaction. The chemical reaction allows discharge of 'electrical' current which liquefies the tissues. Erosion and migration through luminal walls can occur within 2 hours. In the case of chemical charring, the foreign body can become adherent to the tissue, making removal traumatic.

Radiographic findings noted in Table 8.2 can be used to identify the size and location of the foreign object and the recommended clinical strategy.

Chronic Infective Foreign Body

Often easily mistaken for other causes, foreign bodies left in situ can cause an infective or inflammatory response and must be considered during differential diagnosis. These can be expedited transfers rather than completed as an emergency.

In this circumstance, a sample for gram stain and culture should be obtained through the bronchoscope at the time of foreign body removal to guide antibiotic management.

All children with a history of suggested foreign body aspiration should have an urgent airway assessment by a senior anaesthetist, who should discuss the proposed airway management plan before attempting intubation. The biggest risk during intubation is further impaction.

2. Should this child be intubated prior to transfer and, if so, how should the intubation be undertaken?

Intubation of these children will always be a weighted consideration of the risks and benefits.

Any signs of developing, worsening or significant respiratory compromise, however, will necessitate intubation prior to transfer. Airway control prior to transfer should be discussed between the referring and accepting hospitals with a view to minimising patient risk.

In the event the child becomes increasingly tachypnoeic and distressed and needs respiratory support to avoid respiratory arrest, how would you conduct this?

The method of intubation and ventilation of a child with either an aspirated or swallowed foreign body will differ with the exact nature, location and duration of the object.

Aspirated Foreign Body

An aspirated foreign body should be removed either during direct laryngoscopy, or through a bronchoscope under general anaesthesia, as soon as possible and usually by ENT surgeons.

Pre-medication is not usually advised, so as to avoid loss of airway reflexes before control can be achieved by the anaesthetist. Steroids (e.g. dexamethasone 0.4–1 mg/kg IV) can be administered early to help reduce inflammation caused before and during removal.

In the case of a stridulous child without impending airway obstruction, anaesthesia can be undertaken with a gaseous induction (sevoflurane is preferred) or alternatively with smooth IV induction by an experienced anaesthetist. Senior ENT cover should be present in case emergency tracheotomy is needed for complete obstruction and inability to oxygenate or ventilate.

Avoidance of positive pressure ventilation is recommended to reduce further impaction; however, the priority is to ensure oxygenation at all times. Insertion of a ventilating bronchoscope is often preferred to intubation. Maintenance of spontaneous ventilation is preferred to ensure oxygenation and reduce migration of the foreign body by positive pressure ventilation, but neuromuscular blockade may be required if deep bronchoscopy is necessary or to improve the surgical view. Topical lidocaine to the vocal cords can be of use when using a bronchoscope without muscle relaxation.

There is no evidence of superiority of volatile over total IV anaesthesia for maintenance of anaesthesia in this setting.

Once the foreign body has been removed, further examination of the tracheobronchial tree is recommended in case of other foreign body fragments. Once the object has been removed, positive pressure ventilation should be used to improve any established atelectasis.

Swallowed Foreign Body

This can be an equally emergent issue, with case reports of children with swallowed foreign bodies (especially batteries) leading to haematemesis and massive haemorrhage.

Anaesthesia and airway control for oesophageal foreign body is usually less challenging; however, careful management of the child is required to reduce exacerbation of symptoms or distress. Induction of anaesthesia should be based on usual patient factors.

Novel Techniques and Extra Considerations for Removal of Foreign Bodies

Much of the historical literature discusses removal of foreign body by use of rigid bronchoscopy; however, there is increasing use of flexible bronchoscopy. Adjuncts used can include endobronchial blockers, balloon angioplasty catheters or urinary catheters that are passed distal to the foreign body and inflated, and then used to pull back the foreign body. Complications of this technique include dislodging the foreign body and further impaction.

Magnetic extractors have been described for removal of metallic foreign bodies. Diathermy or laser may be needed to clear granulation tissue around a foreign body.

Occasionally thoracotomy may be indicated if the foreign body cannot be retrieved using bronchoscope, and, in extreme cases, cardiopulmonary bypass or extracorporeal membrane oxygenation may be required to facilitate foreign body removal in difficult cases.

Non-pharmacological Methods of Keeping a Child Calm

Keeping the child calm is a key aspect in the management of an aspirated or ingested foreign body. In reality this is difficult, especially if the child requires an emergency transfer whilst conscious and without the use of sedatives.

Options to consider include:

- Play teams/therapy.
- Visual or audio distraction with bubbles, toys, books or more recently, electronic tablets. Television appears to be an effective technique.
- Virtual Reality is becoming more common place.
- Involvement of parents with any therapy and accompanying the child on transfer.
- Transfer in accompaniment with a paediatric nurse if possible.
- Minimising numbers of staff involved.
- Hands off approach.
- Offering rewards such as stickers for remaining calm.

3. Are there any child safeguarding issues to consider?

Paediatricians and clinicians dealing with children are advised to 'Be alert, question behaviours, ask for help and refer' where unsure.

Clinicians should retain a low threshold for considering safeguarding issues or non-accidental injury especially in the presence of features including:

- Delayed presentation
- Differing stories between parents and the child or other family members
- Stories that change over time
- Evidence of poor supervision
- Any child already on a Child in Need or Child Protection Plan.

It is important to remain alert to signs of abuse or neglect and question behaviours if aspects seem unusual.

Management

Most trusts will have their own local policy or guidelines to follow. To start with, ensure the child is in a safe place and consider the safety of other children at the home. E-learning for Health Safeguarding Children Level 2 describes a stepwise approach:

- Make a note of your concerns and observations.
- Discuss with senior medical and nursing colleagues.
- Discuss what you are going to do and why with the child and their parent(s) or carer(s) – as long as this does not put the child or siblings at increased risk.
- Notify and refer to children's social services by phone. In an emergency (e.g. the child absconds or the parent tries to take the child), call the police.
- Participate in a Strategy Discussion with social services, police and other agencies (e.g. school).
- If the Strategy Discussion concludes the young person is at risk of significant harm, a Section 47 Child Protection Enquiry should be called.
- After completion of the enquiry, a case conference is held.
- The case conference decides whether or not the young person should be placed on the Child Protection Register and subject to a Child Protection Plan.

Robust and contemporaneous documentation must be completed. It is good practice to ask for consent to share information in these cases, although protecting a child at risk would outweigh this.

The child in this case remained self-ventilating and unsedated for transfer during a journey time of 45 minutes. By the end of the transfer, it was evident that swallowing secretions was becoming an increasing problem, with the commencement of drooling during the transfer, but the child remained unchanged from a respiratory point of view, and the drooling was managed by placing the child in side-lying position.

Prior to transfer, the ENT surgeons at the accepting hospital had been alerted to the admission and the estimated time of arrival of the retrieval team and child. The chest X ray had been shared with the ENT team, and they had made provision to take the child directly to theatre for endoscopic foreign body removal. To facilitate this, the child was pre-admitted on the hospital electronic health care system by transfer of information from the retrieval team to the PICU admissions clerk, ensuring that the child could be taken directly to theatre, correctly identified on arrival and with the accompanying parent able to sign consent for the procedure.

A coin was successfully removed from the child's oesophagus. On follow-up oesophago-scopy 3 days later, there were no residual signs of previous impaction or trauma, and the child was discharged well, with advice to the parent regarding access of small children to tempting objects.

Further Reading

Bellieni CV, Cordelli D, Raffaelli M et al., Analgesic effect of watching TV during venepuncture. *Arch Dis Childhood* 2006;91(12):1015–17.

Child Protection and the Anaesthetist July 2014. www.rcpch.ac.uk/sites/default/files/2018-03/child_protection_and_the_anaesthetist.pdf.

E-learning for Health Safeguarding Children Level 2. Health Education England website for online learning: https://portal.e-lfh.org.uk/

Farrell PT. Rigid bronchoscopy for foreign body removal: anaesthesia and ventilation. *Ped Anaes* 2004; 14(1):84–9

Kendigelen P. The anaesthetic considerations of tracheobronchial foreign body aspiration in children. *J Thorac Dis* 2016;8 (12):3803–7.

Maconochie I, Bingham B, Skellett S. Resuscitation Council UK www.resus.org.uk/resuscitation-guidelines/paediatric-basic-life-support/#choking

Resus Council UK. www.resus.org.uk/resuscitation-guidelines/paediatric-basic-life-support/#choking

Ruiz FE. Airway foreign bodies in children. Up To Date. www.uptodate.com/contents/airway-foreign-bodies-in-children.

A Child with Facial Swelling

Michael Carter and Shelley Riphagen

A 4-year-old girl presented to the paediatric A&E with her mother and grandmother. Her mother recounted that she had developed facial swelling following a spider bite 2 weeks previously. Prior to the onset of facial swelling, she had seen her GP a week before for new onset noisy breathing. The GP noted normal blood pressure, normal urine dipstick but mild stridor. A short course of prednisolone was prescribed for mild croup and the stridor resolved. A week later the spider bite occurred with worsening associated facial swelling over the next 2 weeks and the stridor recurred. Mother noted the stridor was mainly at night, to the extent that the child found it difficult to lie flat. She was also generally tired but had no other abnormal history.

On examination she was sitting upright on the bed, talking in full sentences, but with capillary oxygen saturation of 92% in room air and dull bases especially on the left. Cardiovascular examination revealed normal rate, rhythm and blood pressure, but grossly engorged jugular veins and upper abdominal and chest veins.

Initial blood results from full blood count are noted in Table 9.1.

Her CXR is shown in Figure 9.1.

She was referred to the regional retrieval service due to the concern regarding her widened mediastinum on CXR and for ongoing investigations at a tertiary centre.

Questions

1. What are your primary concerns for the cause of this child's symptoms and radiological findings?
2. What are the potential respiratory and cardiovascular emergencies that arise due to mediastinal masses?
3. What are the prime considerations of management of children with this problem, including during transfer?

1. What are your primary concerns for the cause of this child's symptoms and radiological findings?

The combination of the respiratory symptoms, specifically clinical history and examination consistent with airway obstruction, facial swelling with evidence of upper body venous engorgement and a widened mediastinum evident on CXR is highly suggestive of a mediastinal mass, most likely of malignant origin. This is not an acute problem, but has been symptomatic for at least 3 to 4 weeks. The spider bite is likely incidental but something concrete that parents might use to rationalise the non-specific symptoms of the child.

Table 9.1. Presenting full blood count

Haemoglobin	116 g/l
White cell count	10.5 (10^3/mm^3)
Neutrophils	5 (10^3/mm^3)
Lymphocytes	4.5 (10^3/mm^3)
Platelets	438 (10^3/mm^3)

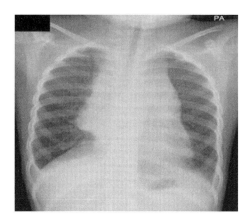

Figure 9.1 Admission chest radiograph.

Mediastinal masses occur in the anterior, middle or posterior mediastinum, dependent on the origin tissue. The mediastinum is cephalad to the heart within the upper thorax. The aetiology of mediastinal masses is typically determined by histological examination of biopsy tissue from the mass itself or an associated lymph node. A recent review of 44 children with anterior mediastinal masses in southern England showed 36% to be secondary to Hodgkin lymphoma, 32% non-Hodgkin lymphoma (of which two thirds were T cell derived, and one third was B cell derived), 20% to be T cell acute lymphoblastic leukaemia and a small proportion (2% each) were lipoblastomas, teratomas, myosarcoma or primitive neuroectodermal tumour. Of these tumours, 25% were diagnosed from biopsy tissue that was not within the mediastinal mass, and eight of the children were treated with steroids 1–3 days prior to biopsy. This highlights the importance of a low threshold of suspicion for anterior mediastinal masses and of very early discussion with tertiary centres to enable optimum treatment in A&E and planning of immediate care in any receiving tertiary unit.

2. What are the potential respiratory and cardiovascular emergencies that arise due to mediastinal masses?

This child has the potential for rapid deterioration from both a respiratory and cardiovascular point of view, and she must be managed with these oncological emergencies in mind.

The child already has evidence of airway obstruction in history and examination.

The presence of stridor in this setting identifies the location of the airway obstruction to the supraglottic, glottic or sub-glottic trachea. This obstruction can occur in the intrathoracic or extrathoracic trachea. Many children with enlarging mediastinal masses will start off with 'wheezing' (expiratory noise) because of intrathoracic tracheal obstruction, that progresses over time to stridor (inspiratory noise) as the obstruction increases or the mass expands outside the chest through the thoracic inlet. Airway obstruction only becomes symptomatic (noisy) at rest when airway diameter is >50% reduced. It is always worse when lying flat, as the heavy tumour burden compresses the trachea further. The history usually supports this, with children reporting worsening orthopnoea. The respiratory reserve in this setting is extremely limited, and children should remain calm with no cause for agitation.

The additional presence of hypoxia should increase the concern. This may be related to the presence of associated malignant pleural effusions or areas of lung collapse, due to airway obstruction, as is seen in this child's CXR (Figure 9.1) with left lower lobe collapse evident (diaphragm not clearly seen on left).

The cardiovascular emergencies associated with mediastinal masses are two-fold.

Tumours originating in the mediastinal lymph nodes encase and may rarely invade the great vessels. The superior vena cava, encased with tumour, becomes partially obstructed, resulting in upper body and facial swelling and in extreme circumstances, in cerebral oedema. Upper body veins become engorged and parents often note the child's face has become swollen and eyes bloodshot (conjunctival engorgement). If the blood flow becomes very sluggish, or there is intravascular tumour invasion, intravascular thrombus formation is also possible and exacerbates the obstruction acutely.

Reduction in venous return from the upper body (representing >50% cardiac venous return in younger children) reduces cardiac output. This is worse, like the airway obstruction, when lying flat. High venous pressures may result in hydrostatic leak into both the pleural and pericardial spaces.

Additionally, the tumour may invade the pericardium and result in a malignant pericardial effusion, which will have the same net effect as superior vena cava obstruction. Pericardial effusions limit diastolic filling, and myocardial infiltration may limit systolic function.

If made to lie flat, in the setting of severe superior vena cava obstruction, the child may lose cardiac output and arrest. In this setting, positive pressure ventilation applied during cardiac arrest will exacerbate the reduction in passive, spontaneous ventilation-associated venous return to the right heart by negative intrathoracic pressure.

3. What are the prime considerations of management of children with this problem, including during transfer?

Paediatricians and anaesthetists are familiar with the respiratory support and control that can be achieved with intubation and ventilation in many sick children.

This is not the case for children with mediastinal masses, where the procedure of intubation and taking over spontaneous ventilation is very high risk.

Initial treatment strategies should try to avoid this scenario.

The child should be left undisturbed and sitting upright in the position of greatest comfort. This is more likely to maintain airway calibre and optimise venous drainage, thereby also reducing intracranial hypertension.

If respiratory compromise appears immediately life-threatening, spontaneous ventilation can be supported non-invasively, initially by mask continuous positive airway pressure, held by a competent airway operator, and then as non-invasive bilevel positive airway pressure for transfer, with the child in a semi-recumbent, semi-prone, left lateral position.

Steroids may be given after urgent liaison with a tertiary oncology team and the retrieval team, who will be responsible for the child's transfer. Discussions regarding the use of steroids should consider the high probability of tumour lysis syndrome in the setting of high tumour burden malignancies like mediastinal masses. This emergency will require acute management of hyperkalaemia related to cell lysis.

Administration of steroids may limit the ability of oncological teams to make a histological diagnosis. For this reason, the use of steroids should be predated by a discussion with the oncology team, including the list of diagnostic blood tests that should be performed prior to steroids. The concomitant risk of tumour lysis syndrome during transfer makes it a strategy of last resort. If steroids are used, the child should be transferred with defibrillation pads already in situ, and careful attention to ECG for signs of hyperkalaemia.

An additional mantra in superior vena cava syndrome is that one must 'resuscitate the inferior vena cava': IV therapy should be given via cannulas in the lower limbs. IV therapy given within the drainage system of the superior vena cava will not circulate effectively. Additional to the airway risk, the risk of complete superior vena cava obstruction and subsequent loss of cardiac output must be predicted. The team must make provision to minimise the risk and duration of obstruction by using higher filling pressures and positioning.

Intubation and positive pressure ventilation are occasionally required. Induction of anaesthesia should be performed with cardiostable drugs, such as ketamine and fentanyl, that do not produce vasodilatation. Avoidance of muscle relaxation, and maintenance of airway tone and spontaneous ventilation during anaesthesia is preferred. Anaesthesia should be supported by judicious volume boluses administered by lower limb vessels, and inotropes should be infusing prior to induction. If a steel coil reinforced/armoured tube is available, this should be deployed. Once intubated and with the endotracheal tube extremely well secured, the child should be turned immediately into a left lateral semi-prone position, bolstered with cushioning, for transfer. Clearly intubation and ventilation is an extremely high-risk procedure and should be undertaken by the most experienced anaesthetist available.

Summary

This case is used to illustrate the importance of careful thought regarding the interpretation of clinical findings, in a child, who at first glance did not appear to be very unwell. If the differential or likely diagnosis includes mediastinal mass, careful evaluation of presenting and possible clinical emergencies related to mediastinal mass must be performed.

Key 'rules of thumb' are

1. The mediastinum is normally less than one quarter of the width of the chest, or twice the width of the child's spinal vertebral body.
2. The thymus is rarely visible in children older than 3 years of age, and although large and potentially confounding in infants, is in the process of involution in the following years.
3. Patients with mediastinal masses should be retrieved sitting upright, with left side down, managing their own airway, and with a cannula in a lower limb vein.
4. The child should not be asked or made to lie down – with computed tomography of the chest contraindicated at presentation if the child is symptomatic.

5. The child should be kept as calm as possible, with procedures minimised, during retrieval to a specialist PICU. The retrievalist should consider the adage 'less is more' when faced with the child with an acute presentation of anterior mediastinal mass.

Further Reading

Malik R, Mullassery D, Kleine-Brueggeney M, et al. Anterior mediastinal masses – A multidisciplinary pathway for safe diagnostic procedures. *J Pediatr Surg* 2019;**54**:251–4.

Pearson JK, Tan GM. Pediatric anterior mediastinal mass: A review article. *Semin Cardiothorac Vasc Anesth* 2015; **19**(3):248–54.

Wilson LD, Detterbeck FC, Yahalom J. Superior vena cava syndrome with malignant cause. *N Engl J Med* 2007;**356**(18):1862–9.

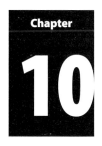

Pneumonia and Empyema

Elizabeth Daisy Dunn and Marilyn McDougall

Retrieval Call

A 3-year-old child attended the local hospital, with her parents, complaining of abdominal pain. This had been ongoing for 2.5 weeks. She had seen her general practitioner on more than one occasion, where the abdominal pain had been managed as constipation. Her parents reported no improvement. Parents had brought her into hospital on this occasion because she had become increasingly sleepy and lethargic. They had also noticed her breathing had changed. On arrival in A&E she was noticed to have severe respiratory distress with clinical observations recorded in Table 10.1.

On admission to A&E a venous cannula was sited, and some initial blood tests including a blood gas were sent. The results are noted in Table 10.2.

In view of her respiratory distress, a mobile CXR was obtained urgently and is shown in Figure 10.1.

Based on her clinical condition, the CXR findings and the blood results, the local team proceeded with the following management:

- IV ceftriaxone 80 mg/kg
- IV crystalloid totalling 80 ml/kg in four separate 20 ml/kg boluses.

Despite the volume resuscitation, there was minimal improvement in the blood pressure or heart rate. They contacted their on-call anaesthetic team, who agreed the child needed intubation and ventilation. The team assessed the CXR together. They noted left lung whiteout with mediastinal shift, probably due to a large left pleural effusion.

Questions

1. What is the background of pneumonia +/- empyema in this clinical context?
2. What advice would you give the local team regarding the ongoing low blood pressure prior to intubating the child?
3. What issues on transfer might you face regarding ventilating this child?

1. What is the background of pneumonia +/− empyema in this clinical context?

Pneumonia is highly prevalent within the paediatric population, with both viral and bacterial pneumonias being a frequent cause of paediatric admissions, in particular during winter. Pneumonia must be suspected in all children with a fever >38.5°C in association with chest recession and tachypnoea.

Table 10.1. Physiological observations

Heart rate	174 bpm
Respiratory rate	56 breaths per minute
SpO_2	92%
Blood pressure	104/57 mmHg
AVPU	Alert but lethargic

Table 10.2. Initial blood tests and venous blood gas

Bloods		Initial blood gas	
Haemoglobin	104 g/L	pH	7.36
White cell count	40 (10^3/mm^3)	pO_2	6.3 KPa
Neutrophils	28 (10^3/mm^3)	pCO_2	3.3 Kpa
CRP	368 mg/L	HCO_3	17 mmol/L
Creatinine	30 U/L	Base excess	−9.5 mEq/L
Urea	4 mmol/L	Lactate	4.31 mmol/L
Na	118 mmol/L	Glucose	1.9 mmol/L

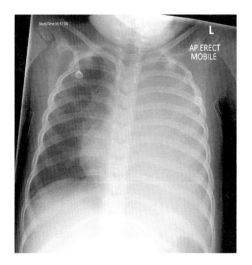

Figure 10.1 Admission chest radiograph.

All patients with suspected pneumonia should be treated with antibiotics initially. It can be difficult to differentiate viral from bacterial pneumonia. The degree of derangement of inflammatory markers may be helpful, but not definitive. Dual causation, with primary viral and secondary bacterial pathogens is not uncommon. There is a well-known link between influenza virus and secondary invasive bacterial infection with *Streptococcus pneumoniae*.

IV therapy should be provided to all those who are critically ill and requiring PICU intervention, and those who are experiencing complications associated with pneumonia. It is appropriate to manage these children in the category of sepsis, and perform the septic bundle, including blood cultures and IV antibiotic administration, within 1 hour of diagnosis of sepsis.

Children with predisposing conditions leading to vulnerability to pneumonia (e.g. any form of immunodeficiency including oncological diagnoses, congenital heart disease, sickle cell disease) should be aggressively managed early, as they are more likely to deteriorate rapidly.

The most common organisms to cause pneumonia are streptococci, in particular *Streptococcus pneumoniae* with many emerging serotypes not covered by the current vaccine strategy. Public health reports show that staphylococcal infections and Group A streptococcal infections have increased in prevalence in the last decade, with these pneumonias more likely to be complicated by empyema and require PICU admission. Some children may present with toxic shock from either of these bacteria. This should be managed as per toxic shock guidelines, with early consideration of IV clindamycin and immunoglobulin, both with toxin-modifying effects.

National and local guidelines should be followed regarding antibiotic choice for community-acquired pneumonia. In most cases, broad spectrum, appropriate antibiotics should be selected to cover Group A strep and *Staphylococcus* as well as *Streptococcus pneumoniae* if pneumonia complicated by empyema is suspected. In children who acquire nosocomial pneumonia or who are immunocompromised, an infectious diseases specialist should be consulted regarding broader antibiotic coverage.

Complications of Pneumonia (including Para-pneumonic Effusion and Empyema)

Para-pneumonic effusions and empyema should be diagnosed clinically with percussion and auscultation of the chest and confirmed radiologically (CXR and ultrasound if possible). Empyema has an incidence of 3.3 per 100,000 children, therefore complicating a reasonable number of admissions to hospital. Non-infective para-pneumonic effusions are rarer, only complicating 1% of pneumonias.

Effusions and empyemas should always be ruled out in children with pneumonia and persistent fever after a 48-hour period of treatment with IV antibiotics. Ultrasound is the most useful modality to define both effusions and empyemas. There is a higher incidence in males and younger children, which increases over the winter period – likely in association with the rise in bacterial prevalence.

The definition and in-depth management of para-pneumonic effusions and empyemas is detailed in the British Thoracic Society (BTS) guidelines. Management requires IV antibiotics and in the case of empyema or significant fluid collection, insertion of a chest drain. Microbiology (+/- cytology) sample analysis should guide further management. Rarer causes, for example, TB, should also be considered where appropriate. Travel, immunisation status and TB contacts are an important aspect of the history-taking in these cases.

Specific caution must be applied prior to drainage of large effusions or those under tension (in this case with mediastinal shift), or in those children who have pre-existing cardiovascular compromise. The sudden changes in intravascular volume associated with drainage may result in profound destabilisation and even cardiovascular collapse. Children should be volume loaded before drainage, and for large effusions or those under tension, release of fluid must be controlled by intermittent clamping and controlled volume release from the thoracic cavity.

Early usage of urokinase following insertion of a chest drain has been recommended by BTS guidelines in treatment of empyema. Video-assisted thoracostomy surgery (VATS) may be required at a later stage in the minority of children if medical management and simple drainage plus urokinase is ineffective. The recovery from empyemas and effusions is generally excellent in children.

2. What advice would you give the local team regarding the ongoing low blood pressure prior to intubating the child?

The most important step in the management of this child is to identify the presenting clinical emergencies. This child has evidence of respiratory failure with shock and is at risk of rapid decompensation when exposed to anaesthetic drugs. Despite having already received 80 ml/kg of IV fluids, and IV antibiotics, there is no significant or sustained improvement in shock.

Ongoing volume resuscitation provided it is still resulting in benefit (decreased heart rate and improved blood pressure and clinical appearance) should continue. It is clear, however, after already receiving equivalent to total circulating blood volume, that additional measures are now required to resuscitate this child.

As per APLS guidelines, once over 40 ml/kg of crystalloid fluid boluses have been given, inotropic support should be started as quickly as possible, while continuing other resuscitation measures. Dopamine can be initiated peripherally as can dilute adrenaline. There is documented profound hyponatraemia (Na 118 mmol/l) commonly seen in toxic shock and exacerbated by respiratory illness. In this situation, hypertonic saline may be effective as both volume expander and to increase the sodium to a level less likely to cause seizures.

Good IV access prior to anaesthetic induction is a necessity (minimum two cannulas). This must be attained and secured prior to commencing induction. If IV access is too difficult, intra-osseous access must be established. It is not always possible to completely stabilise a critically ill child prior to anaesthesia, but the team should be advised of the risks of the situation and active resuscitation should be in progress before, during and after intubation and ventilation, with the awareness that positive pressure ventilation reduces right-sided cardiac filling.

If central access is available, either via central line or intra-osseous, commence adrenaline or noradrenaline as per local guidance. Rapid treatment of shock is in the best interest of the patient and will reduce end organ injury.

Local PICU guidelines will give you guidance and support in the preferred first line choice of vasopressors and inotropes. Dosage calculations in children based on weight are available in drug calculator applications. An overview of initial vasopressor and inotropic options can be found in Chapter 57.

Prior to induction of anaesthesia in this child, there should be:

- A combined paediatric and anaesthetic team brief: the possibility of cardiac arrest is high. Team members should all have clearly defined roles. A team leader must be identified. The anaesthetic team cannot usually fulfil this role during induction, as they need to remain focused on safe anaesthesia and securing intubation and ventilation.

- All relevant precautions to prevent cardiac arrest must be in place with volume boluses and cardiac arrest drugs drawn up and ready. A syringe of pressor agent (dilute adrenaline, phenylephrine or metaraminol) should be part of the suite of drugs immediately available to the anaesthetist.
- Full monitoring must be in place with end tidal CO_2 connected and blood pressure cuff cycling at least every 2 minutes. Heart rate bips should be audible, and a team member designated to watch the monitor and report and record events if possible.
- Drug choice and dose must be open for discussion, and the non-anaesthetic team members must be aware of the likely side effects of drugs to be used. Ketamine with aliquots of fentanyl to desired effect, would be ideal, due the improved cardiostable nature of ketamine. Remember that shock in itself causes a reduced level of consciousness and delayed onset of action of drugs due to prolonged circulation time, thereby warranting a smaller dose of induction agent, expecting the anaesthetic to take longer to achieve effect. Both of these factors should be considered during induction of anaesthesia.

3. What issues on transfer might you face regarding ventilating this child?

There should be consideration of the effect that the fluid collection around the lung will have on the ability to ventilate the patient following induction of anaesthesia. Adequate preparation with pre-oxygenation and positive end-expiratory pressure (PEEP) is essential. Anticipation of desaturation following induction is also important. The efficiency of spontaneous breathing should not be underestimated. The move from negative to positive pressure ventilation does not only impact ventilation but also causes profound blood pressure changes. The patient may require high peak pressures and an increased level of PEEP to optimise oxygenation. A cuffed tube should be chosen in anticipation of high ventilatory requirements. If optimisation of oxygenation and ventilation cannot be achieved despite this, urgent drainage of the pleural fluid should be undertaken. The operator identified to undertake this procedure, should be scrubbed and ready with sterile set and correct instruments and drain.

Chest drain insertion (See Chapter 54 for full insertion guidance)

The BTS guidelines strongly suggest small chest drains should be used. There is no evidence that larger drains confer any advantage, and therefore minimising patient discomfort will be significant in future care (e.g. analgesia and sedation).

When inserting a drain, consideration of rapid fluid shifts should be noted – there is a risk, however small, of re-expansion pulmonary oedema (RPO). Slow drainage of a very large pleural effusion, such as in this case, with regular clamping of the drain after each 10 ml/kg of fluid loss, in a similar manner to 'controlled bleeding', and replacement of like-for-like intravascular losses is suggested. In view of this theoretical risk (well reported in adults), the BTS guidelines suggest that 10 ml/kg of fluid from an effusion should initially be removed, and then the drain clamped for 1 hour. This may not be possible where oxygenation and ventilation is severely compromised after intubation, and despite high ventilatory pressures.

Further Reading

Advanced Paediatric Life Support – Chapter 6, The Child In Shock – ALSG.

British Thoracic Guidelines for Management of Community Pneumonia. www.brit-thoracic.org.uk/document-library/guidelines/pneumonia-in-children/bts-guideline-for-the-management-of-community-acquired-pneumonia-in-children-update/.

British Thoracic Guidelines for the Management of Pleural Infection in Children. thorax.bmj.com/content/60/suppl_1/i1.

British Thoracic Guidelines for the Management of Community Acquired Pneumonia in Children: Update 2011. www.brit-thoracic.org.uk/document-library/guidelines/pneumonia-in-children/bts-guideline-for-the-management-of-community-acquired-pneumonia-in-children-update/.

Health Protection Report, Public Health England – Surveillance of Streptococcus pneumoniae: 2015. https://assets.publishing.service.gov.uk/government/uploads/system/uploads/attachment_data/file/570792/hpr4016_strp-pnmnae.pdf.

Public Health England Report – Group A Streptococcal Infections: Third Report on Seasonal Activity 2018/19. https://assets.publishing.service.gov.uk/government/uploads/system/uploads/attachment_data/file/800932/hpr1619_gas-sf3.pdf.

Surviving Sepsis Guidelines – 8th February 2020. https://journals.lww.com/pccmjournal/Fulltext/2020/02000/Surviving_Sepsis_Campaign_International_Guidelines.20.aspx.

The Child with a Cough and Concerning White Cell Count

Jo Dyer and Maja Pavcnik

A 4-week-old baby had been an inpatient for 3 days being treated for bronchiolitis. He was being managed on high flow nasal cannula (HFNC) with minimal oxygen requirement and a mild increase in work of breathing at rest. On the third day after an oral feed, he had marked intercostal recession, nasal flaring and tachypnoea so had been changed to nasogastric feeds.

The district general hospital team called as they were concerned that he had not improved clinically during his admission and in the previous 4 hours, prior to referral, had developed increasingly frequent coughing episodes with associated fleeting desaturations into the mid 80s. His CXR on admission had been clear but a repeat X-ray showed bilateral infiltrates. His white cell count (WCC), which was high at presentation, had also increased markedly. At the time of referral, he had been placed nil by mouth and was being started on continuous positive airway pressure (CPAP).

The baby had been commenced on co-amoxiclav on the day of admission. Nasopharyngeal aspirate was positive for rhinovirus. The parents reported that the older sibling had a cough and coryzal symptoms. The repeat blood tests and his physiological observations at the time of referral are shown in Tables 11.1 and 11.2, respectively.

CXR is shown in Figure 11.1.

Questions

1. Given the above information, what concerns would you have with the child's current diagnosis and management?
2. Thirty minutes later, the referring team call to say the baby is now having significant colour change when coughing. What would be your advice to the local team?
3. The parents have asked to speak to you. They are concerned as they overheard someone speaking about organ support and their other child also has a cough. What information do you need to communicate with parents?

1. Given the above information, what concerns would you have with the child's current diagnosis and management?

This neonate has a clear history of a respiratory infection and evolving CXR changes. The clinical deterioration is not unremarkable in bronchiolitis where symptoms usually peak between 3 and 5 days after onset of illness. The escalation of respiratory support from HFNC to CPAP is an appropriate strategy to meet the clinical need.

Table 11.1. Initial laboratory and blood gas results

Bloods		Initial blood gas (venous)	
Haemoglobin	110 g/L	pH	7.43
White cell count	106 (10^3/mm^3)	pO$_2$	5.8 KPa
Neutrophils	40 (10^3/mm^3)	pCO$_2$	5.3 KPa
Lymphocytes	62 (10^3/mm^3)	Lactate	1.1 mmol/L
CRP	32 mg/L	Glucose	4.6 mmol/L
Creatinine	22 U/L	Base excess	2 mEq/L
Urea	3.5 mmol/L		
Na	132 mmol/L		
K	4.1 mmol/L		

Table 11.2.

Heart rate	168 bpm
Respiratory rate	62 breaths per minutes
SpO$_2$	98% on FiO$_2$ 0.25
Blood pressure	107/54 mmHg
AVPU	Alert
Temperature	36.5°C

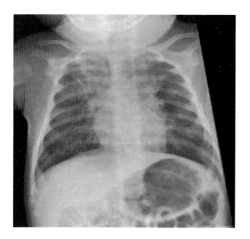

Figure 11.1 Chest X-ray at time of referral.

The laboratory findings, however, are concerning. There is a marked leucocytosis (high WCC) with a predominance of lymphocytes. Leucocytosis can occur in response to physiological, inflammatory, malignant or infective processes in the body. Physiologic leucocytosis is well recognised in the neonate but counts rarely exceed 30,000.

Table 11.3.

Factors associated with increased morbidity & mortality in pertussis
Age ≤3 months
Unvaccinated
Leucocytosis $\geq$50 (10^3/mm^3)
Pneumonia
Cardiovascular instability
Pulmonary hypertension
Rapidly progressive course

Hyperleucocytosis, defined as WCC >100,000 mm^3, usually occurs in leukaemia and other myeloproliferative disorders. In neonates, this is a rare clinical finding which can be associated with congenital malignancy/leukaemia, transient abnormal myelopoiesis (TAM, reported in about 10% of children with trisomy 21), and as a response to an infectious stimulus. In a young child, unimmunised or incompletely immunised, and presenting with a respiratory illness, especially with coughing in spells, there must be a high suspicion that leucocytosis is in response to **pertussis** (infection with *Bordetella pertussis*). This is particularly true where there is either leucocytosis with **lymphocytosis** (a total WCC $\geq$20 with $\geq$ 50% lymphocytes) or an isolated lymphocytosis. Neonates up to 2–3 months are particularly at risk, as they are too young to have received any immunisations against the disease.

Pertussis is a highly contagious respiratory illness caused by the *Bordetella pertussis,* a gram-negative coccobacillus producing potent endotoxins. It results in a toxin-mediated leukocytosis, hyperviscosity syndrome, endotoxin-mediated vascular endothelial damage, lymphocyte deformity with abnormal rolling, and organisms attaching to and multiplying among the cilia of the respiratory epithelium. There is a **broad spectrum of disease severity**, from mild respiratory symptoms to fulminant multi-organ dysfunction. Severe disease occurs predominantly in infancy and can include necrotising bronchiolitis/pneumonia with respiratory failure/apnoea and pulmonary hypertension, myocardial dysfunction, and encephalopathy/seizures. Pathophysiology is mediated by endotoxin and microvascular slugging with thrombosis. This is particularly prominent in the lungs and cerebral microvasculature.

Factors associated with severe disease are outlined in Table 11.3.

This baby has multiple markers for poor prognosis namely age, vaccine status, WCC, pneumonia and sustained tachycardia. Advice to the referring team would be that this is a potentially three- or-four pronged emergency involving respiratory failure, likely cardiovascular collapse, hyperleucocytosis and an evolving encephalopathy.

Urgent transfer to paediatric critical care is required with the aim to reduce WCC rapidly and the associated likelihood of developing complications associated with leukocytosis.

Leucodepletion via double-volume exchange transfusion or leukofiltration is a first-line management strategy to attenuate the disease severity of critical pertussis patients with hyperleukocytocis. Success of this treatment relies on the procedure being carried out before the infant is severely compromised and the priority here is facilitating a timely transfer in a stable and supported manner in order to commence this therapy.

As demonstrated by this case, many infants with pertussis will initially present with a relatively mild illness but may progress to severe disease. Clinicians frequently underestimate severity of illness in this age group, resulting in delayed transfer and admission to intensive care and contributing to increased morbidity and mortality.

It is widely agreed that all young infants (3 months old and younger) with suspected pertussis, should be admitted to monitor their WCC, regardless of the severity of their presenting symptoms. The exact relationship of duration of symptoms to cardiopulmonary instability and evolution of critical illness is not well described. Initial investigations should include testing for pertussis (as per Public Health England guidelines, most appropriate specimen is the nasopharyngeal swab) and regular monitoring of the WCC. Those with any markers of severe disease should be referred early for discussion about the need for retrieval to a paediatric intensive care unit. This infant presented with a WCC of 30 with a marked lymphocytosis. This should have alerted medical practitioners to the possibility of pertussis.

2. Thirty minutes later, the referring team call to say the baby is now having significant colour changes when coughing. What would be your advice to the local team?

Stabilisation of this child for transfer would include **assessing the need for intubation**. This should be flagged early in discussions between the local team and transport team as the baby has deteriorated significantly in the last few hours. The blood gas is falsely reassuring. Assessment of need for intubation should be based on the infant's clinical examination and the predicted course of events based on known disease evolution, not on a blood gas result – in fact, a normal blood gas result may detract from clinical judgement.

A baby having episodes of profound desaturation, even if normally saturated between times, is not safe to transfer self-ventilating or on non-invasive respiratory support. This baby needs urgent anaesthetic support for intubation and ventilation. Expediting the transfer of this baby is a priority and intubation of the infant prior to the arrival of the retrieval team will aid this. The most appropriate person to intubate will depend on the skills and experience of the local team available at the time of the referral. As well as the anaesthetic team, consideration of utilising the experience of paediatricians who have worked in neonatal units or calling the neonatal unit for assistance may be appropriate.

The process of induction of anaesthesia and intubation and ventilation is likely to be challenging from a number of aspects. The baby clearly has significant lung disease and lung compliance should be anticipated to be reduced. Once muscle relaxed, it will be difficult to manually ventilate the baby and the two-person technique of bag valve mask ventilation (BVM) should be employed. Because of the reduced lung compliance, it is likely that BVM will result in gastric distension. A helper should be tasked solely with keeping the stomach decompressed by regular nasogastric tube aspiration with a 50 ml syringe. This baby is already tachycardic, which in this situation may indicate myocardial dysfunction or reduced cardiac filling due to reduced lung compliance or a combination. One requires filling, the other inotropic support. Before induction of anaesthesia, both resuscitation modalities – fluid and inotropic support – should be in progress. Additionally, pulmonary hypertension, secondary to leucostasis and endotoxin has the potential to cause life-threatening instability. As well as the most appropriate personnel, there should be careful consideration of appropriate anaesthetic agents. Emergency drugs must be available and the team must be prepared for this eventuality prior to induction.

Consideration must be made as to the most appropriate centre for this infant's ongoing treatment. Multiple factors will need to be considered as this child will require an isolation room and the potential for multiorgan support. Deterioration of the infant's condition and the need for escalation of supportive therapies should be anticipated. Many centres no longer offer extracorporeal membrane oxygenation (ECMO) for this condition because of the poor outcome if the condition deteriorates this far; however, the national ECMO referral pathway should be followed and relevant discussion undertaken.

Macrolide antibiotics should be used if pertussis is suspected. They are effective in eliminating *Bordetella pertussis* from the nasopharyngeal secretions within 5 days. After the cough is established, antibiotics may not alter the course of the illness but are recommended to limit the spread of organisms to others.

Pertussis is **a notifiable disease** under the Health Protection Legislation (England) Guidance 2010. The local Health Protection Team must be notified of all suspected as well as confirmed cases. They will then provide the team caring for the child with guidance. **Contacts** of confirmed cases will need tracing and may require **chemoprophylaxis and/or immunisations** as per current guidelines. In order to minimise risk, the medical team must take appropriate **infection control precautions**. PPE should be worn for all aerosol generating procedures. Staff who have been in contact without suitable protective equipment may need chemoprophylaxis and/or immunisation if deemed to have had significant contact risk or to be in a vulnerable category.

3. The parents have asked to speak to you. They are concerned as they overheard someone speaking about organ support and their other child also has a cough. What information do you need to communicate with parents?

Pertussis in childhood has a broad spectrum of disease. The highest morbidity and mortality rates are seen in the youngest patients. This neonate is presenting with many markers of poor prognosis and is likely to have a complex PICU stay. Conversations with the parents need to reflect this and you would be unable to reassure them that there will be a positive outcome. **Mortality rates are reported as 40–70% for infants requiring PICU care** and there is significant morbidity in many survivors.

In this scenario the older sibling also has a cough and coryzal symptoms. It is important to elicit from the parents whether **family members** have been immunised. The current **UK vaccine schedule** includes pertussis in the 8, 12 and 16 week vaccines, with recognition that after the second vaccine most infants have good immunity. Children receive a further pertussis booster in the pre-school vaccinations. It is well recognised that the effectiveness of the pertussis vaccine decreases with time. Older siblings of this baby should have been vaccinated and therefore would unlikely to be at risk of severe disease. The mother should have received **a vaccine booster during her pregnancy**. Pregnant women can help protect their babies from developing pertussis in the first few weeks of life by getting vaccinated – ideally from 16 weeks up to 32 weeks gestation.

Discussions around vaccine uptake and health promotion are difficult in this scenario as the baby is acutely unwell; however, they need to be had in a timely and sensitive manner.

Further Reading

Berger JT, Carcillo JA, Shanley TP, et al. Critical pertussis illness in children: A multicenter prospective cohort study. *Pediatr Crit Care Med* 2013; 14:356–65.

Carbonetti NH. Pertussis leucocytosis: mechanisms, clinical relevance and treatment. *Pathog Dis* 2016;74(7):ftw087.

Domico M, Ridout D, McLaren G, et al. Extracorporeal membrane oxygenation for pertussis: predictors of outcome including pulmonary hypertension and leukodepletion. *Pediatr Crit Care Med* 2018;19:254–61.

Ganeshalingham A, McSharry B, Anderson B, et al. Identifying children at risk of malignant *Bordetella pertussis* infection. *Pediatr Crit Care Med* 2017; 18:e42–7.

Pertussis – guidelines for public health management: www.gov.uk/government/publications/pertussis-guidelines-for-public-health-management.

Rowlands HE, Goldman AP, Harrington K, et al. Impact of rapid leukodepletion on the outcome of severe clinical pertussis in young infants. *Paediatrics* 2010;126:e816–27.

Winter K Zipprich J, Harriman K, et al. Risk factors associated with infant deaths from pertussis: A case-control study. *Clin Infect Dis* 2015;61:1099–1106.

Worsening Stridor, to Intubate … or Not to Intubate

Joanna Davies and Shelley Riphagen

A 10-month-old boy, previously fit and well, presented to his A&E at 4 o'clock in the morning with severe respiratory distress. He had a barking cough and inspiratory stridor and was diagnosed with croup. On admission he was treated with two back-to-back adrenaline nebulisations and oral dexamethasone. His work of breathing improved and he was admitted to the paediatric ward for observation. A few hours later, his work of breathing became laboured with increasing stridor, tracheal tug and significant subcostal recession. His respiratory rate was 40 breaths per minute and his heart rate was 170 bpm. He was given a budesonide and adrenaline nebuliser and again his work of breathing and stridor settled.

A few hours later his work of breathing increased again, now with loud stridor and significant recession. He was given a further dose of oral dexamethasone and his fourth adrenaline nebuliser with good effect.

At 1 o'clock that afternoon, the referring hospital called the transport service as a forewarning, advising that the baby may need retrieving due to increasing work of breathing.

Observations at the time of referral are noted in Table 12.1.

Up to this point the baby had received six adrenaline nebulisers and 300 mcg/kg oral dexamethasone. He had been seen by the anaesthetists who had assessed that he did not need intubation.

Questions

1. What advice would you give to the referring team about the management of the baby's airway as a forewarning call at 1 o'clock?
2. What advice would you give to the referring team about the management of the baby's airway in case of further deterioration?
3. If, as a retrieval team, you arrive at the above clinical scenario with a marginally improved clinical picture in an unintubated child, would you proceed with transfer and under what conditions?

1. What advice would you give to the referring team about the management of the baby's airway as a forewarning call at 1 o'clock?

When taking referral calls in a paediatric emergency retrieval service, there are a number of prime responsibilities of the team. Firstly, is the child being referred critically unwell and does the referring team need emergency management advice ? Secondly, is the proposed

Table 12.1.

Heart rate	150 bpm
Respiratory rate	37 breaths per minute
SpO_2	96% in room air
Capillary refill time	<2 sec
AVPU	Alert

problem list or diagnosis by the referring team most likely or correct? Thirdly, if the child is not critically unwell now, is deterioration or improvement more likely? Finally, does the child require transfer considering the responses to the first three questions.

Croup (laryngotracheobronchitis) is a common illness in childhood and usually affects children between six months and three years. Up to 5% of children with croup are admitted to hospital and of those, 2–3% will require intubation. Croup is caused most commonly by Parainfluenza (types 1 and 3) or Influenza A and B but also by respiratory syncytial virus, rhinovirus, human metapneumovirus, adenovirus and coronavirus. It is characterised by a barking cough, hoarse voice, respiratory distress, wheeze and stridor due to inflammation and oedema of the upper airway mucosa.

Nebulised adrenaline is recommended for severe croup. It is thought to stimulate α-adrenergic receptors in the subglottic membranes causing vasoconstriction and reducing mucosal oedema. This has been associated with a transient reduction in the symptoms of croup and is given to allow the **steroids time to act.**

It is helpful to categorise severity of symptoms of croup. Although the initial presentation described above was severe, according to NICE guidance at the point of referral, it may appear that the severity has fallen to moderate. It is important to note, when evaluating severity, that the baby had just received the sixth adrenaline nebulisation, the clinical effect of which is sustained for around 1 hour. Additionally no information was given about the baby's level of activity, or whether they were lethargic or agitated or calm and responsive.

Children with croup, treated with nebulised adrenaline may develop re-emergence of the symptoms of croup, but they are less pronounced in children who had concurrent treatment with oral glucocorticoids. In the clinical situation described above, it would appear that the baby is not improving despite maximal therapy. The district general hospital anaesthetists, having evaluated the child, did not feel that the child needed intubation at the time of evaluation. When evaluating need for intubation and ventilation in this setting, it is important to attempt to predict whether the baby or child will be able to maintain the level of work of breathing in the following hours. The level of alertness may be the clue to how likely this is. It may be prudent to make the baby/child nil by mouth at this stage and make plans for further deterioration to the point of requiring intubation.

2. What advice would you give to the referring team about the management of the baby's airway in case of further deterioration?

The indications for intubation in a child with croup follow 'failure of medical therapy' with progression to:

- Exhaustion due to increased work of breathing
- Respiratory failure due to hypoxia or hypercapnia
- Decreased level of consciousness
- Imminent airway obstruction.

Once it has been recognised that the child's condition *may* warrant intubation, advanced planning should occur.

Intubation of a child with impending critical airway obstruction should not be undertaken as an emergency if possible. Advance planning allows provision for the likely potential of difficult airway access.

This baby falls into this category where plans for intubation should be made.

COMET is a useful acronym in upper airway obstruction:

C Call for help – the most senior airway doctor/anaesthetist in the hospital and ENT surgeon, who can perform an emergency tracheostomy in case of an 'unable to intubate' scenario. If ENT is not on site, then this call for help should be activated with allowance for travel time.

O Optimise treatment – high flow oxygen avoiding causing distress to the child. Nebulised adrenaline if required, whilst setting up to intubate. Ensure maximum dose of dexamethasone has been given. Anaesthetic cream on cannulation sites but do not cannulate if this will distress the child.

M Monitoring – this should be prepared and at the minimum an oxygen saturation monitor should be on the child, but preferably also heart rate and blood pressure and have end tidal CO_2 monitoring ready for use.

E Equipment – a range of endotracheal tube (ETT) sizes – starting with an appropriate sized uncuffed ETT. There must also be several smaller sizes as the airway is narrowed. (If croup tubes are available use these – they are longer than usual ETTs in smaller sizes so that a smaller than age-appropriate ETT will be sufficient length). Two laryngoscopes with working bulbs and a range of blades, bougie, introducer, laryngeal mask airway, suction, anaesthetic circuit, ENT surgeon with tracheostomy kit prepared on hand.

T Technique – anaesthetic technique should achieve the optimal intubating conditions in the shortest period of time. The child should be accompanied by the most senior airway doctor with their parent/carer to theatre self-ventilating with oxygen if required. Various anaesthetic techniques may be used. Inhalational gas (sevoflurane) can be used to induce anaesthesia with the maintenance of spontaneous ventilation. IV induction of anaesthesia is occasionally utilised, usually where IV access is already in situ. It is ideal to establish that bag valve mask ventilation can be performed after induction of anaesthesia before a muscle relaxant is given

Cautions regarding tubes in small children should be noted.

Do not pre-cut tubes.

The smallest tube that can be used for transfer is 2.5 mm, and it is difficult to clear secretions through this. Saline lavage may be required prior to suction.

If the 2.5 mm ETT does not fit down on primary laryngoscopy, the small orange bougie can be used to 'intubate' the trachea. The 2.5 mm ETT is then rail-roaded over the bougie under direct vision, using two operators.

The usual duration of stay in PICU is a few days.

If the tube size and associated resistance to breathing allows, the child is allowed to wake up and either will require minimum ventilation or in the case of bigger children with bigger diameter ET tubes, may self-ventilate through a Swedish nose (small airway humidification device) during the day and require minimum ventilation at night.

Extubation is usually planned for 48 hours post admission to allow oral steroids to take full effect before extubation.

At 4 o'clock in the afternoon, the referring hospital called the retrieval team to request transfer to a paediatric intensive care unit and informed the team that the baby was about to be intubated with the ENT surgeon accompanying the anaesthetist to theatre.

The retrieval team activated transfer. On arrival at the hospital an hour later, they discovered the baby asleep, self-ventilating, on his mother's lap with intermittent stridor and moderate work of breathing.

The local team were adamant the transfer to PICU went ahead.

3. If, as a retrieval team, you arrive at the above clinical scenario with a marginally improved clinical picture in an unintubated child, would you proceed with transfer and under what conditions?

Observations are noted in Table 12.2.

The referring team reported they had prepared theatre to intubate and then the baby had fallen asleep. They now felt he did not require intubation.

When the baby awoke, he sat on Mum's knee and engaged happily, playing 'Peepo' but had moderate to severe work of breathing still evident.

Considerations:

- The baby had presented more than 12 hours ago and still had moderate to severe work of breathing despite optimal therapy.
- The referring hospital team wanted the retrieval team to transfer the baby but did not think the baby warranted intubation.
- The retrieval team did not want to compromise the safety of the baby by transferring him, self-ventilating in case of deterioration during the ambulance journey potentially requiring intubation, but also did not want to intubate the baby for the purpose of transfer alone.
- The baby had been nil by mouth for almost 6 hours and had had no IV fluids as he did not have IV access.
- It was early evening and there was a large team on standby including ENT awaiting a decision.

Table 12.2.

Heart rate	152 bpm
Respiratory rate	42 breaths per minute
SpO_2	97% in room air
Blood pressure	150/69 mmHg
AVPU	Alert

This is a team decision involving the local anaesthetic consultant, the local paediatric consultant, the ENT consultant, the local paediatric nursing team and the retrieval team including the retrieval consultant by telephone if necessary.

A clear plan must be developed with all in agreement.

This is the plan that was developed for this baby:

- Attempt IV access (anaesthetic cream in situ) almost as a stress test, to test ability to cope with increased respiratory demands of crying, in anaesthetic room environment close to theatre.
- The rationale for this, when all advice is usually to avoid causing stress is that the baby would either need to receive milk from a bottle or need IV fluids as he had been nil by mouth for 6 hours.
- If the stress causes the baby to deteriorate, the baby and team are in the ideal environment in theatre including ENT, in case of 'can't' intubate scenario, to proceed to intubation.
- If the cannula can be sited without problem, and the baby managed the stress of cannulation, then it would probably be safe to remain at the district general hospital.

In this case:

- The IV cannula was sited, but in the process, the baby had increased work of breathing and stridor and it was felt he was nearing exhaustion.
- The decision was made to proceed to intubation. Intubation was recorded as grade 1; however, the anaesthetist was only able to pass a 3.0 uncuffed endotracheal tube through the vocal cords.
- This was secured, a CXR used to confirm the correct length at T2, further IV access was obtained and the baby was uneventfully transferred to PICU with parents in the ambulance.

Further Reading

Geelhoed G. (2019) Chapter 6.4 Croup. In P Cameron, G Browne, M Biswadev, et al., eds. *Textbook of Paediatric Emergency Medicine*. 3rd ed. London Elsevier.

Bijornson CL, Johnson DW (2013) Croup in children. *CMAJ* 185, 1317–23.

National Institute for Health and Care Excellence (2019) Clinical Knowledge Summary: Croup. https://cks.nice.org.uk/topics/croup.

Sakthivel M, Elkashif S, Al Ansari K, Powell C. (2019) Rebound stridor in children with croup after nebulised adrenaline: does it really exist? *Breathe* 15, e1–e7.

Nickson C. (2020) Life in the Fast Lane: Croup. https://litfl.com/croup.

Difficult Asthma

Christopher Hands and Andrew Nyman

A 12-year-old girl, weighing 35 kg, was referred to your service at 22:00. She had presented with an acute exacerbation of asthma and despite emergency management had deteriorated. She had been diagnosed with asthma 4 months previously when she had developed a nocturnal cough. She noticed breathlessness at school whilst doing exercise and since, had seen her GP and was using prescribed regular beclomethasone and as required salbutamol.

She had presented to A&E at 07:00. Treatment had been initiated with hourly salbutamol and 6-hourly ipratropium nebulisers and a bolus of magnesium sulphate. She was commenced on IV hydrocortisone. She had initially improved but later continued to deteriorate during the evening with increased work of breathing and an increasing oxygen requirement. She was given a further bolus of IV magnesium sulphate and was commenced on a salbutamol infusion at 1 mcg/kg/min.

At the time of referral her clinical status was reported as:

RR 40 and unable to complete sentences; SpO_2 90% on high-flow nasal cannula oxygen (HFNO) 100% 45 L/min.

Blood gas: pH 7.37; pCO_2 3.7; lactate 4; BE −6; HCO_3^- 22.6.

CXR from 08:00 that morning showed hyperinflation to nine posterior rib spaces; bilateral streaky infiltrates; no collapse, consolidation, or pneumothorax and a noticeably small cardiac shadow.

Her heart rate was 145 bpm with no palpable pulsus paradoxus. She was flushed with brisk capillary refill. Blood pressure was 135/75 mmHg.

She was anxious and hypervigilant.

Questions

1. What advice would you give to the referring team regarding this child's stabilisation?
2. What are the possible complications that may occur at stabilisation?
3. What approach would you take to mechanical ventilation in this patient on retrieval?
4. What precautions would you take and what possible rescue measures might you consider/employ during retrieval?

1. What advice would you give to the referring team regarding this child's stabilisation?

This child is in respiratory failure and requires urgent senior anaesthetic attendance. She is likely to need intubation for ventilatory support imminently. An urgent repeat mobile CXR would help determine whether there was another cause for this deterioration, such as a lobar collapse or pneumothorax. It is also unusual to have a new diagnosis of asthma in a previously well child, with no family history, and while this is possible, differential diagnosis should include an anterior mediastinal mass (especially in view of the worsening at night when lying down), which will be ruled out on CXR.

The child also has evidence of salbutamol toxicity (tachycardia, hypervigilance/ anxiety and high lactate). The nebulised therapy should be stopped, and the IV therapy reduced to a maximum rate (maximum for adults as well) of 20 mcg/min. She has had a marked deterioration despite optimal and potent bronchodilator therapy. The lack of effectiveness of the potent bronchodilators (salbutamol and magnesium) suggests that her deterioration is not due to bronchospasm, but now most likely secondary to mucus plugging. Consider advising stopping the bronchodilators altogether as the negative side effects may be exacerbating the clinical picture (tachycardia – increased cardiac oxygen demand, tachypnoea – increased air trapping and hyper-inflation) and they are clearly now ineffective. The focus of treatment now should be control of inflammation (appropriate dose steroids), diagnosis and management of small airway plugging (as seen via CXR and lack effectiveness of bronchodilators) and advanced support of breathing.

2. What are the possible complications that may occur at stabilisation?

Her work of breathing indicates that she has a non-compliant chest and you should anticipate that mechanical ventilation will require high pressures to move the chest. She is hyper-inflated and air trapped with a compressed cardiac shadow on CXR, which means she will appear relatively 'volume depleted' because of the air trapping causing reduction in right sided cardiac filling and thus cardiac output. She is already hypoxic. Once she is anaesthetised and spontaneous effort no longer contributes to ventilation, , she is likely to deteriorate quickly. This will be a high-risk induction of anaesthesia. It is important that the most senior anaesthetist available attends the patient. Consider the safest environment in which to anaesthetise and intubate the patient and whether it is safe to transfer the patient to theatre. This may provide a better environment, but the un-intubated, unsupported transfer may be too destabilising, and transferring on HFNO can be challenging and lack complete control.

The relative 'volume depletion' will put the child at risk of circulatory collapse on induction when vascular tone falls and positive pressure mask ventilation is applied to the hyper-inflated lung, further reducing right sided filling. To prevent this, the child should have volume bolus prior to induction and additional fluid boluses, vasopressors and arrest drugs drawn up before induction.

It is important to choose the correct endotracheal tube, aiming for the largest possible diameter with a cuff, to allow high pressure ventilation and minimise the leak. Once the tube is in place, and the cuff inflated, it may be very difficult to ventilate the patient. Manual ventilation with high pressures to achieve chest movement may be the only way to achieve oxygenation. Remember that the pressure you apply at the hub of the tube will be dissipated by the airway obstruction en route to the alveoli. Cardiac arrest is likely to be secondary to hypoxia or relative hypovolaemia, but also consider hypokalaemia, as the patient has been given high doses of salbutamol.

3. What approach would you take to mechanical ventilation in this patient on retrieval?

Take complete control of ventilation. Use regular muscle relaxation and ventilate using a pressure control mode to achieve adequate chest movement. This sometimes requires alarmingly high peak pressures. Use a slow rate, between 10 and 15 bpm to avoid further air trapping and complete lung emptying during expiration. If possible, it is useful to measure the plateau pressure during an inspiratory hold. The plateau pressure should be no higher than 35 cmH$_2$O, and the positive end-expiratory pressure (PEEP) should be fixed at 5 cmH$_2$O to avoid de-recruitment of any normal lung. There is no need to measure auto-PEEP. The difference between peak and plateau pressure will be a good indicator of the degree of small airway obstruction, and reassurance that the peak pressure generated does not reflect the pressure at the alveolus. The peak to plateau (or pause) pressure difference will allow tracking of improvement of mechanical obstruction.

The child should remain muscle relaxed and sedated while disease control is achieved. Consciousness and air hunger will drive tachypnoea, exacerbate air trapping and patient-ventilator dysynchrony. Ensure ventilator settings provide adequate minute ventilation. Tidal volumes should be between 8 and 10 ml/kg. Allow permissive hypercarbia as long as the pCO$_2$ is trending downwards during treatment. Remember severe V:Q mismatch means that the end-tidal CO$_2$ will not reflect the pCO$_2$ accurately. During transfer, 10 kPa is a reasonable target for ETCO$_2$, but it may not be achievable. Driving ventilation to achieve a normal pCO$_2$ in acute severe asthma is likely to lead to barotrauma and aggravate gas-trapping.

4. What precautions would you take and what possible rescue measures might you consider/employ during retrieval?

Physiotherapy: As the main pathophysiology is now likely to be mucus plugging, moving mucus plugs is likely to yield a larger improvement in oxygenation than any other intervention. Whilst the mucus plugs found in asthma are extremely tenacious and deep in the small airways, basic percussion and suctioning with saline lavage may improve oxygenation for long enough to facilitate transfer.

Mechanical decompression: Even with slower respiratory rates, there is a high risk of breath-stacking in this patient group, causing worsening hyper-inflation and eventually allowing no tidal ventilation. If it becomes impossible to ventilate the patient due to breath stacking, it may be necessary to fully disconnect the patient from the ventilator to allow full expiration. Manual decompression may be indicated if the expiratory time is too long, but there is a risk of circulatory collapse, and this manoeuvre should be undertaken with caution, complete cardiorespiratory monitoring in place and resuscitation ready. Development of pneumothorax in this situation is a significant risk

Methylxanthine and beta-2 agonist infusions: Aminophylline infusion has been shown to improve diaphragmatic function and oxygen saturation in children with severe asthma, although with no improvement in any other clinical outcomes. Aminophylline has a narrow therapeutic range with a daunting side-effect profile. The risks and benefits should be carefully weighed before introducing this drug with consideration of the fact that if two potent bronchodilators (salbutamol and magnesium) have not been effective, bronchos-pasm is probably *not* the main problem, and mucus plugging is not improved by aminophylline. There is very little data to support the clinical efficacy of IV salbutamol infusions in this context, although its use is indicated in many guidelines.

Ketamine infusion: There is some low-level evidence that ketamine infusion may improve outcomes in severe asthma, and although it has some adverse effects, the side-effect profile is favourable compared to methylxanthines and beta-2 agonists. One important side effect is the bronchorrhoea (bronchial hypersecretion), which may assist by washing out mucus plugs from the distal airways.

Volatile anaesthetics: Whilst volatiles, such as sevoflurane, have been used to treat severe asthma, their use remains controversial, and there is as yet no evidence to indicate that they improve clinical outcomes. This management strategy is also not possible on transfer. The additional cardiovascular side effects of this group of drugs are not well tolerated in 'volume depleted' settings.

Extra-corporeal membrane oxygenation (ECMO): Some children with refractory severe asthma may need to be supported with ECMO. In cases where oxygenation is rapidly deteriorating, it is appropriate to consider whether the patient should be transported to a centre that can deliver ECMO. In this case veno-venous ECMO is ideal.

Intratracheal rhDNase: This patient is being treated with supra-maximal bronchodilator therapy and was commenced on corticosteroids more than 12 hours ago. It is unlikely that her further deterioration this evening is due to refractory bronchospasm. Mucus plugging of her airways is the likely pathophysiology. Intratracheal instillation of rhDNase, with subsequent physiotherapy-directed pulmonary toilette has been demonstrated to break down the mucus plugs that form in asthma, resulting in improved oxygenation, but should only be undertaken by those familiar with the procedure.

Further Reading

BTS/SIGN Asthma guideline: www.brit-thoracic .org.uk/quality-improvement/guidelines/ asthma/.

Durward A, Forte V, Shemie S. 'Resolution of mucus plugging and atelectasis after intratracheal rhDNase therapy in a mechanically ventilated child with refractory status asthmaticus'. *Crit Care Med.* 2000;28(2):560–2.

Stather D, Stewart T. 'Clinical review: mechanical ventilation in severe asthma'. *Crit Care* 2005;9:581–7.

Wong J, Lee J, Turner D, Rehder K. 'A review of the use of adjunctive therapies in severe acute asthma exacerbation in critically ill children'. *Expert Rev Respir Med* 2014;8(4):423–41.

Chapter 1

Transfer of Child with Pulmonary Hypertension

Kenneth MacGruer and Alison Pienaar

A large district general hospital has called to request a transfer of a 4 kg, 6-month-old ex 25-week premature infant, who is an inpatient in their level 3 NICU. The baby has not left hospital since birth and had a difficult neonatal course. He was intubated at birth and was not successfully extubated until 10 weeks of life. He has significant bronchopulmonary dysplasia (BPD) as a result of his extreme prematurity with secondary pulmonary hypertension diagnosed on echocardiogram. Although he has been relatively stable on high flow nasal cannula oxygen (HFNC) 8 L/min of flow and FiO$_2$ 0.4, he has deteriorated today. His usual medications are sildenafil for pulmonary hypertension; furosemide and spironolactone for chronic lung disease; and weaning doses of clonidine and chloral hydrate for agitation.

The team are calling now because the baby has had a significant deterioration over the last 4 hours with high temperatures (39.8°C), increasing oxygen requirement (now on continuous positive airway pressure [CPAP] of 8 cm H$_2$O with 60% O$_2$), and tachycardia with dropping blood pressure requiring IV access and two 10 ml/kg fluid boluses. The NICU team has commenced initial shock management and started appropriate IV antibiotics. The concern is that the child has sepsis and they are keen to intubate him as soon as possible, but are exceedingly nervous in view of the pulmonary hypertension and the already significant oxygen requirement. They have called the retrieval service to seek advice around intubation and request transfer to PICU as the baby has outgrown NICU and they feel this problem will be ongoing. Before referral some basic blood tests and gas have been performed as shown in Table 14.1.

Questions

1. How might this patient's condition affect where you choose to transfer him and what treatment options might there be in PICU.
2. What advice would you give the local team regarding the intubation of this baby, both from a clinical and human factor standpoint?

1. How might this patient's condition affect where you choose to transfer him and what treatment options might there be in PICU?

This patient has an acute history, clinical examination and blood results consistent with shock possibly due to infection. Sepsis in itself can be managed in most PICUs depending on severity of disease and support required. The background of BPD and pulmonary

Table 14.1. Blood tests and venous gas

Blood gas		Bloods	
pH	7.29	Haemoglobin	132 g/L
pCO$_2$	10.2 KPa	White cell count	28.1 (10^3/mm^3)
HCO$_3$	40.1 mmol/L	Pits	445
Base excess	+11	Urea	10 mmol/L
Lactate	2.3 mmol/L	Creatinine	29 U/L
Glucose	3.8 mmol/L	CRP	135 mg/L

hypertension makes this case more complicated and should be considered when deciding on an accepting unit for this patient. Note the classic compensated respiratory acidosis picture of the blood gas – typical of ex-premature neonates with any chronic lung disease.

Pulmonary Hypertension

The largest numbers of children with pulmonary hypertension (PH) are those with transient disease processes including persistent PH of the newborn and systemic-to-pulmonary shunts, accounting for up to 82% of paediatric patients with this condition. PH secondary to pulmonary disease accounts for 10% of cases, which includes 5% of all children with BPD, and 1.5% of children with obstructive sleep apnoea will have PH. The overall incidence of PH in children is low. The classification of PH is generally based on the location of the pathology in the pulmonary vascular bed and the underlying aetiology.

In PH, the structure and function of the pulmonary vasculature is abnormal. PH increases the right ventricular (RV) afterload and therefore leads to RV hypertrophy as the heart tries to maintain adequate cardiac output. RV failure may develop with deleterious effects on left ventricular function and cardiac output.

In the case of our patient, he had been difficult to wean from mechanical ventilation and had an on-going significant oxygen requirement. To investigate this issue, he had an echocardiogram done which showed RV hypertrophy and tricuspid regurgitation with a peak velocity of 2.91 m/s but with preserved RV function. Additionally, signs of RV hypertrophy were seen on ECG.

Treatment of Pulmonary Hypertension

Coordination of treatment of children with PH should be multidisciplinary. The evidence for treatment strategies in children is poor and is extrapolated from adult data and consensus of expert opinion. Treatment options include:

Oxygen and respiratory support: oxygen is a powerful vasodilator and should be used to treat hypoxia or as an adjunct to other pulmonary vasodilators. Respiratory support can be considered to optimise oxygen delivery or treat hypoventilation – but the decision to start this should not be taken lightly, this is discussed in question 2.

Phosphodiesterase type-5 inhibitors (PHE5): e.g. Sildenafil™. PHE5 degrades cGMP in smooth muscle cells. Inhibition of this increases intracellular cGMP resulting in pulmonary vasodilation.

Inhaled nitric oxide (NO): NO is produced endogenously and regulates vasodilation by increasing cGMP levels. Given by inhalation NO diffuses through the vascular endothelium and causes relaxation of pulmonary vascular smooth muscle generally without other side effects.

Prostacyclins: Cause vasodilation by increasing cAMP. Some difficult to manage patients can end up on long-term infusions of synthetic prostcyclins, e.g. epoprostinol, and as such are at risk of line infections and pump failure.[5]

Bearing all of this in mind our patient would be best managed in a PICU that has an associated paediatric cardiology service so that he can have regular echocardiograms to monitor his PH and so that treatment decisions can be made jointly between cardiology and PICU.

2. What advice would you give the local team regarding the intubation of this baby, both from a clinical and human factor standpoint?

The local team correctly identified that the child was deteriorating and required resuscitation for shock and then intubation and ventilation. In patients with PH the decision to intubate should not be taken lightly. While intubation and ventilation offers clinical benefits including maximising inspired oxygen, controlling ventilation, reducing respiratory workload and facilitating delivery of inhaled of NO, induction of anaesthesia and intubation is a high-risk procedure and could result in an acute pulmonary hypertensive crisis, loss of cardiac output and cardiac arrest.

Oxygen is a potent pulmonary vasodilator and increasing $PaCO_2$ causes pulmonary vasoconstriction. Acidosis in itself also contributes to pulmonary vasoconstriction.

Intubation may result in a period of hypoxia (or less oxygen delivery) and/or hypoventilation and respiratory acidosis. This can trigger the abnormal pulmonary vasculature to undergo exaggerated vasoconstriction, resulting in an acute rise in the pulmonary vascular resistance (PVR). This can lead to a reduction in cardiac output as the right ventricle struggles to eject against increasing pulmonary pressures and venous return to the left atrium is acutely diminished. This can lead to cardiopulmonary arrest.

In children who have a cardiac shunt (patent foramen ovale, atrial septal defect, ventricular septal defect or patent ductus arteriosus) cardiac output may be somewhat preserved by a right to left shunt when the pulmonary pressure becomes supra-systemic, albeit with significant desaturation. If the patient has had a previous echocardiogram it is useful to ascertain the presence of a potential shunt.

When discussing an intubation plan with the local team, highlighting and being clear about the risks is important, but should be done without causing unnecessary alarm. Advice surrounding intubation may include the following, bearing in mind the baby is in a level 3 NICU where personnel are experienced in intubating infants.

Preparing the Patient

- Inform parents of requirement to intubate and the specific associated risks.
- Ensure adequate venous or intra-osseous access is in place.

- Commence peripheral inotropes to augment the systemic blood pressure, for example, dopamine or noradrenaline prior to induction.
- Pre-oxygenate optimally with 100% oxygen. Do not disconnect from respiratory support (e.g. HFNC oxygen, CPAP until induction has commenced).

Gather All Necessary Resources

In addition to standard intubation equipment the team should also prepare:

- Cardiac arrest drugs
- Short acting alpha agonists e.g. phenylephrine to support blood pressure
- Fluid boluses
- Capnography
- Inhaled NO circuit if available
- Additional intra-osseous needle, if vascular access is not optimal.

Personnel and Anticipation of Problems

- Select an experienced anaesthetic colleague to support the neonatal team (or vice versa) as this is no longer a tiny premature.
- Identify specific roles for each member of the team for the intubation, including a team lead who is not the intubator.
- Ensure intubation conditions are optimised to maximise chances of the first attempt being successful, including choosing the right equipment.
- Anticipate and discuss potential problems. Everyone should be allocated a role for the cardiopulmonary arrest scenario.

Intubation Plan

- The team should use their standard induction for a shocked child. The following exceptions to this should be applied:
    - Avoid the use of atropine (which is often a standard part of NICU induction) as a faster heart rate may impair RV filling and cause a resultant reduction in cardiac output. This child is no longer within the neonatal period and a severe bradycardia secondary to vagal stimulation is less likely to occur at this age especially if the child is adequately anaesthetised.
    - Avoid the use of propofol in this patient as the child is shocked. Moderated doses of cardiostable induction agents should be used (ketamine and fentanyl). Fluid bolus should be prepared no matter the agent chosen. All anaesthetics will reduce endogenous sympathetic drive.
- Preload should be optimised for RV filling – suggest a fluid bolus peri-intubation.
- End-tidal CO_2 monitoring for intubation should be followed as standard for induction of anaesthesia. This is not available in all NICUs, but should be brought from theatres on portable monitoring. Remember and remind the team that $ETCO_2$ will diminish during periods of acutely elevated PVR because of a reduction in pulmonary blood flow. This should not be misinterpreted as endotracheal tube (ETT) dislodgement.

- Given the patient has severe BPD, anticipate that the lungs will be poorly compliant and require high mean airway pressures to achieve adequate minute ventilation. Placement of an appropriately sized cuffed ETT should be advised.
- Hyperventilation can be used acutely in the settling of suspected pulmonary hypertensive crisis and can be done easily using the bag; however, caution should be used to not over-ventilate as this can cause decreased venous return, alveolar distension and lung damage as well as cerebral vasoconstriction.
- Highlight to the team that an acute deterioration may occur sometime after intubation as a result of an increasing CO_2 on the initial ventilator settings applied. As such, careful attention should be paid to the CO_2 after intubation and appropriate adjustments to the ventilator should be made. $ETCO_2$ and blood gases should correlated and used to confirm adequate ventilation.
- Following intubation, commence appropriate sedation. Inadequate sedation may precipitate pulmonary hypertensive spells. The child should be kept muscle relaxed for transfer.

Further Reading

Berger RM, Beghetti M, Humpl T, et al. Clinical features of paediatric pulmonary hypertension: A registry study. *Lancet* 2012;379(9815):537–46.

Galiè N, Humbert, M, Vachiery J-L, et al. Guidelines for the diagnosis and treatment of pulmonary hypertension. *Eur Respir J* 2015; 46:903–75.

Haddad F. Right ventricular function in cardiovascular disease. *Circulation* 117(13):1717–31.

Nichols DG, Shaffner DH, (eds). *Rogers' Textbook of Pediatric Intensive Care.* 5th Ed. 2016.

van Loon RL, Roofthooft MT, Hillege HL, et al. Pediatric pulmonary hypertension in the Netherlands: Epidemiology and characterization during the period 1991 to 2005. *Circulation* 2011;124(16):1755–64.

Chapter 5

A Blue Baby

Joanna Davies and Shelley Riphagen

A term, 'newborn baby', with normal antenatal scans was referred to the transport service with severe cyanosis. There were no maternal risk factors for infection and the baby weighed 3.0 kg. The baby was born by caesarean section and after birth was noted to have ongoing cyanosis with saturations variable between 50% and 60%, although she appeared otherwise vigorous. There was mild subcostal and intercostal recession with tachypnoea. Due to the ongoing significant cyanosis despite oxygen, she was intubated and ventilated in 100% oxygen, with only marginal improvement in saturations. No murmur could be heard. The clinical examination prior to intubation is noted in Table 15.1.

The baby had been started on broad spectrum antibiotics and the referring team were considering the potential differential diagnosis at the time the referral call was made. The CXR was shared electronically at the time of referral and is shown in Figure 15.1.

Questions

1. What tests could be easily performed to help establish whether this baby is likely to have congenital heart disease (CHD)?
2. If CHD is suspected, what management principles should be applied?
3. When dealing with a baby with this condition what are the transport priorities?

1. What tests could be easily performed to help establish whether this baby is likely to have congenital heart disease (CHD)?

When dealing with the triage of acutely unwell children, it is important to identify whether the presentation would classify as emergency. As described in other chapters, this evaluation should always be undertaken in a systematic manner, using a progressive A B C approach.

In this baby, the main clinical problem is severe cyanosis. The baby is unable to oxygenate blood. The inability to oxygenate may be related to a pulmonary problem or cardiac pathology associated with inadequate pulmonary blood flow or mixing, causing deoxygenated blood to bypass the lungs. Severe cyanosis is a life-threatening condition and identifies this as an emergency. It would fit into the category of neonatal collapse. In all emergency conditions, there should be a rapidly applicable set of management steps that can be instituted immediately, without needing to establish the definitive underlying aetiology. We will discuss these steps in the response to question 2.

However, when trying to differentiate between cardiac and pulmonary causes of cyanosis, there are some simple clinical tests and examination features which can be determined.

Table 15.1. Examination before intubation

Respiratory rate 75 breaths per minute saturations 50%	Minimal respiratory distress
Heart rate 150 bpm Blood pressure 59/38 mmHg	Weak femoral pulses, heart sounds normal
AVPU Alert	Blood sugar 3 mmol/L

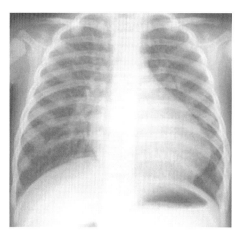

Figure 15.1 Chest radiograph prior to intubation.

In a baby with lung disease causing this degree of cyanosis, the clinician should expect to discover significant clinical pathology on examination and CXR evaluation. With this degree of cyanosis, we would expect the lung parenchyma to be so abnormal as to not be able to exchange gas. The parenchymal involvement would make the chest non-compliant and the baby would be working hard to breathe. In this baby, besides the cyanosis and significant tachypnoea, there are no other signs of respiratory distress, and the parenchymal evaluation of the CXR reveals no pathology. Additionally, even in the worst lung disease, the application of 100% oxygen will usually result is a some increment in oxygen saturations (positive hyperoxia test) which is not usually the case for cardiac disease. The ability to clear carbon dioxide may be an additional factor to differentiate respiratory from cardiac causes of hypoxia.

Cardiac causes of newborn cyanosis fall into one of three main groups.

The first, and arguably most common is pulmonary hypertension (either secondary or primary) where the supra-systemic pulmonary pressures prohibit transit of deoxygenated blood through the right heart and pulmonary circulation into the left heart and the systemic circulation. Blood shortcuts via the foramen ovale and ductus arteriosis directly from right to left with deoxygenated blood supplied to the systemic circulation. Depending on the cause of the pulmonary hypertension, the lungs may be very abnormal on CXR or completely oligaemic. Until the pulmonary vascular resistance can be normalised, these babies may be minimally responsive to oxygen.

The second group is those babies with congenital heart defects causing right-sided obstruction, with blood unable to transit normally through the right heart. This obstruction may be at valvar level, at the tricuspid or pulmonary valve, or in the

Table 15.2. Comparison of clinical and radiological findings

	TGA	TAPVD
Clinical	Cyanosis $\pm$ shock	Cyanosis $\pm$ shock
Saturations	Pre ductal (right hand) lower than lower body saturations	Equally low everywhere
CXR – lungs fields	Clear and normal	Engorged, interstitial and alveolar oedema, pleural effusions
Cardiothoracic ratio (heart size)	Normal	Small
Mediastinum	Narrow	Widened (supracardiac TAPVD)

pulmonary outflow tract. Either has the effect of causing diversion of blood across the foramen ovale. The lung fields on CXR are extremely oligaemic, and the cardiac shadow in some cases is abnormal with the 'empty' pulmonary arteries causing a boot-shaped left heart border. Supplemental oxygen makes no difference to saturations as there is no normal pulmonary blood flow to pick up oxygen. The right-to-left shunt at atrial level sustains cardiac output, and initially, despite the hypoxia, the baby usually retains a good cardiac output with no evidence of shock.

The third group of newborns with cyanosis of cardiac origin fall into a group of conditions which are the most commonly missed antenatally because of their normal intracardiac anatomy on screening fetal ultrasound. Two main congenital heart lesions are Transposition of the Great Arteries (TGA) and Total Anomalous Pulmonary Venous Drainage (TAPVD) both presenting with profound cyanosis and progressive shock, if left untreated. Luckily, despite their almost identical clinical presentation, they are relatively easily differentiated with bedside examination, investigations and CXR as seen in Table 15.2.

In our neonate, on further questioning of the referring clinicians we were able to establish that the baby had post ductal saturations in the 60s, higher than the measured right hand saturations, and in conjunction with the CXR evaluation, TGA is significant possibility in this baby.

2. If CHD is suspected, what management principles should be applied?

As soon as CHD is suspected in an unwell neonate, along with usual resuscitation procedures for a collapsed neonate, an IV infusion of prostaglandin E_2 should be commenced at the earliest opportunity.

Early senior support should be recruited from both the paediatric and anaesthetic teams. Resuscitation of the collapsed neonate should be approached in a systematic manner. The baby should be placed in oxygen-targeting saturations in the 70–85% range. Respiratory support should be applied using an anaesthetic circuit with positive end-expiratory pressure, in an attempt to minimise work of breathing and optimise oxygen delivery. After IV access is established, if the child is not shocked, prostaglandin should be started at 10 nanograms/kg/min.

For those neonates who are shocked, a small volume bolus challenge of 5–10 ml/kg can be attempted, and repeated or not, depending on the response. In those who respond unfavourably to volume, early application of inotropes should be instituted – either dopamine or low dose adrenaline.

Paediatric retrieval team and specialist cardiology advice should be sought regarding escalation of prostaglandin, dependent on initial response to the infusion, and the clinical picture with most likely diagnosis.

As soon as some degree of improvement has been achieved, the baby should be intubated taking all precautions to avoid cardiac arrest – with arrest drugs available, good team debrief prior to anaesthesia and cautious anaesthetic drug administration, with dosing based on the level of acuity of the baby.

Higher doses of up to 50–100 ng/kg/min may be necessary when the ductus has closed and needs to be reopened; however, this should only be escalated with senior specialist advice. Prostaglandin E_2 relaxes vascular smooth muscle and will maintain patency of the ductus arteriosus.

The use of prostaglandin in self-ventilating babies is acceptable, as long as the neonate is fully monitored and observed at all times. Prostaglandin-related apnoea, hypotension and flushing are most likely in the first hour of starting the prostaglandin, and apnoea is associated with higher doses in sicker neonates. This is not relevant in the ventilated baby.

3. When dealing with a baby with this condition what are the transport priorities?

In a neonate with a 'duct dependent lesion' with cyanosis and shock, transfer is an emergent issue. Although prostaglandin may improve the clinical situation to some degree in TGA, it may make no difference in those with TAPVD.

These are the two congenital heart lesions requiring transfer without delay to a cardiac interventional centre.

There must be no delay because of trying interminably to secure IV or intra-arterial access. Umbilical access may still be relatively easy in this group and if not a low threshold for intra-osseous access should be maintained if peripheral or central IV access is difficult.

Non-invasive blood pressure monitoring is perfectly acceptable, if access is delaying transfer.

Cardiology and potentially cardiac surgery should be placed on standby at the receiving institution and the transfer process should be made safer by preparing for cardiovascular instability en route.

Remember during transport that these are extremely sick unstable babies who can neither maintain temperature nor glucose homeostasis, and both need active management.

Congenital Heart Disease

CHD is the commonest birth defect, affecting approximately 6–10/1000 live births, and is also the leading cause of death in children with congenital malformations. It is thought up to 58% may be diagnosed antenatally but this leaves a large proportion who present without a cardiac diagnosis, and potentially as collapsed neonates.

Transposition of the great arteries is the most common cyanotic heart lesion and constitutes around 5% of CHD. It is more common in males than females with a ratio of

3:1, and maternal risk factors include diabetes, age over 40, alcoholism and viral illness during pregnancy.

In TGA, the great vessels are transposed from their normal position, so the aorta arises from the morphological right ventricle and the pulmonary artery from the left ventricle. Deoxygenated systemic blood returning from the body enters the right heart and is pumped via the aorta back around the body. In parallel, the oxygenated blood from the lungs enters the left atrium and ventricle and is pumped back to the lungs via the pulmonary artery transposed into the aortic position. Unless intra- or extracardiac mixing between the two parallel circulations is achieved, survival is impossible. In approximately 30% of patients with TGA, there are also coronary artery abnormalities. Unfortunately, this is not always a 'simple lesion' and there may be other associated defects including ventricular septal defect, and left ventricular outflow tract obstruction.

In simple TGA (with intact ventricular septum which accounts for about 60% of all TGA), the neonate presenting in this manner is likely to need urgent balloon atrial septostomy to improve intracardiac mixing of oxygenated blood with deoxygenated blood to achieve oxygen saturations of around 80%, before definitive surgery to switch the great vessels and reimplant the coronary arteries is undertaken. Ductal patency will usually be maintained until the definitive surgery.

Before transfer, a senior clinician should speak to the parents together explaining the critical nature of the condition and the high suspicion of congenital heart defect.

As the baby may need an emergency intervention, if at all possible, one of the parents should accompany the baby for surgical consent purposes.

In this case it is very difficult, with the father asked to decide to accompany the newborn or remain with the mother, who is post-operative caesarean section. It is acknowledged that this will be an incredibly stressful and upsetting time for the parents especially as antenatal scans did not highlight any CHD, and the necessary separation between mother and baby will amplify the sadness (until, she can be relocated to the same hospital site, if at all possible). Ensure that the mother has photographs of her baby and if the condition of the baby is stable on the prostaglandin infusion, it may be possible for the transfer team to transfer the baby to see the mother before departure to the tertiary centre, but not if this compromises the baby's condition by delaying transfer.

Further Reading

Browning Carmo KA, Barr P, West M, et al. Transporting newborn infants with suspected duct dependent congenital heart disease on low-dose prostaglandin E1 without routine mechanical ventilation. *Arch Dis Child Fetal Neonatal Ed* 2007; 92: F117–19.

Kemper AR, Mahle WT, Martin GR, et al. Strategies for implementing screening for critical congenital heart disease. *Pediatrics* 2011;128: e1259–67.

Meckler GD, Lowe C. To intubate or not to intubate? Transporting infants on prostaglandin E1. *Pediatrics* 2009;123: E25–30.

Saris GE, Balmer C, Bonou P, et al. Clinical guidelines for the management of patients with transposition of the great arteries with intact ventricular septum. *Eur J Cardio-Thorac Surg* 2017;51:(1)e1–e32.

A Shocked Blue Baby Who Won't Improve

Jenny Budd and Shelley Riphagen

A baby girl was referred at 18 hours of age. She had presented due to parental concerns of poor feeding and change in colour. She had been seen by the neonatal team and taken to the NICU where her referral observations were recorded as below in Table 16.1.

Clinical assessment of the baby revealed that she was lethargic, with moderately increased work of breathing and obvious cyanosis. Central pulses were palpable; however, peripheral pulses were more difficult to feel and her peripheral perfusion was poor. The anterior fontanelle was soft. There were no maternal or pregnancy concerns to suggest any infectious risk, and repeated routine antenatal scans had all been unremarkable.

By the time of the referral call, the baby had been given IV antibiotics and a fluid bolus of 10 ml/kg of normal saline. High flow oxygen via face mask had also been commenced. The neonatal team had sent some baseline blood tests, obtained a blood sugar and CXR displayed in Table 16.2 and Figure 16.1.

The saturations had increased from 72% to 84% in response to the facemask oxygen and the fluid bolus had decreased the heart rate from 190 bpm to 178 bpm, but the blood pressure and peripheral perfusion had not improved. The baby was intubated and ventilated. Urgent retrieval was requested because despite escalation of ventilation and maximising the amount of oxygen being delivered, the baby had worsening saturations.

Questions

1. What is the most likely diagnosis for this baby?
2. What measures can be taken prior to transfer to optimise the condition of this baby?
3. What information are you going to give to the parents?

1. What is the most likely diagnosis for this baby?

This baby has presented as a 'collapsed neonate' with the most common causes for this state being vertically transmitted infections, congenital heart disease, space occupying lesions in the chest (including diaphragmatic hernia), some inborn error of metabolism and occasionally trauma (including non-accidental injury) or other serious abdominal emergencies. All possibilities should be considered and positively excluded as soon as possible with easy to perform investigations including CXR; head ultrasound and where relevant, abdominal X-ray/ ultrasound along with baseline blood tests including blood gas, glucose and ammonia.

In the setting of cyanosis with shock, the possibilities are immediately narrowed down to heart and lung problems, with most space occupying lung problems easy to exclude on

Table 16.1.

Heart rate	190 bpm
Blood pressure	53/42 mmHg
Saturations	74%
Respiratory rate	65 breaths per minute

Table 16.2.

Initial blood results

Na	132 mmol/l
K	4.1 mmol/l
Urea	2.7 mmol/l
Creatinine	51 U/l
Haemoglobin	156 g/l
Glucose	3.2 mmol/l
CRP	<1 mg/l

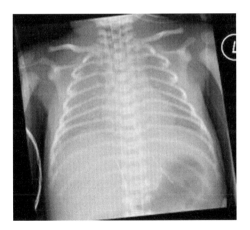

Figure 16.1 Admission chest radiograph.

CXR. This baby most likely has a congenital heart lesion causing this presentation due to the CXR showing no space-occupying lung lesion, persistent hypoxia despite ventilation and oxygen and developing shock.

There are two main congenital heart lesions which are difficult to pick up antenatally because of the normal intracardiac anatomy, and both present with worsening shock and progressive cyanosis: transposition of the great arteries (TGA) and total anomalous pulmonary venous drainage (TAPVD).

Of the two, TGA is the more common lesion with 60% of infants with this condition having the lesion with an intact ventricular septum. In this setting, the circulation is divided into two: one of deoxygenated blood and the other of oxygenated blood. The circuits run parallel to each other, and because the great arteries are transposed, the aorta and systemic circulation see progressively desaturated blood, with the coronary arteries and myocardium becoming more and more hypoxic with progressive myocardial dysfunction and shock. In this situation, the lung fields are normally perfused and at first the heart size is also normal; however, the shape of the cardiac silhouette may be the pathognomonic 'egg on the side' because of the orientation of the great vessels in the upper mediastinum.

In TAPVD, the circulation is normal until the pulmonary venous drainage which does not empty, as usual, into the posterior aspect of the left atrium. The four veins often form a confluent chamber, which collects all the oxygenated pulmonary venous blood and then decompresses by a superior, inferior or intracardiac vein into the systemic circulation, joining the systemic venous return in the right atrium. This leaves the left side of the heart relatively 'empty' with extremely diminished left-sided cardiac output and rapid progress to profound shock with progressive desaturation. In this case, because the pulmonary venous return is obstructed, the lungs become progressively engorged with worsening pulmonary venous hypertension, as is the case in this baby.

No amounts of volume or inotropes or even prostaglandin will improve the situation, and the baby needs emergency surgery once a definitive echocardiogram has confirmed the diagnosis.

2. What measures can be taken prior to transfer to optimise the condition of this baby?

Optimisation of the clinical condition of a baby with obstructed TAPVD is extremely difficult if not impossible without surgery. The main focus should be maximising support and minimising delay of transfer to a cardiac surgical centre.

Intubation and ventilation with maximum oxygen was a correct and appropriate course of action. At the time of referral to the retrieval service, the baby's saturations were 70–80%. By the time the retrieval team met the baby, 90 minutes after the initial referral was made, the best saturations that could be achieved were 71%. By this point, inhaled nitric oxide had been commenced in an attempt to improve her saturations, with no response.

Dopamine and adrenaline infusions had been commenced to address the hypotension. This improved the baby's blood pressure from 53/42 mmHg to 60/40 mmHg. The blood pressure readings from this baby clearly demonstrated hypotension and needed intervention. The commencing of inotropes cannot be avoided, but needs to be done with an awareness that both dopamine and adrenaline will increase the heart rate in an already tachycardic baby and increase myocardial oxygen utilisation. Increasing tachycardia may be counterproductive to improving cardiac output.

Support of the respiratory and cardiovascular systems are essential to the baby's survival, but ultimately may not improve her clinical condition. The obstruction within the circulation means that her condition will progressively deteriorate. The focus of this baby's management must remain the urgent need for cardiac surgery. Ensuring the baby is well sedated and muscle relaxed will reduce metabolic demand which is important given that cardiac output is compromised.

For the referring teams, measures can be taken to ensure that the baby can be transferred as quickly as possible once the retrieval team arrives. Ensuring that the endotracheal tube is in an optimum position (position confirmed on CXR) and safely secured, there is adequate and reliable IV access, ideally central access (umbilical venous and arterial lines are quick and easy to establish in a young baby) are important contributions to ensuring that the retrieval is as swift as possible.

A prostaglandin infusion was commenced early on in the initial treatment. This was entirely appropriate. The aim of this was to open up or indeed maintain patency of the ductus arteriosus, enabling arterial and venous blood to mix. In any collapsed neonate, where cardiac disease is suspected, prostaglandin should be commenced and in most cases is a life-saving intervention. An obstruction to either the systemic or pulmonary circulation requires the ductus arteriosus to be patent for the baby to survive. Even in a situation where the exact nature of the cardiac lesion is unclear, a prostaglandin infusion is indicated to preserve life until an accurate diagnosis is obtained.

It is possible that in the setting of obstructed TAPVD, opening up the patent ductus arteriosus (PDA) with the use of prostaglandin may result in a greater degree of cyanosis. This could be attributed to blood shunting right to left (from pulmonary artery to aorta) through the PDA as the pulmonary pressures may well be supra-systemic. The risks of not commencing prostaglandin in a baby who has collapsed as a result of an undiagnosed cardiac lesion far outweigh the risk of increasing hypoxia in an already hypoxic baby.

In summary, optimisation of a baby such as this one requires intubation and ventilation with a high oxygen concentration. Inhaled nitric oxide was started in this infant, not unreasonably, but will likely have no beneficial effect. Cardiovascular support is required through the use of inotropes. Recognition that this condition will not improve without surgical intervention and rapid transfer to a cardiac surgical centre will optimise the outcome.

By the time this baby reached the operating theatre 4 hours after the initial referral call, the best oxygen saturations that could be achieved were 54%.

3. What information are you going to give to the parents?

This baby is clearly critically ill. It is important that the parents are given this information in an honest and empathic manner. There is very little chance that any parent in a situation such as this will be able to retain much information, so clear, concise information is most beneficial. It is important that they understand the gravity of the situation, and that they know that there is a surgical option for their baby. The parents need to understand that urgent transfer to a cardiac surgical centre by a specialist transport team is essential. Generally, the use of language such as 'open heart surgery' helps parents to have some understanding of the situation they are facing.

Most parents will want to accompany their baby on the transfer. Having had a caesarean within the last 24 hours, consideration had to be given to the best way to transfer this baby's mother. This mother was obviously in significant discomfort. Travelling in the ambulance at speed can be uncomfortable and more so for someone who has recently had major abdominal surgery. The postnatal ward at the referring hospital deemed the mother fit for discharge, but the retrieval team took the decision that the mother should not travel with the baby in the ambulance, but rather she should be taken in a car by a friend or family member to the destination hospital.

The retrieval team clarified the marital status of the parents. This can have implications for the consent for the surgical process. Currently, if parents are not married, the father must be named on the child's birth certificate to be able to give consent. Obviously at only 18 hours of age, this baby's birth had not yet been registered.

There are many publications regarding mortality and morbidity for TAPVD. Assuming the baby survives until surgical intervention, mortality in the immediate postoperative period is low. Those with TAPVD as an isolated defect have a much better prognosis. Some patients develop recurrent pulmonary vein stenosis which carries a significant risk of morbidity and mortality. At presentation, however, it is impossible to tell if this baby will be in this category, and there would be little advantage in imparting this information in any detail to the parents at the time of retrieval.

Further Reading

Akkinapally S, Hundalani SG, Kulkarni M, et al. Prostaglandin E1 for maintaining ductal patency in neonates with ductal-dependent cardiac lesions. *Cochrane Database Systematic Rev* 2018, Issue 2. Article no. CD011417. DOI: 10.1002/14651858.CD011417.pub2.

STRS Neonatal Collapse Guidelines. www.evelinalondon.nhs.uk/resources/our-services/hospital/south-thames-retrieval-service/neonatal-collapse-nov-2017.pdf.

STRS TAPVD Guidelines. www.evelinalondon.nhs.uk/resources/our-services/hospital/south-thames-retrieval-service/total-anomalous-pulmonary-venous-drainage.pdf.

Yong MS, Zhu MZ, Konstantinov IE. Total anomalous pulmonary venous drainage repair: redefining the long-term expectations. *J Thorac Dis* 2018;10(Suppl 26):S3207–10. doi: 10.21037/jtd.2018.08.05

Under a Spell

Catia Pinto and Miriam Fine-Goulden

A 2-month-old baby has presented to A&E at her local district general hospital with severe frequent episodes of cyanosis. She had been diagnosed antenatally with Tetralogy of Fallot and was known to the tertiary hospital paediatric cardiology team.

The local team referred her for transfer to tertiary care because her saturations were occasionally dipping down to 50% although for the majority of the time, they were maintained above a baseline of 80% with high-flow oxygen. Her parents also reported she has been a little snuffly for the previous 2 days and that her breathing had changed. It was faster than they had noticed previously, and she had some evidence of subcostal recession.

The parents mentioned that they understood that, due to her condition, she would remain 'blue' until she had her surgery, which was yet to be scheduled. She was not on any regular medication. They had tried placing her in the 'knees-to-chest' position, as advised by cardiology, but it only helped briefly.

A rapid nasopharyngeal aspirate sample taken in A&E was negative for viruses.

The paediatric team were calling for advice regarding what would be the next steps in this child's management, and to seek advice regarding transfer in a safe manner to cardiology.

At the time of referral her clinical examination revealed a respiratory rate of 30–46 breaths per minute, oxygen saturations of 76–83% in air, heart rate of 156 bpm, blood pressure of 110/60 mmHg and liver palpable 4 cm below the costal margin.

The results of a capillary blood gas are shown in Table 17.1 and CXR in Figure 17.1 which showed the typical 'boot-shaped' cardiac shadow and normal-looking lung fields, with no pulmonary cause of desaturation evident.

Questions

1. What causes 'spelling' in Tetralogy of Fallot?
2. What would you advise the local team regarding the further management of the child?
3. When should the child be transferred to a paediatric cardiac centre?

1. What causes 'spelling' in Tetralogy of Fallot?

Tetralogy of Fallot (ToF, sometimes referred to as 'Tet') is the most common of the cyanotic congenital heart diseases and, as the name implies, consists of four component defects including:

Table 17.1. Capillary gas results

pH	7.35
pCO$_2$	5.6 KPa
pO$_2$	3.4 KPa
HCO$_3$	21 mmol/L
Base excess	−2.5 mEq/L
Lactate	2 mmol/L
Glucose	4.5 mmol/L
Na	138 mmol/L

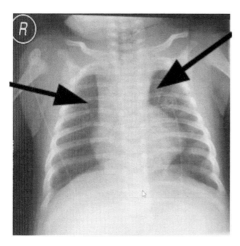

Figure 17.1 Admission chest radiograph.

- Right ventricular outflow tract obstruction (RVOTO) usually in the form of sub-pulmonary infundibular muscles with or without pulmonary valve and pulmonary artery branch involvement, with a broad spectrum of severity
- Right ventricular muscle hypertrophy secondary to RVOTO
- Overriding aorta straddling the ventricular septum
- Ventricular septal defect (size and position of which determines the degree of shunting possible between left and right).

'Spelling', when associated (ToF, refers to sudden onset profound cyanosis related to change in right to left intracardiac shunting. The baseline degree of cyanosis in ToF depends on the severity of obstruction to pulmonary blood flow. In most cases, there is some blood flow across the pulmonary valve. 'ToF', 'Tet', cyanotic or blue spells occur periodically. They may be unprovoked or occur following episodes of abnormal crying or distress. The spells are thought to be caused by spasm of the right ventricular infundibular muscle but may be precipitated or exacerbated by a reduction in right ventricular preload, for example with systemic vasodilation caused by a rise in temperature, or as a result of dehydration. These hypercyanotic spells cause acute severe hypoxia and can lead to a loss of cardiac output, due to a lack of pulmonary blood flow, and subsequent loss of consciousness. In many cases, the spells can be managed successfully at home by parents or carers who are taught to place the baby in knees-to-chest position to increase systemic vascular resistance and to force blood through the right ventricular outflow tract.

The parents had brought in this baby, who was known to spell, but they had felt the spells were becoming more frequent and they were less successful in managing them.

It is important in children with cyanotic spells to exclude other causes of worsening cyanosis including airway obstruction, respiratory infections, anaemia, seizures with hypo-ventilation and breath-holding episodes, amongst others.

2. What would you advise the local team regarding the further management of the child?

Pre-operative cases of ToF would be expected to have a degree of cyanosis. The ongoing management would depend on the baseline level of cyanosis and the presence or absence of spells.

Definitive management is surgical repair, which involves either relieving or bypassing the obstruction to pulmonary blood flow and closing the ventricular septal defect. This is usually delayed beyond the neonatal period as results are improved when children have had an opportunity to grow and mature to some degree before surgery, with most children operated between 3 and 12 months of age.

A child suffering from either increasingly frequent and/or non-self-resolving spells needs immediate attention, employing a standard ABCD approach. It would be important to support the local team in ensuring the following are considered:

A. Some cases of ToF may be associated with tracheomalacia. This is best managed in the acute stage by applying positive end-expiratory pressure (PEEP) or **continuous positive airway pressure** (CPAP) especially if there is an intercurrent respiratory trigger, which has precipitated the spelling.

B. **Administer oxygen** to improve oxygen delivery. In cases of severe cyanosis, intubation and mechanical ventilation may be required.

C. In the acute emergency with a cyanotic baby known to have ToF, the baby can be placed in a **knees-to-chest position**: This causes an increase in systemic vascular resistance (SVR) relative to pulmonary vascular resistance (PVR) and forces pulmonary blood flow.

Beta-blockers are used to reduce spells by at least two mechanisms. They relax the muscular infundibulum, thereby relieving spasm and dynamic outflow tract obstruction; and reduce the heart rate, which facilitates longer filling time, better right ventricular filling and thereby reduced RVOTO. Beta-blockers may also contribute by increasing SVR by blocking peripheral vasodilatation. In the acute phase, beta-blockers are given intravenously, but many children are managed at home on oral propranolol, awaiting surgery, so it is important to check the medication history before administering in the acute setting.

Phenylephrine increases SVR almost immediately without causing further pulmonary infundibular contraction. Other drugs with a similar effect may also be used, e.g. metaraminol and noradrenaline. Adrenaline should be avoided as this can cause pulmonary vasoconstriction and tachycardia, which could exacerbate the cyanosis.

DEFG

Avoid agitation. Crying and breath-holding can increase PVR and increase intrathoracic pressure, thereby reducing cardiac preload.

Sedation/analgesia may be required to decrease heart rate, oxygen consumption and catecholamine response, all of which contribute to worse clinical condition in these children. Ideally, IV access should be obtained for low dose morphine; however, alternative opiates and ketamine can also be administered via other routes including the enteral, intranasal, subcutaneous or intramuscular routes.

Acidosis increases PVR further. Attempt to address the cause.

Electrolyte abnormalities may impact on cardiac rhythm and myocardial function and must be addressed.

Review fluid status: If dehydrated, the hypertrophied RV may be underfilled, impairing cardiac output.

If these measures do not resolve the issue, then the advice would have to be to proceed to intubation and ventilation; however, this can be extremely challenging in a spelling child.

In this case, the child was started on oxygen, but not intubated. Induction drugs and equipment were prepared. Furthermore, phenylephrine and fluid boluses were also made available. Good IV access was also obtained prior to the transfer and oral propranolol was initiated earlier as per cardiology advice. The child was given time to 'stabilise' prior to making the decision to transfer self-ventilating.

If intubation and ventilation are necessary, then precautions should be taken against:

1. Induction drugs causing vasodilation and loss of preload, with acute profound cyanosis. Ketamine should be used with phenylephrine and volume boluses ready to be administered in the case of desaturation not associated with problems with ventilation.

2. Positive pressure ventilation will reduce preload by positive intrathoracic pressure and loss of spontaneous breathing. Preload should be adequate, and volume bolus may be required to establish positive pressure ventilation.

Intubation and ventilation of children with congenital heart defects is not without problems, and before undertaking these procedures, a good understanding of the anatomy and likely physiology must be discussed with the entire team. Expert help should be sought from retrieval teams (who will have access to paediatric cardiac anaesthetists) if possible, prior to undertaking these procedures.

3. When should the child be transferred to a paediatric cardiac centre?

This child was known to the paediatric tertiary cardiology team and the parents were aware and understood his cardiac condition. He had become worse over the previous few days and there should have been no delay in expediting his transfer to the right team.

As part of the retrieval team, you will encounter pre-operative ToF cases who have been diagnosed and are being followed up at home, awaiting surgery. Occasionally you may also encounter a child as yet undiagnosed.

The carers of children with a ToF diagnosis receive counselling and are mostly prepared to manage a spelling episode, and traditionally have been advised to 'keep their baby happy' as a preventive measure. They will usually seek medical attention when the frequency of spells increases, or when the previously advised measures are not successful in resolving the episodes.

Undiagnosed cases typically present with severe cyanosis or with reported episodes of loss of consciousness, sometimes associated with periods of becoming grey or blue. The paediatric cardiology team should always be contacted where a congenital heart defect is suspected or known and there is a change in the child's condition.

In the case of ToF, where the measures listed above have failed to improve the cyanosis and condition of the child, this is a medical emergency and the child needs to be transferred by the retrieval team to a cardiac surgical centre as soon as possible.

If the child is unventilated, the parents should always be encouraged to travel alongside the team as it is beneficial for everyone. It is known that carers can reduce the level of agitation/anxiety experienced by the children. Furthermore, this type of early discussion and involvement is also beneficial for the long-term 'relationship triangle' formed by the child, family and multidisciplinary team, and if urgent surgery is needed the parents will be required for consent.

Outcome

This child was successfully transferred (with difficulty due to ongoing desaturations) but the spells could not be terminated in PICU and the child was operated 24 hours after transfer.

Further Reading

Apitz C, Anderson RH, Redington, AN. Tetralogy of Fallot with pulmonary stenosis. In: Anderson, RH, Baker EJ, Penny D, et al. (eds). *Pediatric Cardiology* 3rd ed. Philadelphia: Churchill Livingstone, 2010:753–73.

Fanous E, Mogyorosy G. Does the prophylactic and therapeutic use of beta-blockers in preoperative patients with tetralogy of Fallot significantly prevent and treat the occurrence of cyanotic spells? *Interact Cardiovasc Thorac Surg* 2017;25:647–50.

Leung AKC, Leung AAM, Wong AHC, Lon KHL. Breath-holding spells in paediatrics: a narrative review of the current evidence. *Curr Pediatr Rev* 2019;15:22–9.

A Decline in Function

Shelley Riphagen

A referral call was received regarding an 11-year-old boy who had presented to the A&E of his local hospital about 2 hours earlier. The boy, who appeared well grown, had been on a school rugby trip the week before and had broken his finger during a tackle. During the tour he felt he had performed disappointingly, and admitted that his running seemed 'heavy'. The week following the tour, he had developed increasingly severe abdominal pain and become breathless playing on the trampoline with his sister. His parents felt he had also become pale and quieter than usual.

On the morning of admission, he had begun complaining of severe arm and leg pain and they had noted that his arms and legs had become discoloured. He was assisted in to A&E by his parents as he was in severe pain on walking.

At triage he was afebrile, with a respiratory rate of 36 breaths per minute and saturations of 95% in air. He was able to answer questions appropriately in only two-word phrases due to breathlessness. His heart rate was 130 bpm and blood pressure 146/118 mmHg. It took repeated attempts to obtain the blood pressure measurement because of the pain the blood pressure cuff caused him, when inflated. The triage nurse moved him to 'Resus' because of the alarming 'rash' over his arms and legs, which were all extremely cold with capillary refill time over 5 seconds peripherally.

At the time of referral, the medical team had assessed him and were worried about cardiac failure. He had a gallop rhythm and displaced apex beat with 3 cm hepatomegaly. They had only been able to site one cannula because the child was in severe and unbearable pain with any compression of his arms or legs. On siting the cannula they had only been able to obtain a venous gas which is shown in Table 18.1 and a mobile CXR, shown in Figure 18.1. Due to the extreme pain in his limbs, lack of peripheral pulses and worrying rash the referral team felt he needed transfer as soon as possible.

The referral hospital was over an hour transfer time from the regional paediatric intensive care and cardiac centre.

Questions

1. Is this an emergency and if so, what would you advise as initial management of this child?
2. What features are unusual in this setting and how would it alter your decision making?
3. Based on the echo [described after question 2 below] performed locally by the adult intensive care consultant, what advice would you give in terms of transfer advice, and what is said to the child and parents?

Table 18.1. Venous blood gas

pH	7.21
pCO_2	6.9 kPa
HCO_3	14 mmol/L
Base excess	−9 mEq/L
Lactate	6.9 mmol/L
Glucose	13.1 mmol/L
Na	129 mmol/L

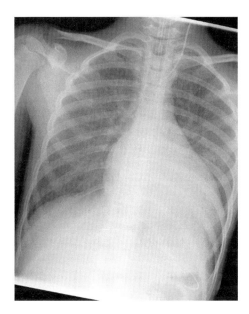

Figure 18.1 Admission chest radiograph.

1. Is this an emergency and if so, what would you advise as initial management of this child?

What constitutes a clinical emergency? When identifying whether a presentation constitutes a clinical emergency, it is important to develop a structured, systematic evaluation to ensure that nothing is missed. A clinical emergency situation has the potential to deteriorate immediately or within a short period of time, to threaten a patient's life or long-term health, if not remediated emergently by various levels of intervention.

This child had cardiogenic shock with clinical signs of cardiac failure (tachycardia, tachypnoea, cardiomegaly, hepatomegaly, hyponatraemia, CXR) and lactic acidosis. This required emergency intervention instituted in a stepwise manner with repeat re-evaluation of intervention.

To start with, the child should be placed in oxygen, and if tolerated positive pressure respiratory support, including high flow nasal cannula oxygen.

His blood pressure is preserved; however, the clinical presentation suggested that his cardiac function was not. While it is not therapeutic, a baseline ECG and echocardiogram performed locally will help guide treatment choices while the retrieval team are en route. He is old enough for the adult cardiac services to undertake the echo, to at least give some idea of valve competence, presence or absence of pericardial effusion and cardiac function.

The child was in severe pain. From the description over the phone, his limbs sounded poorly perfused – cold, discoloured and painful. Adequate analgesia would allow him to co-operate better, and potentially reduce his tachycardia and cardiac oxygen demand. A low-dose morphine infusion should be started via the single cannula.

From description of the initial difficulty with IV cannulation attempts, efforts to site a second cannula should be avoided until the child's pain can be brought under control and if possible, more information is available regarding cardiac function.

All the above interventions should be instituted and response evaluated while awaiting the retrieval team.

2. What features are unusual in this setting and how would it alter your decision making?

This child had a relatively short history of illness and up to a week ago was playing competitive sport. On presentation, he was shocked with lactic acidosis; however, his blood pressure was unusually well preserved. Noticeably the pulse pressure was very narrow. Despite the 'good' systolic blood pressure, there was evidence of intense peripheral vaso-constriction with cold, mottled, discoloured and almost pulseless limbs. There was a suggestion of ischaemic limb pain by the response of the child to attempts at cannulation or blood pressure measurement.

There was significant cardiomegaly on CXR.. The CXR supported the impression of cardiac failure with 'bat wing' increase in perihilar vascular markings with upper lobe venous diversion and evidence of pleural fluid with blunting of the costophrenic angle and fluid in the horizontal fissure.

The question had to be asked whether the high blood pressure was responsible/was the aetiological factor for the cardiac failure, progressing to cardiogenic shock and hence the child was able to function well until a week before presentation, and if so, what was the aetiology of the hypertension.

Arrival of the Retrieval Team

While the retrieval team were en route, an ECG was performed and the local adult intensive care consultant was able to perform a basic echocardiogram. The local team asked to handover away from the child who was sat up in the bed, on 2 L/min nasal cannulae oxygen and morphine 10 mcg/kg/min. Saturations were 97% but his heart rate remained largely unchanged. He was calm, co-operative and settled, though very anxious not to be touched, and when left alone was not in as much pain. Both parents were sitting anxiously beside him.

The Echo report was very alarming, noting a hypertrophic heart with very, very poor ejection (less than 5%) with autocontrast visible in both ventricles due to blood 'swirling' within the cavity.

3. Based on the echo performed locally by the adult intensive care consultant, what advice would you give in terms of transfer, and what is said to the child and parents?

The echo findings were very alarming to the clinical team and the adult intensivist was surprised how 'well' the child looked. Extreme physiologic abnormalities can be masked by a teenager who 'soldiers on' despite feeling very unwell.

With regard to transfer, could this child be moved safely to a higher level of care in the current condition? In this situation, one needs to balance the risk of any intervention with the possible benefit. This child would need better IV access, to start some inotropic support and start heparin in view of the very poor function.

The risks of transfer relate to the risk of arrhythmia and cardiac arrest en route. The acceleration and deceleration effects of transfer can be extremely challenging to compromised cardiac output. The ambulance journey would need to be steady rather than high speed. To minimise the risk of arrhythmia, electrolytes including magnesium, calcium and potassium should be optimised; however, there were no ectopics visible on the ECG, so the chance that they were severely deranged was reduced and with only one IV access, replacing electrolytes would be difficult. With adequate explanation, would the child tolerate siting an external jugular line with some local anaesthetic, while sitting up? Neck veins will probably be extremely engorged and it will likely be easy to establish this access without causing significant pain to the child. This would allow checking of electrolytes and correction if necessary. Defib pads should be sited prior to transfer.

Should milrinone and intravenous heparin be started before transfer? The transfer time is not significant, and delaying starting both these medications until a definitive paediatric cardiac assessment is available in a stable, supported paediatric intensive care environment, is likely the preferable option. It is difficult to anticipate the response to inodilators like milrinone, and this child is critically stable at present. Dropping the blood pressure by excessive dilation may reduce myocardial perfusion and precipitate acute decompensation. Heparin is used to reduce clot formation in the poorly contractile heart with blood at risk of stagnating in the atrial appendices. This infusion can wait as the time delay is not significant. To run milrinone, heparin and morphine for transfer will require more vascular access than the child currently has in situ, so unless external, or internal jugular access can be achieved with the child sitting up and calm, this may shift the transfer decision to morphine alone for transfer.

This child will be an enormously high risk intubation, thus any procedure which will require intubation and ventilation, should be reserved until the child is safely in intensive care with the right personnel and the right equipment, including the option of extracorporeal haemodynamic support. Keeping the child self-ventilating for transfer, supported with oxygen or non-invasive ventilation is preferable.

The parents and child would need to be informed of the clinical assessment of heart failure and planned management for the child. This needs to be done in a manner that is honest but calm and positive in the communication with the child. You need the child to remain co-operative and not be frightened. It is of no benefit at present, until you have more definitive information, to detail the intense gravity of the cardiac dysfunction to the child. He will need to know as soon as the right psychological support is in place, in the

PICU. His parents, on the other hand, need to be fully informed of the gravity of the problem and the intense concern about the child's safety during transfer. They will certainly want to know what is causing the problem, and you will not be able to provide these answers. You can at least provide them with a clear plan of action and the measures necessary to ensure safe transfer. You will need to ensure they are aware that you need their and the child's full co-operation and calmness to achieve the best outcome.

Outcome

This child was safely transferred self-ventilating on oxygen and morphine to PICU. He had a jugular central line inserted under local anaesthetic, while sitting up, after a gentle conversation by the retrieval team lead. Electrolytes were all checked and within normal limits. He had an uneventful transfer.

On admission to PICU the cardiology team confirmed a hypertrophic cardiomyopathy with extremely poor function. Milrinone was started at low dose without loading. Heparin was also started once in PICU. He tolerated continuous positive airway pressure over the first night in PICU and felt slightly less breathless the next morning before he had a sudden onset focal seizure, which was later correlated with a small cerebral infarct.

The day after admission and in view of the extremely poor cardiac function, he was presented to cardiac transplant team, and accepted in principle while investigations were outstanding. Two days after admission he had a renal ultrasound which precipitated an urgent CT abdomen, where a large phaeochromocytoma was detected. The family were found to carry the Von Hippel Lindau mutation.

Over the next month, and once blood pressure control had been achieved, the child had the tumour successfully removed and by 6 months had entirely recovered cardiac function and returned to school well. The family remains under surveillance to date.

Further Reading

Agrawal G, Sadacharan D, Kapoor A, et al. Cardiovascular dysfunction and catecholamine cardiomyopathy in pheochromocytoma patients and their reversal following surgical cure: results of a prospective case-control study. *Surgery* 2011;150(6):1202–11.

Waguespack, SG, Rich T, Grubbs E, et al. A current review of the etiology, diagnosis, and treatment of pediatric pheochromocytoma and paraganglioma. *J Clin Endocrinol Metab* 2010;95(5):2023–37.

Chapter 19

Rash, Tachycardia and Irritability

Shelley Riphagen

The parents of a 4-week-old baby brought her in to the A&E after an unsettled night of high-pitched crying and high temperature with an inability to settle her and a refusal to feed. They had noted a progressive rash from the day before involving redness of her hands and feet and a fine, red papular rash over her body. She had had coryzal symptoms and a low-grade temperature the whole week, but had been otherwise well, as had her 2-year-old sibling.

On examination in the A&E she was mottled peripherally with a diffuse red blanching rash. She was irritable during examination with a high-pitched cry but no significant increase in work of breathing. Her observations are noted in Table 19.1. She had a distended, slightly tender abdomen and was reported to have been vomiting. She had had no stool that day. A peripheral cannula was sited and a venous blood gas and baseline blood tests, including blood culture were sent. The blood gas results are displayed in Table 19.2.

By the time she was referred, she had received 40 ml/kg volume resuscitation on arrival in A&E, but had not improved significantly enough for the local team to be reassured enough to admit her to the paediatric ward. They had ongoing concerns about her abdomen and had performed a CXR (Figure 19.1) and abdominal X-ray (Figure 19.2). The abdominal X-ray did not clearly identify any pathology, however they were concerned regarding the possibly enlarged heart size and 'wet' looking lung fields on the CXR and were seeking advice regarding further volume resuscitation and ongoing management

They reported the baby had had good response initially to the volume with heart rate reducing to 188 bpm temporarily, but it had gradually increased over the last hour to 204 bpm with blood pressure slightly worse now at 72/30 mmHg, although the baby had good central capillary refill of 2 sec and pulses were easily felt. The rash had also become more diffuse and more obvious.

Questions

1. The district general hospital team was seeking advice. They were unsure of how to proceed. How would you manage this referral?
2. Having clarified the situation, how would your structure your advice?
3. Following admission to PICU an ECG and echo performed shows small voltage complexes with some non-specific ST changes. Echo demonstrated significant globally reduced function with normal intracardiac anatomy and a small rim of pericardial fluid. How would you tailor your therapy and investigations?

Table 19.1. Initial observations

Temperature	38.6°C
Respiratory rate	40 breaths per minute
Saturations	100%
Heart rate	208 bpm
Blood pressure	76/36 mmHg
Capillary refill time	4 secs
AVPU	Irritable

Table 19.2.

pH	7.33
CO_2	4.4
HCO_3	22 mmol/L
Base excess	−2 mEq/L
Lactate	2.5 mmol/L
Na	132 mmol/L
K	4.9 mmol/L

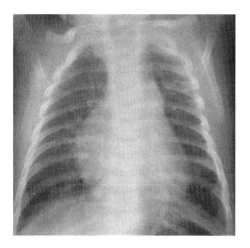

Figure 19.1 Admission chest radiograph.

1. The district general hospital team was seeking advice. They were unsure of how to proceed. How would you manage this referral?

Nearly 50% of referral calls to paediatric emergency retrieval services in the UK are made as calls for 'advice'. As a team or individual taking referrals, it is important to take all the relevant referral details and review the case with 'fresh eyes', with the luxury of not being in the heat of the clinical moment or having to manage multiple demands in A&E and elsewhere.

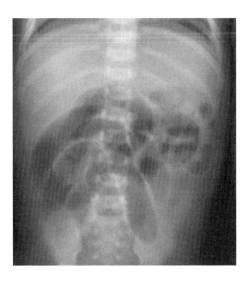

Figure 19.2 Admission abdominal.

Referral is an opportunity for a senior clinician to make a considered evaluation and opinion of the case being referred. Once that opinion has been formulated, it may not necessarily be that the outcome of the call is only advice. Part of that advice may be that the baby needs transfer.

Multiple factors affect clinical judgement in a busy acute environment. These include:

- Staff competencies and skill relating to level of training and personal judgement
- Organisational factors affecting staffing, clinical pathways and pressure in A&E or in the ward
- Communication especially at handover and where multiple individuals are involved in the child's care.

Situational awareness may be compromised by excessive demands on the individual, and the referrer may develop inattentional blindness, where clearly abnormal physiologic parameters or results do not stand out as usual because of the distraction of other surrounding activity. Once a proposed diagnosis has been made, fixation errors may prevent consideration of other scenarios.

Thus it is important during the call to establish:

- What the referrer is requesting
- Why this request is being made
- What specifically is concerning the clinical team and the referrer.

When dealing with sick children, there are certain groups of children who for various reasons are more difficult to evaluate than others. They require special caution to ensure that serious disease has not been missed. These children require specific attention to all details, with any abnormal values or findings interrogated critically despite how the children may appear clinically.

These groups include:

- Neonates and very young babies, who have a relatively generic response to any physiological or pathophysiological challenge
- Teenagers, who will notoriously 'soldier on' despite critical illness

- Children with significant neurodisability, who do not display the usual response to pain or discomfort
- Children with chronic conditions who, with their parents, are used to a chronic burden of being unwell.

Before the end of the call or giving any advice, it is essential to identify whether the presentation is that of a clinical emergency, and if so what clinical emergency is evident, in order to give relevant advice. In this case, it is not advice alone that is required.

2. Having clarified the situation, how would your structure your advice?

How do you establish whether the clinical picture being referred fits the pattern of a clinical emergency? This is best undertaken by developing pattern recognition of the most common paediatric emergencies of which there are only about 10 when grouped as follows in a structured A B C manner:

A Airway obstruction
B Respiratory failure
C Shock (any cause)
D Encephalopathy (with or without raised intracranial pressure)
E Electrolyte and metabolic emergencies
F Renal failure and fluid balance emergencies
G Glucose and endocrine emergencies
H Haemato-oncologic emergencies
I Injuries, trauma and surgical emergencies

Structured, sensible and relevant practical advice cannot be given until the problem for which advice is being offered has been correctly identified, and both the referrer and referred come to an agreement regarding the nature and scale of the clinical problem.

In this case, the baby was shocked with unrelenting tachycardia, not fully explained by pyrexia or discomfort. She was also encephalopathic with irritability and vomiting as a significant historical and examination feature. Where a child is encephalopathic, it is important to look for signs of raised intracranial pressure (RICP). The presence of shock and encephalopathy with RICP makes recognition and clinical evaluation difficult. because the shocked child would normally be tachycardic and hypotensive, and the encephalopathic child with RICP would be bradycardic and hypertensive, thus it is not inconceivable in this scenario that the one is confounding the other, and the numbers may be balanced and 'normalised'. Once the child is anaesthetised, the overwhelming problem will be exposed.

Advice regarding further management should proceed in a structured ABC manner.

- Urgent senior anaesthetic and paediatric support is required.
- The baby should be placed in 100% facemask oxygen. Once anaesthetic support arrives, the anaesthetic team could provide positive end-expiratory pressure support to reduce the work of breathing and support cardiac function.
- Good vascular access must be established. There is obvious concern about volume resuscitation. This must be reviewed with another volume bolus and critical evaluation of response to treatment. Does the heart rate come down and the blood pressure get better? Is the liver size static or enlarging? As long as there is a positive response to fluid,

additional volume can be given, while inotrope infusions are prepared. The baby appeared flushed and vasodilated rather than cold and shut down. In this case, noradrenaline would be ideal, but while central access is obtained dopamine can be started at 10 mcg/kg/min, running peripherally. Noradrenaline, in dilute form, can also be run peripherally over a short period of time if there is good access. If external jugular or intra-osseous access is established, noradrenaline central dosing strength could be started directly.

- The baby appeared irritable and encephalopathic. There may or may not be intracranial hypertension. The fontanelle can be examined as a baseline. In this setting, a dose of 3 ml/kg hypertonic saline will potentially reduce cerebral swelling but will also aid shock resuscitation especially in the setting of low serum sodium (via anti-diuretic hormone secretion secondary to shock).
- Antibiotics and antivirals providing adequate and appropriate CNS cover must be started especially in light of the rash.
- Once treatment for shock and possible intracranial hypertension have begun, the baby will likely be safe enough to ensure adequate anaesthesia prior to intubation and ventilation.
- Other causes of shock and encephalopathy should also be excluded. Although the baby is almost out of the neonatal collapse period, metabolic conditions must be considered, and an ammonia sent urgently.
- A nasogastric tube should be placed on free drainage and the abdomen decompressed until it can be evaluated by a surgeon. A urinary catheter should be inserted in view of the large volume resuscitation already given, and as a means of tracking adequacy of ongoing shock resuscitation and renal perfusion.
- Glucose infusion should be given at a rate to deliver ~ 8 mg/kg/min until the ammonia is known.

It is clear that the baby is very ill, but the 'good colour' may be misleading the team to under-evaluate the baby.

In view of the concerns of possible cardiac involvement, the baby should be transferred to a centre with cardiology on site, so that a full clinical evaluation can be undertaken, including ECG and echocardiogram.

3. Following admission to PICU an ECG and echo performed shows small voltage complexes with some non-specific ST changes. Echocardiogram demonstrated significant globally reduced function with normal intracardiac anatomy and a small rim of pericardial fluid.' How would you tailor your therapy and investigations?

Paediatric surgeons evaluated the abdomen, which although very distended and tender with no bowel sounds, was not peritonitic. The CRP was only 4 with white cell count 4.6. Based on the clinical examination and early special investigations, they did not wish to proceed with surgery.

Because of the clinical and special investigation appearance suggesting a pancarditis, with encephalopathy and gastrointestinal symptoms, a full myocarditis screening panel was undertaken with rectal swab requested urgently from the lab to try and identify enteroviruses.

The rectal swab returned a positive result for parechovirus within 24 hours, which confirmed the PICU clinical suspicion of enteroviral infection, with its enteric origin and predilection for brain and heart muscle infection.

Almost one third of babies with parecho virus infection have gastrointestinal symptoms and signs along with the rash. Approximately 12% have aseptic meningitis or encephalitis and may go on to have seizures and irreversible white matter changes. The acute presentation is usually that of warm shock responding well to volume resuscitation and noradrenaline. In view of this baby's poor function on echo, milrinone was also added to the noradrenaline infusion. The baby recovered well over the next week, was extubated after 3 days and discharged within the week with recovering cardiac function and no apparent neurologic sequelae at PICU discharge.

Summary

Lessons learned from this retrieval included:

1. Always evaluate each referral call with fresh eyes. Make your own clinical judgement regarding what is required and what the outcome of the referral should be.
2. Neonates fall into the group where extra vigilance is required. A reassuring appearance and quiet baby may hide a critically unwell child.
3. Develop a systematic approach to evaluation of the presenting emergency.
4. Develop a systematic approach to sensible and practical resuscitation and stabilisation advice.

Further Reading

Gawronski O, Parshuram C, Cecchetti C, et al. Qualitative study exploring factors influencing escalation of care of deteriorating children in a children's hospital. *BMJ Paediatr Open* 2018:2(1): e000241.

Grosbee J. Handoffs and communication. The underappreciated roles of situational awareness and inattentional blindness. *Clin Obstet Gynaecol* 2010;53(3):545–58.

Olijve L, Jennings L, Walls T. Human parechovirus: an increasingly recognized cause of sepsis-like illness in young infants. *Clin Microbiol Rev* 2018;31(1):e00047–17.

Is the Baby's Heart Rate Supposed to Be Slower than Mine?

Olga Van Der Woude and Shelley Riphagen

A baby boy with a tertiary centre diagnosis of complete heart block was delivered at 34 weeks of gestation via emergency caesarean section at the local hospital because of fetal bradycardia. The mother had been diagnosed with anti-Ro/La antibodies during the pregnancy. The antenatal scans at the tertiary referral centre were normal to date. The baby was born in good condition but developed an increased work of breathing 5 minutes after birth and was intubated after 20 minutes due to desaturations related to a bradycardia of 50 to 60 bpm. The baby was referred to the regional cardiac centre and the paediatric retrieval team for transfer.

At the time of referral, the baby was ventilated on low pressures in air. An echo of the heart was performed and showed a structurally normal heart with a small patent foramen ovale and poor ventricular function and confirmed the low heart rate in the setting congenital heart block. The neonatal team had inserted an umbilical venous cannula for ease of vascular access. An umbilical arterial cannula was attempted but failed. Observations and blood gas at the time of referral are shown in Table 20.1.

Questions

1. Should a bradycardic newborn baby be intubated?
2. What are the best methods to increase the heart rate when transferring a child and when should this be attempted?
3. Where is the best place for a baby with an antenatal diagnosis of complete heart block to be born?

1. Should a bradycardic newborn baby be intubated?

The cardiac output of neonates is mainly dependent on heart rate due to their relatively fixed stroke volume. Significant bradycardias are not well tolerated and lead to low cardiac output state and deterioration of cardiac function. Rates above 55 bpm may be tolerated for some time.

The incidence of congenital heart block is estimated to be about 1 in 22,000 live births.

The most common causes of congenital heart block in neonates are maternal auto-immune disease (about 45%) and congenital heart disease (about 53%). Mothers with auto-immune disease are often asymptomatic but may have anti-Ro or anti-La antibodies. These antibodies can cause irreversible damage to the conduction system of the fetal heart. The risk to the fetus of developing congenital heart block, where the mother has anti-Ro or anti-La antibodies, is about 2%.

Table 20.1.

Observations	Blood gas
Heart rate 50–60 bpm	pH 7.35
Non-invasive blood pressure 57/34 mmHg	pCO_2 5.7 kPa
Capillary refill time <2 seconds	pO_2 6.2 kPa
SpO_2 97–100% in air	HCO_3 22.8 mmol/L
	Base excess −2.4 mEq/L

Congenital complete heart block has a high mortality rate of about 20% and this is even higher in foetuses diagnosed with hydrops in utero, in structural heart disease and in premature birth. Optimal management of newborns with congenital heart block is not well known due to the low incidence of the condition. Most cases need permanent pacemaker implantation in the neonatal period.

The need for intubation depends on the condition of the baby. Both intubating and not intubating have advantages and risks, so it is important to consider both the risks and benefits in each individual patient.

Bradycardias in neonates cause a low cardiac output, which can result in inadequate oxygenation of organs and tissues. Signs and symptoms of low cardiac output include increased work of breathing, low blood pressure, cold extremities, prolonged capillary refill time, reduced urine output, acidosis and lethargy. In babies showing signs and symptoms of low cardiac output, it can be advantageous to reduce oxygen consumption and this can be achieved by intubating and ventilating them. This could prevent further deterioration.

A great disadvantage of intubation and ventilation, however, is the need for anaesthesia and sedation, with sedation potentially leading to even lower heart rate. Anaesthetic drugs can cause hypotension, further reduction of cardiac output, arrhythmias and cardiac arrest in babies in an already low cardiac output state. Careful choice of anaesthetic drugs is important, aiming to not reduce the cardiac output any further and emergency drugs should be preemptively drawn up and available.

2. What are the best methods to increase the heart rate when transferring a child and when should this be attempted?

The transfer of a baby with a low heart rate carries added risks and management can be difficult. The cardiac output of a neonate is dependent on heart rate. Very low rate bradycardias are not well tolerated, causing impairment of cardiac function. Heart rates above 55 bpm in neonates with a structurally normal heart are usually reasonably well tolerated and often do not need urgent intervention. If the heart rate is less than 55 bpm, or if the patient is showing symptoms of cardiac failure or reduced cardiac output, the usual treatment of choice is urgent pacemaker implantation. In neonates with structural heart problems, rates below 70 bpm usually require intervention. Permanent pacemaker implantation can only be performed in hospitals with specialised cardiac services and neonates born in other hospitals need to be transferred. Transferring a neonate with a heart rate of less than 55 bpm (or less than 70 bpm in structural heart disease), or with symptoms of a low cardiac output state are high risk. Attempts to increase the heart rate before or during

Table 20.2.

Drug	Mechanism of action	Dosage
Atropine	Antimuscarinic – parasympatholytic	20 µg/kg
Adrenaline	α1/α2, β1/β2 agonist	0.1–2 µg/kg/min
Dopamine	Main effect dose dependent: DA1/DA2 (lower dose)[a] β1/β2 (intermediate dose)[b] α1/α2 (higher dose)[c]	3–5 µg/kg/min 5–10 µg/kg/min 10–20 µg/kg/min
Isoprenaline	β1/β2 agonist	0.1–1 µg/kg/min (heart block) 0.02–0.5 µg/kg/min (bradycardia)

[a] dopamine receptor; [b] β = beta receptor; [c] α = alpha receptor.

transfer may lead to a more stable clinical situation, but there is no evidence for which treatment works best, with both pharmacological and non-pharmacological methods being tried.

Pharmacological Treatment

The initial cause of low cardiac output in congenital heart block is the low heart rate, and therefore the initial aim of treatment should be to increase the heart rate. Various drugs, including, atropine, adrenaline, dopamine and isoprenaline (Table 20.2), are known for their potential to increase the heart rate, and use of these drugs can be considered. However, their effect in neonates is difficult to predict, and they often do not have the desired outcome. It can be difficult to monitor the effect of the drugs because it is difficult to measure the cardiac output in neonates. Blood pressure alone is not a good surrogate for cardiac output since an increased systemic vascular resistance can lead to a higher blood pressure, but to a reduced cardiac output. The use of inotropes, especially in combination, also gives an increased risk of arrhythmias. Careful titration of the drugs and monitoring of clinical condition is important. Echocardiography, if available, could help in assessing the effect of treatment.

Non-pharmacological Treatment

A non-pharmacological method to quickly increase the heart rate is to start external transcutaneous pacing. This can be achieved by using a pacemaker with external pacing pads, or a defibrillator with pacing capacity and external defibrillator pads applied to the chest. Once the pads are applied and connected to the machine, start at a rate of about 100 bpm and the lowest output current. Slowly increase the current until a capture beat is seen on the ECG and leave the final output setting 5–10 mA above capture. A disadvantage of transcutaneous pacing is that the patient needs to be sedated and a neonate would therefore need to be intubated, with the risk of anaesthetic drugs as mentioned earlier. For this reason therefore, it is less desirable in neonates who are self-ventilating and conscious. Other risks include loss of capture, especially with prolonged pacing, and burns at the site of the pads, especially a risk in fragile newborn or premature newborn skin.

A temporary pacing method often used in adults is transvenous atrial pacing. This method could be used in older children but is contraindicated in neonates due to their small size and the risk of venous occlusion. Case reports about temporary transvenous atrial pacing through the umbilical venous route have shown some potential.

3. Where is the best place for a baby with an antenatal diagnosis of complete heart block to be born?

If a neonate with a bradycardia is in heart failure, and temporary pharmacological and non-pharmacological treatments do not have the desired effect, the baby needs an urgent pacemaker implantation. The question before 'where is the safest place for a baby with antenatally known congenital heart block to be born', is when is the right time for the baby to be born. This assessment is a team effort by the fetal medicine team including the fetal cardiologist, who would be monitoring the baby carefully in the last trimester to pick up the earliest signs of cardiac decompensation which should trigger delivery. Heart rate alone in this setting is not a reason to deliver a baby prematurely, and thus for this assessment the mother and fetus should be transferred to a centre with appropriate fetal cardiac expertise. If the baby needs to be delivered because of fetal or maternal well-being concerns, then the safest place for this baby to be born is in a hospital with facilities for pacemaker implantation in neonates and where cases can be discussed in a multidisciplinary meeting setting. When the diagnosis has been made antenatally, all these plans can be set in motion to cover all eventualities.

Further Reading

Di Mauro A, Caroli Casavola V, Favia Guarnieri G, et al. Antenatal and postnatal combined therapy for autoantibody-related congenital atrioventricular block. *BMC Pregnancy Childbirth* 2013;13:220.

Friedman DM, Duncanson LJ, Glickstein J, Buyon JP. A review of congenital heart block; *Images Paediatr Cardiol.* 2003;5(3):36–48.

Hiren D, Lokare S. Temporary neonatal atrial pacing through the umbilical venous route: A novel technique. *Ann Pediatr Cardiol* 2011;4(2):164–5.

Khanna P, Arora S, Aravindan A et al; Anaesthetic management of a 2-day-old with complete congenital heart block. *Saudi J Anaesth.* 2014;8(1):134–7.

Ng O, Shahani SJ. Anaesthetic management of a premature low-birth-weight neonate with congenital complete heart block for implantation of temporary epicardial pacing wires. *Singapore Med J.* 2014;55(1) e9–e11.

Wang B, Hu S, Shi D et al. Arrhythmia and/or cardiomyopathy related to maternal autoantibodies: Descriptive analysis of a series of 16 cases from a single center. *Fron Pediatr* 2019;7:465.

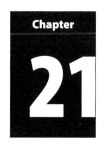
A Pale Lethargic Girl

Maria Gual Sanchez and Shelley Riphagen

An 11-year-old girl, previously fit and well, presented with a 1-week history of feeling unwell, very tired, extremely lethargic and breathless on exertion, on a background of being non-specifically unwell for the previous 2 months. She had no other specific symptoms and was afebrile at the time of presentation. On the morning of presentation, she had an acute onset of severe respiratory distress and was pale, very cold and unable to talk. She reported she had not been to the toilet for most of the previous day and night. Her mother was extremely alarmed by her colour and brought her to her local A&E department by car, although she was unable to walk from the car park and required a wheelchair.

She had been seen three times in the past 6 weeks by her GP due to ongoing fatigue, sleeping in the afternoon after school, not eating properly, with low grade temperatures and sore legs. She had been assessed as possibly depressed, having newly started high school, and had a psychology evaluation booked.

Her only previous visits to her GP were for fainting episodes after starting school at the age of five, which resolved spontaneously during the year.

Prior to this presentation, nothing had changed besides the patient having been on holiday to southern Spain about 3 months previously and having her ears pierced 2 months previously.

Soon after she had arrived in A&E, the referral was made to the retrieval service. At the time of referral the examination findings were reported as follows: she was very pale and mottled and felt cold to her upper arms and mid-thighs. She was awake, alert and co-operative but unable to move independently and she was talking in one-to-two-word phrases due to difficulty breathing. Observations at the time of referral are shown on Table 21.1.

She had bilateral diffuse crackles on auscultation of the chest, an easily audible cardiac murmur and a distended abdomen with tender right upper quadrant. It was difficult to palpate organomegaly because of significant respiratory distress and use of abdominal muscles for breathing. Venous gas result is shown in Table 21.2 and admission bloods in Table 21.3.

Due to the condition of the child, and poor response to oxygen with saturations remaining under 85% in 15 L facemask oxygen, a local emergency call was placed with the plan to intubate and ventilate her to support oxygenation. This was achieved successfully by the local team. After intubation, she had a jugular central line placed and CXR was performed, as seen in Figure 21.1. This was described as showing bilateral perihilar shadowing with small pleural effusions and a relatively normal cardiothoracic ratio.

The local team were extremely worried by her clinical condition and the cardiac rhythm on the monitor. An electrocardiogram was performed as shown in Figure 21.2. This showed

Table 21.1. Observations at referral

Temperature	37.6°C
Heart rate	168 bpm
Blood pressure	128/24 mmHg
Capillary refill time	5 sec
Respiratory rate	54 breaths per minute
Oxygen saturations	71% in air

Table 21.2. Venous blood gas

pH	7.16
pCO_2	6.4 kPa
pO_2	9.1 kPa
HCO_3	13 mmol/L
Base excess	−12
Lactate	9 mmol/L
Na	131 mmol/L
K	6.1 mmol/L
Haemoglobin	71 g/L
Glucose	11.1 mmol/L

Table 21.3. Blood results

White cell count	27.6 (10^3/mm^3)	Na	130 mmol/L	Mg	0.74 mmol/L
Haemoglobin	81 g/L	K	5.9 mmol/L	ALT	997
Platelets	367	Urea	16.4 mmol/L	CPK	538
INR	2.24	Creatinine	128 U/L	CRP	90 mg/L
APTT	1 secs	Phosphate	2.2 mmol/L		

multiple ectopics with some ST depression with short, unsustained episodes of ventricular tachycardia. They were seeking advice and urgent retrieval as she had become worse after the first 20 ml/kg volume resuscitation during intubation.

Questions

1. What is the overwhelming clinical emergency in this child? What is your working differential diagnosis causing this emergency?
2. In this clinical emergency, how would you suggest resuscitating this child and what do you anticipate during resuscitation?

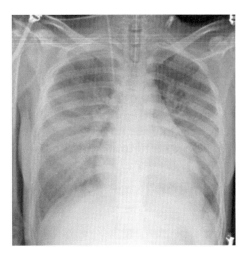

Figure 21.1 Chest radiograph post intubation.

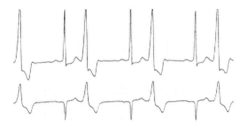

Figure 21.2 Admission electrocardiogram.

3. A 65-minute land transfer is required between the site of presentation at her local hospital and definitive management of this child. What precautions would you ensure are in place to manage the likely instability during transfer?

1. What is the overwhelming clinical emergency in this child? What is your working differential diagnosis causing this emergency?

This child is critically unwell: she is tachycardic, hypotensive, tachypnoeic, hypoxic, poorly perfused and oliguric. Investigations show lactic acidosis, acute kidney injury and acute liver failure. In summary, she is shocked with multi-organ failure and needs immediate resuscitation. Shock is a clinical diagnosis and to recognise and name it early is vitally important for the team performance and the outcome of the child.

Shock is a clinical syndrome caused by a pathophysiological imbalance between cellular oxygen delivery and oxygen utilisation required to meet metabolic demands.

It is classically divided into three phases: compensated, decompensated and irreversible shock.

- In the compensated phase, the body employs compensatory mechanisms in order to maintain perfusion of vital organs (brain, heart, kidneys). Typically, there would be signs and symptoms of reduced perfusion to non-essential vascular beds including skin (cold, pale, prolonged capillary refill), muscle (lethargic, 'weak', muscle aches) and gut (off feeds, nausea, vomiting, loose stools) and may include renal and hepatic hypoperfusion. Additionally, there will be signs and symptoms of early acidosis with appropriate compensatory mechanisms (tachycardia and tachypnoea), but the child would often maintain normal range blood pressure.

- In the second phase, essential organ perfusion is affected, with cellular ischaemia with worsening shock. Clinically there is a worsening of the symptoms previously mentioned, plus altered mental status and early hypotension. Rapidly deployed therapeutic intervention can still reverse the situation.
- In the last phase, cellular ischaemia and necrosis are established with widespread multiorgan failure. Even aggressive intervention at this point may not prevent death.

Prompt shock recognition and treatment are essential in the critically unwell child.

There are various causes of shock, and although the basic principles of resuscitation are the same, each requires refinements, specifics and additions to the basic tenets. A differential diagnosis of aetiology of shock must be made early in order to deliver most appropriate treatment to the child without missing important possibilities. In this case scenario, a possible differential diagnosis would include septic shock and cardiogenic shock.

Septic shock: In the early phases, this is usually a form of distributive shock, with uncontrolled vasodilation and relative hypovolaemia due to capillary leak causing maldistribution of blood flow. However, in paediatric septic shock, it is not rare to observe a component of myocardial impairment. Severe sepsis is one of the most prevalent conditions in the critically ill paediatric population. (In PICUs from all continents, severe sepsis prevalence was 8.2% of all critically ill children, with a mortality of 25%.)

Cardiogenic shock: Cardiac pump failure with inability to distribute and deliver the substrate (blood flow and oxygen) that organs require to continue optimal function. The aetiology of pump failure has various origins including mechanical obstruction to flow from the heart, myocardial failure, valve insufficiency and electrical abnormalities impeding peformance. Each has subtle differences. Currently, cardiogenic shock is increasing in prevalence in the paediatric population as the outcome of congenital heart disease surgery has improved. Additional to congenital cardiac lesions causing outlet obstruction or valve insufficiency, some acute cardiac conditions affect previously healthy children. Although they are rare, a high suspicion index is required.

In this case, there are several clinical details that carefully considered will lead to the correct diagnosis. Septic shock must be suspected in this girl. The child had experienced several days of low-grade fever. White blood cells and inflammatory markers were high at admission. Nevertheless, she presented cold, grey and mottled, making it a less typical picture of early septic shock. Additional to this was the loud heart murmur, bilateral crackles compatible with pulmonary oedema (confirmed with CXR) and significant ECG changes suggesting myocardial or electrical abnormalities. This additional information suggests cardiogenic shock is more likely. Moreover, she had a previous history of atypical 'drop attacks' at a young age, which had not been thoroughly investigated.

Cardiogenic shock can have multiple causes and a cardiac echo performed locally would be of enormous benefit in diagnosis. Nevertheless, if no echo is available, there are several signs that may help with diagnosis. The congestive CXR and hepatomegaly would suggest that both ventricles are affected. In hypertrophic cardiomyopathy, the cardiac output is maintained except in the last stages when the myocardium fails. In myocarditis and dilated cardiomyopathies, the pulse pressure would be narrow. In this case, diastolic pressure is low and there are signs of ischaemia in the ECG. This could all be explained by severe aortic insufficiency where in systole the stroke volume moves anterogradely through the aortic valve, and can maintain a reasonable systolic pressure, but in diastole, part of the stroke volume returns to the ventricle as the valve is incompetent. This retrograde flow 'steals' effective blood flow from the coronaries leading to myocardial ischaemia. The diastolic pressure is lower than expected (usually 60% systolic) leading to a wide pulse pressure shock without being vasodilated. Impaired function, and high left ventricular end diastolic volume leads to pulmonary oedema and subsequent hypoxia, exaggerating the oxygen delivery imbalance of shock.

2. In this clinical emergency, how would you suggest resuscitating this child and what do you anticipate during resuscitation?

In order to resuscitate this child, a systematic A B C approach is recommended.

A: Airway

Securing a definitive airway for ventilation in a critically unwell child is often challenging and can frequently result in decompensation unless carefully managed by an experienced clinician. This is a very sick child with a high risk of deterioration, and senior help and attendance should be sought early. Oxygen should be administered immediately with careful assessment of response to therapy. If the child is unconscious, the airway must be cleared and supported. Actual or anticipated airway compromise, hypoxaemia, compromised ventilation and myocardial support, afforded by positive pressure ventilation, are all indications to proceed to advanced airway management for airway security and mechanical ventilation.

In this case, the patient was clearly hypoxaemic, and ventilation was compromised. The airway was patent and the child still speaking; however, rapid progression of shock might have altered that. There were many reasons to make the decision to intubate early an easy one. Intubation and ventilation would also make managing extreme cardiovascular instability and the risk of cardiac arrest in transit easier to manage.

Anaesthesia required for intubation is a high-risk undertaking in this setting and should be undertaken with all precautions for destabilisation considered and in place. The loss of intense endogenous sympathetic drive would lead to further hypotension even with the most cardiostable anaesthetic. For this reason, the dose and rate of administration of the anaesthetic should be titrated carefully to effect over a more prolonged period of time by an experienced operator. Further hypotension would aggravate myocardial ischaemia and increase the risk of malignant arrhythmias and the risk of cardiac arrest.

B: Breathing

Invasive mechanical ventilation would improve oxygenation and start to remedy the oxygen imbalance of shock. Pulmonary oedema requires high PEEP and the wet, non-compliant lungs also require higher distending pressures. Removing all work of breathing by mechanical ventilation would go some way to redirecting blood from respiratory muscles to heart and brain. The change in intrathoracic pressure from negative pressure in spontaneous breathing to positive pressure with mechanical ventilation and PEEP, changes the ventricular–thoracic pressure gradient, effectively producing afterload reduction and improving cardiac output without the myocardial oxygen cost of inotropes.

C: Circulation

The heart is the source of the problem in this child. Focusing resuscitation here in a thoughtful and carefully reviewed manner will allow titration of treatment to the most effective measures.

Fluid boluses must be considered in all kinds of shock to ensure preload is optimised. This requires careful review of response to treatment to ensure optimal cardiac filling is targeted. In this child with cardiogenic shock, fluid administration must be undertaken extremely cautiously with small aliquots, as excessive volume loading may reduce cardiac performance and output. This child already had bilateral crackles and evidence of pulmonary oedema on CXR, suggesting inability to manage current loading conditions. In this scenario, fluid boluses should not be administered and proceeding to step two by initiating vasoactive drugs would be the better option.

Choice of the most appropriate vasoactive drug is dependent on a good understanding of the likely pathology, the physiological effects of the specific drug and how it can be delivered.

- **Dopamine** (dopaminergic receptors) has dose dependent effects:
  - Low dose 1–5 mcg/kg/min increases sodium excretion via the kidney.
  - Moderate dose 5–10 mcg/kg/min (β agonism) increases heart rate and cardiac contractility.
  - High dose 10–20 mcg/kg/min (α agonism) increases systemic vascular resistance.

- **Adrenaline** (β1, β2 and α1 receptors):
  - Low dose (up to 0.1 mcg/kg/min) with predominant β stimulation achieves increase in heart rate, cardiac contractility and decrease in systemic vascular resistance.
  - At higher doses, the α effect exceeds the β2 effect and there is progressive vasoconstriction.
    - Adrenaline, as infusion, is a good option in cardiogenic shock with low blood pressure and septic shock with impaired function.
    - **Noradrenaline** (predominant α1 stimulation)
  - Increases systemic vascular resistance. In the situation of impaired cardiac function, the increase in the afterload may result in reduced cardiac output.
    - It is the drug of choice in hyperdynamic septic shock presenting as 'warm shock'.
    - **Milrinone** (phosphodiesterase-3 inhibitor)
  - An 'inodilator', with inotropic, lusitropic and vasodilating effects, improves cardiac output by enhancing myocardial relaxation, thus improving ventricular filling and by decreasing the afterload.
  - This makes it a suitable drug to treat heart failure and support cardiogenic shock along with other drugs.

In this case scenario, the ideal drug to choose is one that improves cardiac function and decreases the afterload. Both adrenaline and milrinone would achieve this outcome. In contrast, noradrenaline would be counterproductive, as an increase in systemic vascular resistance would aggravate aortic valve regurgitation and decrease cardiac output, with further clinical deterioration.

3.   A 65-minute land transfer is required between the site of presentation at her local hospital and definitive management of this child. What precautions would you ensure are in place to manage the likely instability during transfer?

Before undertaking transfer, it is imperative to consider the worst-case scenario and likely complications that could be encountered/expected, and prepare for these. The patient should be transferred in the best possible condition; however, there is a limit to what is achievable with the current resources. You must ensure that during transfer, where human resources and equipment are limited, you can still deliver all the expert care required.

This child presented shocked with arrhythmias. It is possible for a malignant arrhythmia to result in cardiac arrest en route. All treatable causes of arrhythmia must be addressed in advance of transfer. Electrolytes must be optimised. Magnesium can usually be assumed low in a critically ill child who has not been eating properly and magnesium top up can usually be given safely without a blood laboratory result. This child must be transferred with defibrillation pads and leads attached and ready to deploy. Cardiac monitoring must be vigilant and immediately responsive. It would be prudent to have an amiodarone infusion ready attached in case it is needed, or to have it running as a slow infusion if the arrhythmia continues to be problematic.

All medication for cardiac arrest must be prepared and ready to use. A team plan for cardiac arrest must be rehearsed and roles specified as there is likely/often only two practitioners during transfer. This would improve team performance in the emergency.

Parents must be fully informed of the severity of the child's condition, that it is a high-risk retrieval, and death is a significant possibility during transfer.

In this case, the patient had acute onset severe aortic insufficiency due to infective endocarditis, against the background of previously undiagnosed bicuspid aortic valve. *Staphylococcus aureus* was the organism identified and possibly introduced at ear piercing. It had completely destroyed the aortic valve, including the septal insertion, producing a large septal abscess responsible for the conduction abnormality. On the morning of presentation, she developed acute pulmonary oedema and shock as the aortic valve leaflet was finally destroyed. She underwent a very difficult transfer with multiple arrhythmias, was admitted to PICU and had an emergency valve replacement with a cadaveric valve, which had to be transferred by police escort from one of the national tissue banks, 3 hours later. The conduction tissue was completely destroyed and the ensuing complete heart block necessitated a permanent pacemaker. She made a superb recovery and was discharged from PICU 11 days later fully recovered.

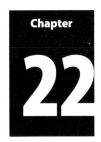

Too Fast for Comfort

Sarah Hardwick and Miriam Fine-Goulden

A 2-month-old baby girl was brought into the A&E of her local hospital by her parents. Their main concern was a change in her breathing and a day's history of feeding less well. She had been born at term and been well until 2 days prior to admission, when she had developed mild coryzal symptoms with a cough. She had not really fed properly on the day of admission and her parents were very concerned. During triage her heart rate was noted to be 270bpm. She was moved to the resuscitation area in A&E for further management. A single-lead ECG showed a narrow-complex tachycardia. The observations in Resus are noted in Table 22.1 with the first blood gas in Table 22.2.

Questions

1. When faced with a child with tachycardia, what should you consider?
2. What are the initial management priorities?
3. Does this child need transfer to a cardiac centre?

1. When faced with a child with tachycardia, what should you consider?

Heart rate in children is affected by a number of factors. It may be a physiological response to a challenge or an abnormal cardiac rhythm secondary to a number of other factors. It is very important to remember that tachycardia in children is one of the main mechanisms to increase or maintain cardiac output and requires very careful evaluation.

Once the heart rate has been identified as excessively fast, the next important step is to determine whether it is broad (usually ventricular) or narrow complex (usually atrial).

Narrow complex tachycardia is either a sinus or an atrial tachycardia with simple supraventricular tachycardia (SVT) being the most common in this group, which also include atrial ectopic tachycardias and atrial flutter.

Sinus tachycardia with a heart rate usually less than 220 bpm is common in children presenting unwell to A&E and differentiating it from a SVT can be difficult. Sinus tachycardia is a common response to multiple triggering factors, with many contributory factors in a very unwell child.

Factors contributing to tachycardia include fever, pain, anxiety, volume depletion, poor cardiac function, anaemia, hypoxia, hypercarbia, drug treatment side effects and some electrolyte imbalances.

Table 22.1. Observations on admission

Temperature	36.9°C
Respiratory rate	38 breaths per minute
Oxygen saturations (in air)	100%
Heart rate	270 bpm
Non-invasive blood pressure	49/28 mmHg
Capillary refill time	<2 secs
AVPU	A

Table 22.2. Venous blood gas

pH	7.35
pCO_2	4.9 KPa
HCO_3	22.9 mmol/l
Base excess	−0.7 mmol/l
Lactate	3.0mmol/l
Na	142mmol/l
K	4.2mmol/l

Table 22.3. Differences between sinus tachycardia and SVT

Feature	Sinus tachycardia	SVT
Rate	Generally slower: Infant <220; Child <180	Generally faster: Infant >220; Child >180
Onset & cessation	Slower/gradual	Rapid/abrupt
Beat to beat variability	Present	Absent
Response to fluid bolus or analgesia	Generally yes	Generally no
P waves	Normal morphology (upright in lead II) & precede every QRS (though may be hard to identify at high heart rates)	Variable depending on aetiology of SVT
Medical history	Consistent with history	May be unexplained

It is therefore important to take a rapid, focused history and complete a thorough physical examination when assessing a tachycardic child. A 12-lead ECG should be performed urgently.

There are also some other recognisable differences between sinus tachycardia and SVT as noted in Table 22.3.

SVT refers to any tachycardia that originates above the bundle of His and is the most common arrhythmia seen in paediatrics. The initial emergency management approach applies to any SVT, though the underlying cause may determine the response to treatment.

SVTs in children are most commonly caused by a re-entry tachycardia involving an accessory pathway, which is either outside the normal atrioventricular (AV) node – AV re-entry tachycardia (AVRT), or within the AV node itself (AVNRT). The accessory pathway has a shorter refractory period than the usual conduction pathway and may be triggered before the normal impulse from the sinoatrial (SA) node has completed its course through the AV node into the ventricle. The premature impulse sets up a re-entry loop which may travel either down the usual pathway and up the accessory pathway (orthodromic) or in reverse (antidromic), stimulating rapid atrial contraction.

The arrhythmia may be terminated by stopping or slowing conduction through the AV node, using vagal manoeuvres, pharmacological therapy or synchronised electrical cardioversion. Once terminated, it may be possible to identify ventricular pre-excitation shown by delta waves on the ECG suggestive of Wolff–Parkinson–White syndrome.

Ectopic atrial tachycardia accounts for about 10% of SVTs in children. An area of cells with enhanced automaticity (outside the normal sinus node) triggers the rapid rate. P waves may be identifiable on ECG, but the axis is often abnormal and is dependent upon the site of origin. This is often refractory to pharmacological or synchronised electrical cardioversion.

Atrial flutter is more common in children with congenital heart disease but can be seen in the infant with a structurally normal heart. It may be well tolerated if there is a degree of AV block slowing the rate of the ventricular response, but cardiovascular compromise will occur when there is rapid AV conduction resulting in a rapid ventricular rate with inadequate ventricular filling time. Vagal manoeuvres or adenosine will not convert the rhythm but may unmask flutter waves (recognisable by the saw tooth appearance on ECG) by temporarily increasing the AV block and slowing the rate.

2. What are the initial management priorities?

The first and most important point when faced with a tachycardic child is to determine whether the presentation is an emergency. If yes, it is important to identify the type of emergency. Once having identified that this is an emergency with tachycardia causing shock (rather than secondary to shock), the assessment and management should proceed following the ABC approach.

This child had no airway concerns and breathing at the time of admission was normal with good oxygen saturations.

In evaluating the cardiovascular status, the most important step is to determine the presence or absence of shock, and further management is dependent on this fact.

In this case, the child had palpable peripheral pulses throughout with good skin colour and was alert – features that are reassuring. Her blood pressure, however, was low and her venous blood gas showed a lactate of 3.0 mmol/l, concerning features that suggest shock. Moving her to A&E Resus and seeking senior help is appropriate due to the high risk of decompensation and further cardiovascular compromise.

Shock is a progressive state and a spectrum of clinical presentation. The presence of any features of shock necessitate urgent escalation of care to address the problem and halt progression. IV access was obtained and baseline blood tests were performed. A fluid bolus of 10 ml/kg 0.9% saline was given to address the tachycardia and hypotension. There was no heart rate response to the volume bolus and minimal improvement in blood pressure. A gradual improvement in heart rate during fluid bolus could indicate hypovolaemia and might suggest the need for further fluid bolus, but the child should be reassessed regularly, with specific attention to heart rate, blood pressure and liver size, and any further fluid administered with caution.

In a child who is haemodynamically stable, vagal manoeuvres – i.e. stimulating the vagal nerve to slow AV node conduction – should be attempted in the first instance. A method commonly used in infants is brief submersion of the face into iced water, or covering the face with an ice-cold cloth, triggering the 'diving reflex'. The Valsalva method is often attempted in older children, by, for example, exhaling forcefully into a 10 ml syringe. Unilateral carotid massage may also be successful. Occasionally insertion of a nasogastric tube, or laryngoscopy for intubation may convert SVT.

In the shocked child, ice cold cloth to the face or nasogastric insertion may also be attempted but should not delay further urgent management steps. These require rapidly establishing IV access and connecting a cardiac defibrillator, via appropriate sized and placed pads, to the child. If there is no response, or no sustained response to limited vagal manoeuvres, further intervention will be required.

Medical Management
Administration of Adenosine

Adenosine slows conduction in the AV node, by causing hyperpolarisation of cell membranes in the AV node, resulting in temporary heart block. When administering the adenosine dose, it is essential to have secure IV access via a large vein on the upper limb or head and neck. This allows for the shortest access time from site to heart. The half-life of adenosine is extremely short as it is metabolised quickly by adenosine deaminase which is abundant in red blood cells. It must therefore be administered and flushed quickly to have a chance of being effective. Using a fully opened three-way tap allows for rapid adenosine administration and flush to be given immediately afterwards. Prior to administration, resuscitation equipment should be readily available, including a cardiac defibrillator. A rhythm strip should be recorded as the drug is given, which will identify response and allow for rhythm interpretation.

Starting dose is usually 100 mcg/kg, and the dose is increased by 100 mcg/kg if no response, up to 500 mcg/kg – to a maximum of 12 mg, (although the neonate maximum dose is 300 mcg/kg). In children over 12 years of age, adult dosing can be used with initial dose of 3 mg, increasing to 6 mg and 12 mg. If conversion back to sinus rhythm is not sustained, then a second agent should be discussed with cardiology.

Response to adenosine is recognised by an almost immediate and short-lived slowing down of conduction as can be seen in Figure 22.1. An apparent lack of response to adenosine may be due to inadequate dose, inadequate or distant IV access or inadequate bolus technique.

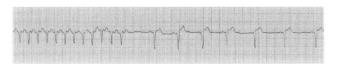

Figure 22.1 Electrocardiogram during adenosine bolus administration

If the child does not respond to adenosine and/or has haemodynamic instability, the anaesthetic team should be asked to attend in case intubation and ventilation is required. An attempt will need to be made to convert the rhythm electrically, however this should not be undertaken until electrolytes have been optimised, any reversible factors addressed and the case discussed with the retrieval team and cardiology service.

Direct Current Cardioversion

If the child is shocked or has failed to respond to adenosine, they may require synchronised direct current cardioversion. Defibrillator pads will have a size guide on the packaging. This is usually paediatric pads <25 kg/<8years and adult pads from 25 kg/8 years. They are usually labelled with pictures to show placement positions. The paediatric positions may be adapted for the neonate to an anterior/posterior placement. Ensure good skin contact without overlapping other monitoring attachments such as ECG dots. Many defibrillators require the ECG electrodes from the defibrillator to be attached for synchronisation of the shock to occur. Energy starts at 1 joule/kg and increases to 2 joules/kg. The synchronising button needs to be pressed before each cardioversion attempt as it resets back to unsynchronised. Normal defibrillator safety is required.

Amiodarone

Amiodarone may be indicated following attempted cardioversion with adenosine and/or synchronous cardioversion. It is a Class III antiarrhythmic drug which acts via potassium channel blockade, slowing repolarisation and prolonging the action potential and refractory period of myocardial cells, thereby reducing the heart rate. It works in all cardiac tissue and so is effective for both supraventricular and ventricular arrhythmias. The APLS guidelines suggest a bolus dose of 5 mg/kg; however, amiodarone should be administered only after discussing with paediatric cardiology, and should be given only where there is full cardiac monitoring in place, as it can precipitate hypotension and bradycardia. An alternative to a bolus dose is a continuous infusion. An initial load is usually administered over 4 hours at a rate of 25 mcg/kg/min, then reduced to 10–15 mcg/kg/min and subsequently titrated to heart rate.

Further Investigation and Management

It may be prudent to administer broad spectrum antibiotics if sepsis cannot be ruled out at initial presentation. If there is any uncertainty over the diagnosis and/or management, the case should be discussed with the retrieval team and paediatric cardiology.

3. Does this child need transfer to a cardiac centre?

Infants and children may present to the A&E with a previously undiagnosed SVT and often the initial concern from the parents is nondescript with variable symptoms that may include irritability, poor feeding or tachypnoea. The majority will respond to initial treatments of vagal stimulation and/or adenosine. Those children who are resistant to treatment, or are unstable and require a greater level of intervention, or are showing signs of heart failure or cardiomyopathy will require retrieval to a PICU. In rare, resistant cases, including forms of atrial ectopic tachycardia, radiofrequency ablation may be required.

All children will require referral to paediatric cardiology to plan ongoing management and follow-up.

Further Reading

Colucci RA, Silver MJ, Shubrook J. Common types of supraventricular tachycardia: diagnosis and management. *American Family Physician* 2010;82(8):942–52.

Esberger D, Jones S, Morris F. ABC of clinical electrocardiography. junctional tachycardias. *BMJ* 2002 324:662–5.

Hannash CR, Crosson JE () Emergency diagnosis and management of pediatric arrhythmia. *J Emerg Trauma Shock* 2010;3(3):251–60.

Chickenpox and Other Bugs

Michelle Alisio and Marilyn McDougall

An 8-month-old boy with chicken pox was admitted to the local paediatric unit for persistent fever and vomiting for 3 days. The rash had started a week prior to presentation (Figure 23.1). He had no diarrhoea, was awake, alert and able to drink from a bottle. He had mild work of breathing and was not hypoxic, self-ventilating in air.

The referring team were concerned by the persistent tachycardia, poor perfusion (prolonged capillary refill time of 3 seconds) and high CRP and thus initiated fluid resuscitation therapy and the relevant antibiotics. He received three 10ml/kg fluid boluses, ceftriaxone and aciclovir after baseline blood tests and cultures were taken (shown in Table 23.1). Initial advice from the retrieval team was given to add clindamycin to his empiric treatment. The initial referral call sought advice for fever management and served as forewarning.

Three hours later the infant was still febrile but looking better. He was comfortable on handling, his vital signs were unchanged, and the CXR had no infiltrates. Repeat blood results were not yet available.

That evening the retrieval team received a second phone call with updated blood results showing the CRP had doubled to 420. The referring team had a new concern regarding a swollen left thigh which resembled cellulitis. The local microbiology laboratory had updated the local team with a positive blood culture showing *Streptococcus* species, which was later confirmed as Group A *Streptococcus* (GAS).

Questions

1. What advice would you give for the persistent fever?
2. Did this patient have septic shock? How do you recognise sepsis?
3. What antimicrobial therapy should be given and why?
4. Can children with a proven viral illness also have a concomitant severe bacterial infection?

1. What advice would you give for the persistent fever?

1a. Fever and Children

Fever is a physiological response to infection. Pyrogens stimulate the hypothalamus to increase the body temperature which inhibits pathogen replication thereby protecting the body. The fever itself is of less importance than the cause for the fever and the main issue is to exclude an underlying dangerous infection rather than treating the fever with antipyretic interventions.

Table 23.1.

Blood tests		Blood gas		Observations	
Haemoglobin	120 g/L	pH	7.39	Heart rate	180 bpm
White cell count	15.6 (10^3/mm^3)	pCO_2	5.1 kPa	Respiratory rate	30 breaths per minute
Platelets	299 (10^3/mm^3)	pO_2	4.7 kPa	Sats	100%
Na	131 mmol/L	HCO_3	23 mmol/L	Blood pressure	93/72 mm/Hg
K	4.9 mmol/L	Base excess	−2 mEq/L	AVPU	A
Urea	2.4 mmol/L	Lactate	3 mmol/L		
Creatinine	15 U/L	Glucose	4.6 mmol/L		
CRP	278 mg/L				

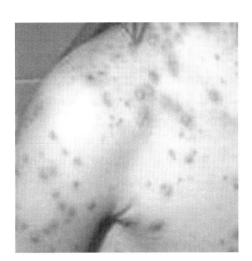

Figure 23.1 Initial presentation of rash. (A black and white version of this figure will appear in some formats. For the colour version, please refer to the plate section.)

Approximately 15–20% of children present to the emergency department with a fever, but only 0.5–1% present with sepsis. When managing a child with fever, focus on the clinical assessment to determine the risk of a serious illness such as pallor or cyanosis, depressed level of consciousness, grunting, tachypnoea, reduced skin turgor and bulging fontanelle. Treat fever in febrile convulsions and in situations such as shock with reduced cardiac output.

It is also important to give confidence-building messages to parents looking after children with fever and to debunk myths, such as high temperatures and rigors indicate severe infection, or antipyretics prevent febrile convulsions and should be used specifically for that purpose. It is also important, however, not to falsely reassure parents when they remain concerned, and to ensure that parents are made aware of the signs of deteriorating clinical condition and the appropriate actions to follow if indeed they have been sent home initially with reassurance.

1b. Non-steroidal Anti-inflammatory Drugs (NSAIDS) and Varicella

Chickenpox is an acute disease caused by varicella-zoster virus and is characterised by a vesicular rash and fever or malaise. Secondary bacterial complications are rare but most frequently involve bacterial infections of the skin and soft tissues caused by GAS and *Staphylococcus aureus*.

It has been suggested that NSAIDs (e.g. ibuprofen) may be a risk factor for severe skin and soft tissue infections with varicella infection in small sample size low-quality evidence papers, but the actual occurrence of necrotizing fasciitis is extremely rare. This may be confounded by the practice that sicker children with higher, more difficult to control fever are more likely to have been given ibuprofen as a second antipyretic. This bias is difficult to tease out. There is no certainty whether there is a real cause or association between NSAID use in chicken pox and severe skin and soft tissue infections. General advice is to avoid using NSAIDs for fever management in children with chicken pox and continue regular safe dosing of paracetamol.

2. Did this patient have septic shock? How do you recognise sepsis?

It was clear from the referral phone call that the local team were concerned and had identified an acutely unwell infant. It is most important as the advice-giving retrieval team to identify if the condition of the child being referred qualifies as an emergency and to ask yourself: Does this child have septic shock? The answer in this case was yes to both: this is an emergency and the child had septic shock. The Surviving Sepsis Campaign defines septic shock as a severe infection leading to cardiovascular dysfunction (including hypotension, need for treatment with vasoactive medication or impaired perfusion).

Four criteria define systemic inflammatory response syndrome (SIRS). These include fever, tachycardia, tachypnoea and high (or low) white cell count. This patient fulfilled all four SIRS criteria as well as cardiovascular organ dysfunction because of impaired perfusion and a high lactate (3mmol/L). Blood lactate levels provide a valuable indirect marker of tissue hypoperfusion and, although not specific (and occasionally affected by the conditions in which the blood was sampled), they can be rapidly obtained by point-of-care tests and are quantifiable surrogates for tissue hypoperfusion. There is no optimal threshold to define 'hyperlactataemia' in paediatrics. In a PICU study, the mortality rate for children with hypotension requiring vasopressors with lactate greater than 2mmol/L was 32% compared with 16% if lactate was less than 2mmol/L.

This patient was poorly perfused and despite having received initial resuscitation of 30ml/kg fluid bolus in 10ml/kg aliquots his systolic blood pressure (SBP) was still on the lower limit of normal (93/72mmHg). He also remained persistently tachycardic despite fluid therapy (165bpm).

Early recognition of sepsis is a challenge and there is no single marker or heart rate threshold that can be applied to diagnose it. There are, however, recommendations to design and implement sepsis screening tools with 'bundles of therapy' tailored to the type of patients, resources and procedures within each institution, driven by the premise that earlier recognition will lead to more timely initiation of therapy and improve morbidity and/or mortality.

3. What antimicrobial therapy should be given and why?

Surviving Sepsis Campaign guidelines recommend the administration of broad-spectrum antibiotics within 1 hour of recognition of septic shock. Those assessed as septic but without clinical signs of shock can allow 3 hours for appropriate blood cultures and investigations to be obtained before starting antimicrobial therapy.

Empiric broad-spectrum antibiotic therapy refers to the use of single or multidrug antimicrobial therapy. The initial choice should take into account the specific clinical history (e.g. age, site of infection, concomitant disease states, indwelling devices, recent hospital exposure). Ceftriaxone, a third-generation cephalosporin, is the recommended antimicrobial for community-acquired sepsis by the National Institute for Health and Care Excellence (NICE). Vancomycin should be added in settings where methicillin resistant *S. aureus* (MRSA) or ceftriaxone-resistant pneumococci are prevalent. Additionally, an aminoglycoside or substitution of a carbapenem is appropriate in settings where ceftriaxone resistance is common in gram-negative bacteria. Recommendations for immunocompromised patients, neonates and intra-abdominal sources of infection to name a few can be found in the latest Surviving Sepsis Campaign guidelines 2020.

In our case, there was an initial suspicion of invasive GAS infection: streptococcal toxic shock syndrome (TSS) or necrotizing fasciitis which was later confirmed by microbiology. The retrieval team advised to give clindamycin to limit toxin production and enhance bacterial clearance. Each regional retrieval service should have agreed antibiotic principles in sepsis management (Figure 23.2).

Streptococcal exotoxins act as superantigens to stimulate T-cell responses and induce cytokine synthesis. This leads to capillary leak, shock and organ failure. Clindamycin is a protein synthesis inhibitor acting as a superantigen inhibitor, suppressing pro-inflammatory cytokine production and is bacteriostatic. Clindamycin should therefore be administered as soon as invasive GAS infection is suspected.

The understanding that invasive GAS infections induce an inflammatory cascade introduces the concept of immunomodulation with the use of intravenous immunoglobulin (IVIG). While IVIG is advocated for use in several sepsis syndromes, there are few randomised control trials and conflicting evidence about its effect in lowering mortality in sepsis. The use of IVIG needs to be weighed against its cost and potential adverse effects including immune-mediated haemolysis and anaphylaxis.

Figure 23.2 Initial interventions for management of sepsis.

Initial Intervention

- Intravenous access x 2 quickly, Intraosseous if IV difficult
- Gas, sugar, B/C, FBC, clotting, U&E, CRP, X match, PCR
- **Antibiotics early (confirm allergy status):**
  - < 1month - IV cefotaxime & IV amoxicillin & aciclovir IV infusion
  - > 1month - IV ceftriaxone 80mg/kg infusion over 30 mins
  - Add IV vancomycin if indwelling line/VP shunt
  - Add IV clindamycin if features of toxic shock
  - Travel outside UK/risk of Abx resistance/allergy-consult ID
- Evaluate level of consciousness and pupils

4. Can children with a proven viral illness also have a concomitant severe bacterial infection?

Yes. Necrotizing fasciitis and TSS are two of the most severe clinical manifestations of invasive GAS. Varicella zoster infection is an important predisposing factor, particularly for soft tissue infection, and there is some evidence that up to 30% of children admitted with varicella have secondary bacterial skin infections.

Necrotising fasciitis is a rare complication of varicella zoster infection but is a serious condition with devastating sequelae requiring prompt diagnosis and emergency plastic surgical management for debridement of necrotic tissue and diagnosis. Necrotising fasciitis is clinically unimpressive, often difficult to recognise and often confused with cellulitis. Symptoms and signs that may suggest necrotising fasciitis are severe pain out of keeping with the skin lesion, persistent tachycardia, rapid progression, poor therapeutic response and blistering necrosis. What is seen externally is the 'tip of the iceberg'. Delay in treatment can be fatal or cause extensive skin and soft tissue loss. Explorative surgery to rule in or rule out definitive diagnosis must be carried out promptly, as an emergency if there is any clinical suspicion.

Diagnosis and appropriate management can be facilitated by immediate emergency access to theatre for intra-operative biopsy and proceed, depending on findings. Specialised radiological investigations, unless immediately accessible, may cause serious delay of definitive surgical treatment.

Further Reading

Mahajan P, Browne LR, Levine D, et al. Risk of bacterial coinfections in febrile infants 60 days old and younger with documented viral infections. *J Pediatr* 2018; 203:86–91.

National Institute for Health and Care Excellence (NICE). Guideline on fever in children. www.ncbi.nlm.nih.gov/pmc/articles/PMC2151818/.

National Institute for Health and Care Excellence (NICE). Chickenpox. www.evidence.nhs.uk/document?id=1643695&returnUrl=Search%3Fps%3D30%26q%3DAciclovir&q=Aciclovir.

National Institute for Health and Care Excellence (NICE). Sepsis: Recognition, Diagnosis and Early Management (NICE Guideline 51). 2016. Available at www.nice.org.uk/guidance/ng51.

Schlapbach LJ, MacLaren G, Festa M, et al. Australian and New Zealand Society (ANZICS) Centre for Outcomes and Resource Evaulation (CORE) and Australian and New Zealand Intensive Care Society (ANZICS) Paediatric Study Group: Prediction of pediatric sepsis mortality within 1 hour of intensive care admission. *Intensive Care Med* 2017;43:1085–96.

Steer AC, Lamagni T, Curtis N, Carapetis JR. Invasive Group A streptococcal disease: epidemiology, pathogenesis and management. *Drugs* 2012;72:1213–27.

UK Medicines Information. www.ukmi.nhs.uk.

Weiss SL, Peters MJ, Alhazzani W, *et al.* Surviving sepsis campaign international guidelines for the management of septic shock and sepsis-associated organ dysfunction in children. *Intensive Care Med* 2020;**46**: 10–67. doi: 10.1097/PCC.0000000000002198.

When Amoxicillin Just Doesn't Cover It

Michael Carter and Marilyn McDougall

A previously healthy 15-year-old boy presented to his local A&E with a 24-hour history of cough, sore throat and difficulty in breathing. He had seen his GP that morning, who had prescribed a short course of oral amoxicillin. He had taken his first dose of amoxicillin 2 hours before presentation to the A&E and subsequently became progressively tachypnoeic and tachycardic, with some suggestion his lips looked more swollen.

He was initially diagnosed with anaphylaxis secondary to amoxicillin and administered intramuscular adrenaline and oral steroids. However, he became increasingly tachypnoeic, tachycardic and peripherally cool. Venous lactate was 5.2mmol/l and a CXR showed bilateral opacity to mid zones with a right-sided pleural effusion. At this stage, a diagnosis of pneumonia with septic shock was made. The local team administered broad-spectrum antibiotics (ceftriaxone, gentamicin and clindamycin), oxygen via nasal cannulae, IV fluid boluses (in 20ml/kg aliquots of crystalloid) and peripheral dopamine (at 5mcg/kg/min) with a target mean arterial blood pressure of 65mmHg.

There was no improvement following this and anaesthetic support for intubation and mechanical ventilation was sought. Referral to the local retrieval team was also made for admission to paediatric intensive care. The child was subsequently anaesthetised and intubated by the local anaesthetic team, without issue, prior to the arrival of the retrieval team.

Questions

1. How is the diagnosis of septic shock made and the disease managed?
2. How is the diagnosis of acute respiratory distress syndrome made and the disease managed?
3. How should you balance an urgent need to retrieve a patient to a tertiary unit (early retrieval) against the need for extended resuscitation?

1. How is the diagnosis of septic shock made and the disease managed?

Until 2016, both paediatric and adult sepsis definitions (collectively known as Sepsis-2) were dependent on meeting two or more criteria for systemic inflammatory response syndrome (SIRS, temperature $\geq 38°C$ or $< 36°C$, tachycardia for age band, tachypnoea for age band or PO_2 $< 43mmHg$, white cell count $> 12 \times 10^3/mm^3$ or $< 4 \times 10^3/mm^3$) in the presence of infection. Severe sepsis was characterised by at least single organ failure, with septic shock characterised by cardiovascular dysfunction.

Table 24.1. Arterial blood tests available on arrival of the retrieval team

Na	142 mmol/L	Albumin	24	APTTR	2.0 secs
K	4.3 mmol/L	ALT	12	pH	7.29
Cl	104 mmol/L	CRP	40 mg/L	pCO_2	5.0 kPa
Urea	5.2 mmol/L	Haemoglobin	166 g/L	pO_2	8.2 kPa
Creatinine	102 U/L	White cell count	5.9 ($10^3/mm^3$)	HCO_3	18.3 mmol/L
Corrected Ca	2.35 mmol/L	Platelet count	229 ($10^3/mm^3$)	Base excess	−8.8 mEq/L
Mg	0.71 mmol/L	INR	1.4	Lactate	3.6 mmol/L

In 2016, the Third International Consensus definitions for Sepsis and Septic Shock (Sepsis-3) defined sepsis in adults as 'life-threatening organ dysfunction caused by a dysregulated host response to infection'. In contrast to previous definitions, Sepsis-3 focused on organ failure in the context of infection as the primary driver of poor outcome, and was defined on the basis of data from large prospective cohorts. Organ failure was defined as an increase in the sequential (or sepsis-related) organ failure assessment (SOFA) score of ≥ 2 points (Table 24.2). Septic shock was defined as a requirement for vasopressors to maintain mean arterial blood pressure ≥ 65mmHg and serum lactate ≥ 2mmol/l despite fluid volume resuscitation. Sepsis-3 had a higher sensitivity and specificity for mortality than Sepsis-2.

The application of Sepsis-3 definitions to children has been attempted, but has been limited by the lack of large paediatric cohorts from which to derive key variables and thresholds, particularly in low and middle income countries. This is especially the case in Africa, where a large randomised trial of fluid resuscitation in severe febrile illness resulted in the surprising observation of increased mortality in children receiving fluid boluses. As a result of this, criteria for the diagnosis of sepsis in children in epidemiological studies typically use Sepsis-2 criteria.

Despite these difficulties, the Surviving Sepsis Campaign has released updated international guidelines on the management of septic shock and sepsis-associated organ dysfunction in children. The UK National Institute for Health and Care Excellence (NICE) has guidance designed specifically for the National Health Service; while a template for this guidance is provided by the Sepsis Trust (https://sepsistrust.org/; Figure 24.1).

2. How is the diagnosis acute respiratory distress syndrome made and the disease managed?

Paediatric acute respiratory distress syndrome (ARDS) is the clinical syndrome of hypoxaemia associated with bilateral pulmonary infiltrates secondary to oedema, as defined by the Paediatric Acute Lung Injury and Sepsis Investigators (PALISI; Table 24.3). Classification is as mild, moderate and severe on the basis of Oxygenation Index (or, in the absence of arterial blood gas measurements, Oxygen Saturation Index). Mortality is high, with 10–12% of patients with mild–moderate disease, and 33% of children with severe disease dying in PICU. Major causes of paediatric ARDS are pneumonia (prevalence 63%, mortality 12%), sepsis (prevalence 19%, mortality 30%) and aspiration (prevalence 8%, mortality 22%).

Table 24.2. Sequential organ failure assessment (SOFA) score

System	Score				
	0	1	2	3	4
Respiration					
PO_2/FiO_2 kPa (mmHg)	≥53.3 (≥400)	<53.3 (<400)	<40 (<300)	<26.7 (<200) with respiratory support	<13.3 (<100) with respiratory support
Coagulation					
Platelets (×10³/L)	≥150	<150	<100	<50	<20
Liver					
Bilirubin (µmol/L)	<20	20–32	33–101	102–204	>204
Cardiovascular	MAP[a] ≥70 mmHg	MAP <70 mmHg	Dopamine <5[b]	Dopamine 5–15 or adrenaline ≤0.1 or noradrenaline ≤0.1[b]	Dopamine >15 or adrenaline >0.1 or noradrenaline >0.1[b]
CNS					
Glasgow Coma Score	15	13–14	10–12	6–9	<6
Renal					
Creatinine (µmol/l)	<110	110–170	171–299	300–400	440
Urine output (ml/day)				<500	<200

[a] Mean arterial pressure.
[b] Expressed as mcg/kg/min IV infusion.

In contrast, adult ARDS is defined on the basis of the 'Berlin criteria', from the original definition of the American European Consensus Conference. The Berlin criteria define ARDS as mild, moderate and severe on the basis of the PO_2/FiO_2 ratio. Mortality for severe ARDS in adults is approximately 45%.

Evidence-Based Management of ARDS

Most evidence for the management of paediatric ARDS is adapted from adult data. Current strategies include the use of 'open lung' ventilation with high PEEP (typically approximately 10cmH₂O) and low ventilation volumes (4–6ml/kg) with a long inspiratory time (1–1.2 secs in children). Such an approach aims to maximise alveolar recruitment and minimise cyclical alveolar collapse and atelectasis. A major contraindication to this approach is dynamic hyperinflation ('breath-stacking'), where end-expiratory volume exceeds functional residual capacity leading to barotrauma and haemodynamic compromise. Dynamic hyperinflation typically occurs in asthma or other obstructive respiratory diseases (including severe bronchiolitis) and requires a separate ventilatory strategy (see Chapter 7 and 13).

SEPSIS SCREENING TOOL TELEPHONE TRIAGE — **UNDER 5**

01 START CHART IF ANY OF THE FOLLOWING ARE REPORTED:
- ☐ Abnormal temperature
- ☐ Appears to be breathing more quickly or slowly than normal
- ☐ Altered mental state – include sleepy, irritable, drowsy or floppy
- ☐ Abnormally pale / bluish skin or abnormally cold hands or feet
- ☐ Reduced wet nappies or reduced urine output

RISK FACTORS FOR SEPSIS INCLUDE:
- ☐ Impaired immunity (e.g. diabetes, steroids, chemotherapy) ☐ Indwelling lines / broken skin
- ☐ Recent trauma / surgery / invasive procedure

NO ▶ SEPSIS UNLIKELY, CONSIDER OTHER DIAGNOSIS

02 COULD THIS BE DUE TO AN INFECTION? YES
LIKELY SOURCE: ☐ Brain ☐ Surgical ☐ Other
☐ Respiratory ☐ Urine ☐ Skin / joint / wound ☐ Indwelling device

NO ▶ SEPSIS UNLIKELY, CONSIDER OTHER DIAGNOSIS

03 ANY RED FLAG PRESENT? YES
- ☐ No response to social cues
- ☐ Doesn't wake when roused / won't stay awake
- ☐ Weak, high-pitched or continuous cry
- ☐ Grunting or bleating noises with every breath
- ☐ Finding it much harder to breathe than normal
- ☐ Very fast breathing / 'pauses' in breathing
- ☐ Skin that's very pale, mottled, ashen or blue
- ☐ Rash that doesn't fade when pressed firmly
- ☐ Temperature <36°C (check 3 times in 10 min)
- ☐ If under 3 months, temperature ≥ 38°C

YES ▶ **RED FLAG SEPSIS START BUNDLE**

04 ANY AMBER FLAG PRESENT? NO
IF IMMUNITY IMPAIRED TREAT AS RED FLAG SEPSIS
- ☐ Not responding normally / no smile
- ☐ Parental concern
- ☐ Wakes only with prolonged stimulation
- ☐ Significantly decreased activity
- ☐ Having to work hard to breathe
- ☐ Poor feeding in infants
- ☐ Reduced urine output
- ☐ Leg pain
- ☐ Cold feet or hands

YES ▶ **FURTHER INFORMATION AND REVIEW REQUIRED: - ARRANGE URGENT FACE-TO FACE ASSESSMENT USING CLINICAL JUDGEMENT TO DETERMINE APPROPRIATE CLINICAL ENVIRONMENT**

NO AMBER FLAGS : GIVE SAFETY-NETTING ADVICE:
CALL 111 IF CONDITION CHANGES OR DETERIORATES.
SIGNPOST TO AVAILABLE RESOURCES AS APPROPRIATE

CALL 999 IF ANY OF:
Is breathing very fast
Has a 'fit' or convulsion
Looks mottled, bluish or pale
Has a rash that does not fade when you press it
Is very lethargic or difficult to wake
Feels abnormally cold to touch

TELEPHONE TRIAGE BUNDLE:
THIS IS TIME-CRITICAL – IMMEDIATE ACTION REQUIRED: **DIAL 999**
AND ARRANGE BLUE LIGHT TRANSFER
COMMUNICATION: Ensure communication of 'Red Flag Sepsis' to crew
Advise crew to pre-alert as 'Red Flag Sepsis'

THE UK SEPSIS TRUST
UKST 2020 TT3.2 PAGE 1 OF 1

The controlled copy of this document is maintained by The UK Sepsis Trust. Any copies of this document held outside of that area, in whatever format (e.g. paper, email attachment) are considered to have passed out of control and should be checked for currency and validity.

The UK Sepsis Trust registered charity number (England & Wales) 1158843 (Scotland) SC050277. Company registration number 8644039. Sepsis Enterprises Ltd. company number 9583335. VAT reg. number 293133408.

Figure 24.1 Sepsis Trust. Acute Hospital Inpatients: Screening and Action Tool for Under 5s. Used with permission. Similar templates for alternative age bands are also available. (A black and white version of this figure will appear in some formats. For the colour version, please refer to the plate section.)

SEPSIS SCREENING TOOL - THE PAEDIATRIC SEPSIS SIX

UNDER 5

PATIENT DETAILS:

DATE:

TIME:

NAME:

DESIGNATION:

SIGNATURE:

COMPLETE ALL ACTIONS WITHIN ONE HOUR

01 ENSURE SENIOR CLINICIAN ATTENDS
NOT ALL PATIENTS WITH RED FLAGS WILL NEED THE 'SEPSIS 6' URGENTLY. A SENIOR DECISION MAKER MAY SEEK ALTERNATIVE DIAGNOSES / DE-ESCALATE CARE. RECORD DECISIONS BELOW
NAME: GRADE:

TIME

02 OXYGEN IF REQUIRED
START IF O₂ SATURATIONS LESS THAN 92% OR EVIDENCE OF SHOCK

TIME

03 OBTAIN IV / IO ACCESS, TAKE BLOODS
BLOOD CULTURES, BLOOD GLUCOSE, LACTATE, FBC, U&Es,
CRP AND CLOTTING, LUMBAR PUNCTURE IF INDICATED

TIME

04 GIVE IV / IO ANTIBIOTICS
MAXIMUM DOSE BROAD SPECTRUM THERAPY
CONSIDER: LOCAL POLICY / ALLERGY STATUS / ANTIVIRALS

TIME

05 CONSIDER IV / IO FLUIDS
IF LACTATE IS ABOVE 2 mmol/L GIVE FLUID BOLUS 20 ml/kg WITHOUT DELAY
IF LACTATE >4 mmol/L CALL PICU. (10ml/kg neonates, REPEAT IF REQUIRED)

TIME

06 CONSIDER INOTROPIC SUPPORT
CONSIDER INOTROPIC SUPPORT IF NORMAL PHYSIOLOGY IS NOT RESTORED AFTER ≥20 mL/
kg FLUID (10 mL/kg IN NEONATES), CALL PICU OR A REGIONAL CENTRE URGENTLY

TIME

RED FLAGS AFTER ONE HOUR - ESCALATE TO CONSULTANT NOW

RECORD ADDITIONAL NOTES HERE:
e.g. allergy status, arrival of specialist teams, de-escalation of care, delayed antimicrobial decision making, variance from Sepsis Six

Figure 24.1 *(cont.)*

Table 24.3. Definition of paediatric ARDS according to PALISI criteria

Age	Exclude patients with perinatal lung disease		
Timing	Within 7 days of known insult		
Origin of oedema	Respiratory failure not fully explained by cardiac failure of fluid overload		
Chest imaging	Chest imaging findings of new infiltrate(s) consistent with acute pulmonary parenchymal disease		
Severity	Mild	Moderate	Severe
OI[a]	$4 \leq OI < 8$	$8 \leq OI < 16$	$OI \geq 16$
OSI[2]	$5 \leq OSI < 7.5$	$7.5 \leq OSI < 12.3$	$OSI \geq 12.3$
Special populations	Not explained by cyanotic heart disease, chronic lung disease and/or left ventricular dysfunction		

[a] OI* = $(FiO_2 \times$ mean airway pressure $\times 100)/PO_2$. [b] OSI* = $(FiO_2 \times$ mean airway pressure $\times 100)/SpO_2$.
* Mean airway pressure in cmH_2O, PO_2 in mmHg.

Other strategies for ARDS include permissive hypercapnia (target pH of ≥ 7.2, or ≥ 7.3 if there is documented evidence of pulmonary arterial hypertension) and mild hypoxia (target $SpO_2 \geq 85\%$, or $\geq 90\%$ in pulmonary arterial hypertension). Pulmonary arterial hypertension may also be treated with nitric oxide. Prone positioning has also been supported by high quality evidence. There are currently few data to support the use of high-frequency oscillatory ventilation.

The role of veno-venous extracorporeal membranous oxygenation (VV-ECMO) for ARDS is controversial. The largest randomised controlled trial of VV-ECMO for ARDS (in adults) showed no significant difference in mortality in intention-to-treat and per-protocol analyses. However, interpretation of the results was controversial due to the near statistical significance, early stopping of the trial for futility and diverging pre-existing views on ECMO for ARDS. The role of ECMO in the retrieval of patients with ARDS is discussed more widely in Chapter 26.

3. How should you balance an urgent need to retrieve a patient to a tertiary unit (early retrieval) against the need for extended resuscitation?

A major challenge for a retrieval specialist is deciding whether to invest time and resources treating patients in the referral hospital, or whether to stabilise the child and move to the receiving unit as quickly as possible. This decision must be made on the basis of the clinical features of the patient and the difference in equipment and human resources between the referring and receiving units. Maximisation of the resources available to the retrieval team can be achieved through judicious use of the skills of the team at the local hospital. Anaesthetic colleagues are competent and experienced at procedures such as central line insertion but may need guidance on decision-making regarding inotrope selection and ventilation strategies for children. Structured discussion with colleagues at the receiving unit is often an excellent way to step back from an acute situation and analyse whether patient outcome is likely to be improved by either further stabilisation or by a swift transfer to a unit where definitive care with higher specification equipment, an expert paediatric intensive care team and multi-specialty input can be given. In this case, the referring anaesthetic team were able to rapidly place venous and arterial lines whilst the retrieval team optimised ventilation in preparation for swift transfer to the receiving unit.

Retrieval

On arrival of the retrieval team, the patient was ventilated by the consultant anaesthetist using a Mapleson C circuit in the A&E, with an FiO_2 of 1.0 achieving peripheral oxygen saturation of 65–80%. His heart rate was 180 beats per minute, with a non-invasive blood pressure of 90/60mmHg following fluid resuscitation of 60ml/kg crystalloid, a dopamine infusion of 5mcg/kg/min and frequent boluses of metaraminol.

Dopamine was increased to 10mcg/kg/min and an adrenaline infusion was added. A detailed telephone discussion between the on-site retrieval team and retrieval consultant (at base) followed. A decision was made to transport the patient to the tertiary paediatric centre without further delay. He was ventilated with a PEEP of 8 and pressure control of 26 during transport. On arrival, he was reviewed immediately by the PICU and Extra-Corporeal Membranous Oxygenation (ECMO) team and placed on veno-venous ECMO within 6 hours of admission. He received 13 days of ECMO therapy, 3 additional days of mechanical ventilation, 7 days of haemofiltration and 4 weeks of high dose flucloxacillin for Panton-Valentine Leukocidin (PVL) positive *Staphylococcus aureus* infection producing pneumonia with empyema, progressing to ARDS and fulminant septic shock. He made a full medical recovery.

Further Reading

Acute Respiratory Distress Syndrome Network. Ventilation with lower tidal volumes as compared with traditional tidal volumes for acute lung injury and the acute respiratory distress syndrome. *N Engl J Med* 2000;**342**:1301–8.

ARDS Definition Task Force, Ranieri VM, Rubenfeld GD, et al. Acute respiratory distress syndrome: the Berlin Definition. *JAMA* 2012;**307**, 2526–33, .

Briel M, Meade M, Mercat A, et al. Higher vs lower positive end-experiatory pressure in patients with acute lung injury and acute respiratory distress syndrome. *JAMA* 2010;**303**: 865–73.

Combes A, Hajage D, Capellier D, et al. Extracorporeal membrane oxygenation for severe acute respiratory distress syndrome. *N Engl J Med* 2018;**378**:1965–75.

Goldstein ., Giroir ., Randolp, A, & International Consensus Conference on Pediatric, S.

International pediatric sepsis consensus conference: definitions for sepsis and organ dysfunction in pediatrics. *Pediatr Crit Care Med* 2005;**6**:2–8, doi:10.1097/01.PCC .0000149131.72248.E6.

Goligher EC, Tomlinson G, Hajage D, et al. Extracorporeal membrane oxygenation for severe acute respiratory distress syndrome and posterior probability of mortality benefit in a post hoc Bayesian analysis of a randomized clinical trial. *JAMA* 2018;**320**:2251–9.

Griffiths MJD, McAuley DF, Perkins GD, et al. Guidelines on the management of acute respiratory distress syndrome. *BMJ Open Respir Res* 2019;**6**:e000420.

Khemani RG, Smith L, Lopez-Fernandez YM, et al. Paediatric acute respiratory distress syndrome incidence and epidemiology (PARDIE): an international, observational study. *Lancet Resp Med* 2019;**7**:115–28.

Levy MM, Fink MP, Marshall JC, et al. SCCM/ ESICM/ACCP/ATS/SIS International Sepsis

Definitions Conference. *Intensive Care Med* 2001;**29**: 530–8, doi:10.1007/s00134-003-1662-x.

Maitland K, Kiguli S, Opoka RO, et al. Mortality after fluid bolus in African children with severe infection. *N Engl J Med* 2011;**364**:2483–95.

Matics TJ, Sanchez-Pinto LN. Adaptation and validation of a Pediatric Sequential Organ Failure Assessment Score and evaluation of the Sepsis-3 definitions in critically ill children. *JAMA Pediatr* 2017;171:e172352.

National Institute for Health and Clinical Excellence (NICE). Sepsis: recognition, diagnosis and early management (NG51). (NICE, London, 2016).

Obonyo NG, Schlapbach LJ, Fraser JF. Sepsis: changing definitions, unchanging treatment. *Front Pediatr* 2018; 425.

Pediatric Acute Lung Injury Consensus Conference Group. Pediatric acute respiratory distress syndrome: consensus recommendations from the Pediatric Acute Lung Injury Consensus Conference. *Pediatr Crit Care Med* **16**, 428–39, doi:10.1097/PCC.00000000000003502015.

Raith EP, Udy AA, Bailey M, et al.Prognostic accuracy of the SOFA score, SIRS criteria, and qSOFA score for in-hospital mortality among adults with suspected infection admitted to the intensive care unit. *JAMA* 2017;**317**:290–300.

Schlapbach LJ, Straney L, Bellomo R, et al. Prognostic accuracy of age-adapted SOFA, SIRS, PELOD-2, and qSOFA for in-hospital mortality among children with suspected infection admitted to the intensive care unit. *Intensive Care Med* 2018;**44**:179–88.

Sepsis Trust. *The UK Sepsis Trust: Clinical Tools*, https://sepsistrust.org/professional-resources/clinical-tools/ (2020).

Shankar-Hari M, Harrison DA, Rowan K M. Differences in impact of definitional

elements on mortality precludes international comparisons of sepsis epidemiology-a cohort study illustrating the need for standardized reporting. *Crit Care Med* 2016;**44**:2223–30, doi:10.1097/CCM.0000000000001876

Shankar-Hari M, Harrison DA, Rubenfeld GD, Rowan K. Epidemiology of sepsis and septic shock in critical care units: comparison between sepsis-2 and sepsis-3 populations using a national critical care database. *Br J Anaesth* 2017;**119**:62636.

Shankar-Hari M. Phillips GS, Levy ML, et al. Developing a new definition and assessing new clinical criteria for septic shock: For the Third International Consensus Definitions for Sepsis and Septic Shock (Sepsis-3). *JAMA* 2016;**315**:775–87, doi:10.1001/jama.2016.0289.

Singer M, Deutschman CS, Seymour CW, et al. The Third International Consensus Definitions for Sepsis and Septic Shock (Sepsis-3). *JAMA* 2016;**315**:801–10.

South Thames Retrieval Service. 2020 Clinical Guidance. Paediatric Critical Care: Acute Respiratory Distress Syndrome (ARDS). (www.evelinalondon.nhs.uk/resources/our-services/hospital/south-thames-retrieval-service/acute-respiratory.pdf, 2019).

Weiss SL, Peter MJ, Alhazzani W, et al. Surviving Sepsis Campaign international guidelines for the management of septic shock and sepsis-associated organ dysfunction in children. *Pediatr Crit Care Med* 2018;**21**:52–e106.

Writing Group for the Alveolar Recruitment for Acute Respiratory Distress Syndrome Trial, I. et al. Effect of lung recruitment and titrated positive end-expiratory pressure (PEEP) vs low PEEP on mortality in patients with acute respiratory distress syndrome: A Randomized Clinical Trial. *JAMA* 2017;**318**:1335–45.

Chapter 25

Tumour Lysis

Jo Dyer and Shelley Riphagen

A 10-year-old boy presented with shortness of breath, hepatosplenomegaly, bleeding gums and a spreading petechial rash. He had non-specific complaints including lethargy for the previous 3 months but had not required hospital treatment and had no specific diagnosis. The week before admission he had developed a petechial rash and low-grade fever, but otherwise felt well, and was reviewed by his GP who sent routine bloods. His parents confirmed with his GP that it was acceptable to continue their holiday plans while awaiting the blood results. He had a proposed review scheduled after return from holidays a week later. He presented to the local A&E department at the holiday destination after a flight to visit his grandparents abroad. During the flight, his symptoms had worsened with onset of breathing difficulties, and his parents brought him to the local A&E after landing.

The local paediatric team from abroad called as the parents informed them that your service is the tertiary children's service for their home region. The referring team were worried about the blood results which showed hyperleucocytosis, thrombocytopenia and metabolic derangement. They suspected a diagnosis of acute lymphoblastic leukaemia (ALL) and felt the child needed urgent transfer home before the situation deteriorated.

He required flight retrieval to a paediatric oncology centre with a PICU facility and arrangements for fixed-wing transfer commenced. However, even under the most favourable circumstances, this would not result in immediate transfer.

The local team were concerned about managing the child for the next 24 to 36 hours and were looking for advice on treatment and management of potential acute deterioration. His observations and investigations are shown in Tables 25.1 and 25.2 and his CXR is displayed (Figure 25.1).

Questions

1. What are the presenting clinical emergencies and what therapies should be instigated prior to retrieval?
2. What complications should be anticipated during the flight retrieval?
3. How could treatment of this child be managed if flight retrieval was delayed?

1. What are the presenting clinical emergencies and what therapies should be instigated prior to retrieval?

This child had a new diagnosis of ALL with respiratory compromise, petechial haemorrhage secondary to thrombocytopenia, anaemia, hyperleucocytosis (WCC >100,000) and was at

Table 25.1.

Respiration rate	32 breaths per minute with mild work of breathing
SaO_2	90% in air 98% in 5 L O_2
Heart rate	85 bpm
Blood pressure	128/82(93) mmHg
AVPU	A

Table 25.2.

Haemoglobin	72 g/L	Calcium	2.4 mmol/L
White cell count	340 (10^3/mm^3)	Phosphate	4.8 mmol/L
Platelets	18 (10^3/mm^3)	Urea	3.5 mmol/L
Na	134 mmol/L	Creatinine	22 U/L
K	4.8 mmol/L		

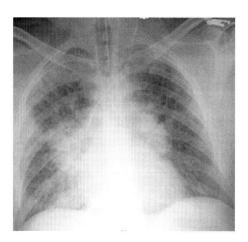

Figure 25.1 Admission chest radiograph.

risk of tumour lysis syndrome. **Hyperleucocytosis** and **tumour lysis syndrome** present two oncologic emergencies which can deteriorate rapidly and need urgent management.

Respiratory symptoms need to be monitored carefully in this child. His respiratory distress may be secondary to stasis of blood in the pulmonary vasculature (see below), anaemia, or a combination of these factors. In the scenario of new presentations of ALL, respiratory distress can also be as a result of airway compression by a mediastinal mass due to tumour. If a CXR had not been taken then this would need to be ordered to rule out a mediastinal mass which could present very different management challenges (see Chapter 9). Careful assessment of his CXR, his response to oxygen therapy, and close monitoring of his symptoms and response to treatments must be undertaken.

He presented with signs of new petechial haemorrhage and thrombocytopenia. Platelet transfusion should be administered, and response monitored. The decision making regarding transfusion of red cells to treat the anaemia is more complex and is discussed below.

The clinical emergency in this case is the hyperleucocytosis, which can cause leukostasis and hyperviscosity syndrome, coagulopathy and tumour lysis syndrome resulting in significant morbidity and mortality. High count leukaemias (WCC >100) are considered a haemato-oncological emergency, requiring prompt and urgent transfer to a primary treatment centre (PTC) where definitive treatment can be initiated after initial investigations. Aggressive early management of this child could not wait for a retrieval team to arrive. Treatment must be initiated under guidance of the PTC.

Hyperleucocytosis results in increased plasma viscosity, vascular endothelial damage, intravascular thrombus and anaerobic metabolism secondary to infarction and haemorrhage. The result is cell trapping in the microvasculature with microthrombi leading to poor tissue perfusion and acidosis. In hyperleucocytosis secondary to leukaemia, the risk of thrombosis is increased as blasts are inflexible. It is most commonly seen in ALL and acute myeloid leukaemia (AML) but occurs at lower white cell cell (WCC) counts, in AML than in ALL. AML cells have larger corpuscular volume and more surface adhesion molecules than those of ALL. This increased blood viscosity is dependent on both the white cell volume and the packed red cell volume. Therefore, blood transfusion for anaemia should be avoided in this scenario unless it is seriously compromising clinical condition. The decision to transfuse would be best made in discussion with the oncology team.

The most frequent complications of leukostasis are respiratory and neurological but multiple systems can be affected. Ongoing close monitoring at the local hospital must look for any of the following signs or symptoms from Table 25.3.

Management strategies for reducing the WCC will need to be discussed between the three teams involved: the local team, team at the PTC and retrieval team. The definitive treatment is urgent commencement of chemotherapy. Other holding therapies to transiently reduce the WCC are exchange transfusion and leukapheresis. These are all usually instigated in a PICU setting as there are high risks for life-threatening complications. In this scenario, if significant delay in transferring the child is anticipated or if his condition worsens, it may become necessary for the local team to start treatment with one of these

Table 25.3.

Respiratory:
- Dyspnoea, tachypnoea
- Low oxygen saturations
- Diffuse bilateral infiltrates on CXR

Cardiovascular:
- Cardiac failure

Neurological:
- Headache, retinal haemorrhage, papilloedema
- Fluctuating or depressed level of consciousness
- Focal signs, seizures, stroke

Renal:
- Renal dysfunction or failure

Other systems:
- Ischaemic change to limbs and digits

therapies. Commencement of any treatments prior to transfer would require careful consideration of risk vs benefit and should be led by the PTC consultant.

Tumour lysis syndrome (TLS) is a life-threatening oncological emergency caused by spontaneous or induced tumour cell death, resulting in a sudden release into the blood stream of intracellular products (nucleic acids, potassium and phosphate). It is characterised by acute life-threatening metabolic abnormalities including hyperuricaemia, hyperphosphataemia and hyperkalaemia. Potential clinical manifestations include renal insufficiency, arrhythmias, seizures, neurological complications and sudden death. Hypocalcaemia is an indirect consequence of TLS and is associated with hyperphosphatemia as the excess phosphate binds available serum calcium.

TLS may occur spontaneously before treatment with chemotherapy or radiation, but more often after the start of therapy. Severe TLS is most commonly associated with malignancies with high rate of cell turn over and or high tumour burden, particularly Burkitt lymphoma, lymphoblastic lymphoma and ALL with high presentation WCC. Patients with hyperleucocytosis associated with leukaemia are always considered candidates for TLS prophylaxis with allopurinol or rasburicase to decrease serum uric acid levels in addition to aggressive IV hydration

Recognition that this child is at risk of TLS is key and management strategies are focused on prevention:

- Hyperhydration with dextrose saline (no added potassium) 3 L/m²/day
- Ensure hyperdiuresis (minimum 3 ml/kg/hr). May require cautious low dose frusemide to achieve this, but should be discussed with PTC as increased risk of leukostasis with dehydration
- Strict monitoring of fluid balance
- Rasburicase as first line, or allopurinol if no rasburicase available locally
- Minimum 8 hourly laboratory testing of urate, potassium, urea and creatinine, phosphate, calcium.

Unrecognised deterioration could lead to life threatening emergency. If TLS develops, management strategies will need to become focused on closer monitoring and active treatment of electrolyte and biochemical abnormalities:

- Urgent re-discussion with PTC and transfer team
- Cardiac monitoring looking for evidence of hyperkalaemia and hypocalcaemia
- Observation for other clinical signs of metabolic derangement

  ○ Vomiting, cramps, seizures, spasms, altered mental state, tetany (hypocalcaemia)
  ○ Weakness, paralysis (hyperkalaemia)

- Emergency management of hyperkalaemia
- Cautious calcium supplementation only if symptomatic hypocalcaemia
- Renal replacement therapies including haemofiltration or haemodialysis requires insertion of a vascath or permacath by an appropriately skilled clinician. Before insertion of vascath, vessels must be imaged to ensure they are not surrounded by tumour, increasing risk of vascular trauma during insertion.

In this setting, these scenarios must be anticipated and planned for as this child cannot be quickly moved to a PTC.

2. What complications should be anticipated during the flight retrieval?

There are numerous physical, physiological and psychological stressors associated with flight retrieval.

The logistics of co-ordinating air transfers are covered in Chapter 3. The length of flight, coordination of land transfers each end, and potential for delays in team mobilisation due to weather and availability of aircraft, contribute to a significant period of time between initial recognition of the severity of this child's condition and his arrival at an appropriate PTC.

Broadly, the need to ensure the child is stable enough for the journey, anticipation of and being prepared for potential complications, relates to all critically ill children being retrieved. There are considerations specific to this case that must be recognised by the teams involved.

- Anaemia and therefore poor oxygen-carrying capacity in an increasingly hypoxic environment:

  o Anticipate worsening of respiratory symptoms and therefore elect to transport in a higher level of inspired oxygen or consider need for escalation of respiratory support prior to transfer to maintain safety. This also needs to be factored into your oxygen requirement calculations.

  o Cabin pressure results in a fall in partial pressure of alveolar oxygen (pO_2) – hypobaric hypoxia. 'Sea level cabin' discussion with flight team if anticipate child will not tolerate hypoxia.

  o Oxygen is a pulmonary vasodilator. It improves blood flow, decreases potential for sludging and thrombi formation, as well as increasing oxygen-carrying gas exchange. Poor delivery of oxygen will result in the reverse of this.

- Ensure you have a recent set of blood results to check improvement/stabilisation. Any deterioration in results will have to be weighed up against delay in reaching centre for definitive treatment.
- If there is significant renal insufficiency or renal failure then this would need to be treated and stabilised locally as limited number of treatments can be continued during transfer.
- Hyperhydration resulting in increased urine output. In this setting catheterisation will be necessary to increase comfort during transfer.
- Calculation of oxygen requirement, equipment battery life, communication tools as per flight retrieval case study/flight tasking (see Chapter 3).

3. How could treatment of this child be managed if flight retrieval was delayed?

Involvement of the expertise of the oncology centre should be sought as early as possible. This child would be deemed an urgent/time critical transfer, and prioritised as such, if the referring centre was within the UK. The need to organise longer distance fixed-wing transfer unavoidably delays this, increasing the chance of complications developing locally, prior to retrieval.

The potential need to instigate complex therapies, such as haemofiltration, leukapheresis and exchange transfusion, requires discussion between all teams involved. The most appropriate place for the child to be managed whilst awaiting retrieval depends upon the expertise of the clinicians, availability of drugs, equipment and monitoring facilities. If any of the treatments are deemed urgent, or it is evident that there will be significant delay in flight retrieval, potential options may include:

- Utilising local adult HDU, ICU or oncology facilities
- Transfer to an alternative centre within the country that can offer appropriate therapies.

Ongoing communication is essential between the referral team, oncology centre and retrieval team base whilst the team are on their outward journey.

There is potential for communication errors with the involvement of three teams, complexity of the case and language barriers. It is essential to identify key people in each team, avoid conflicting advice, multiple handovers of information, repetition, frustration of local clinicians having to repeatedly give information to multiple individuals.

This child underwent successful transfer self-ventilating in oxygen with hyperhydration within 24 hours of the referral. Allopurinol had been started locally, however, the retrieval team brought rasburicase on the transfer and added it to treatment. The child was initiated on definitive treatment on arrival at the PTC and was improving until day 11 when he had a sudden onset acute loss of consciousness associated with a low platelets and a massive intracranial bleed. On post mortem he had significant tumour burden in the brain.

Further Reading

Cheung D. 2018. Oncological emergencies. In *Paediatric Haematology and Oncology: Supportive Care Protocols,* 4th ed. GOSH, UCLH, RMH. www.georgespicu.org.uk/wp-content/uploads/bsk-pdf-manager/2018/10/Oncology-Supporitve-Care-Guidelines-Ed4-v2.0-2018.pdf.

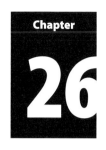

Respiratory Insufficiency on Maximal Support
Is That It?

Federico Minen and Jon Lillie

An 8-week-old baby girl born prematurely had been transferred and admitted to PICU after presenting to her local hospital with respiratory failure due to bronchiolitis. She was born at 30 weeks gestational age in good condition and had a straightforward course without any complications of prematurity. She was discharged home at 36 weeks weighing 2 kg. After 2 weeks at home, she developed respiratory symptoms, was brought to A&E and then admitted to her local PICU where she was intubated and ventilated for RSV bronchiolitis. By 5 days after PICU admission she had improved to such an extent that ventilation could be weaned to minimal support. Over the next 24 hours, however, she deteriorated rapidly with evolving four quadrant opacification on CXR (Figure 26.1), necessitating escalation of ventilation and cardiovascular support. Ventilation was further escalated to high frequency ventilation (HFOV). Piperacillin-tazobactam and gentamicin had been started.

After 8 hours of HFOV, she was not making any improvement and continuing to deteriorate and thus a referral was made from PICU to the regional ECMO centre. At the time of referral she was nasally intubated with a size 3.0mm microcuffed endotracheal tube (ETT), saturating 85–90% with FiO_2 1.0, HFOV mean airway pressure (MAP) 23cmH$_2$0, delta P 60 and inhaled nitric oxide (iNO) at 20ppm. She had been proned for the previous 8 hours to improve ventilation. She was on dopamine infusion 15mcg/kg/min and noradrenaline 0.2mcg/kg/min achieving mean BP of 45mmHg and remained tachycardic 145–170bpm.

On these settings her arterial blood gas at the time of referral was: Ph 7.15, pCO_2 12.6, pO_2 7.9, HCO_3 27.1, BE 5, lactate 0.7, Hb 97.

Questions

1. What would you suggest to improve the current ventilation strategy?
2. Should this baby be transferred for extracorporeal membrane oxygenation (ECMO)?
3. Is there anything in the history to exclude this child from ECMO?
4. The decision was made to transfer the child to the ECMO centre. What investigations and management should be completed prior to transfer?

1. What would you suggest to improve the current ventilation strategy?

The patient was being mechanically ventilated on high settings. The combination of infiltrates on CXR and hypoxia despite oxygen and high MAP meant that she clinically fitted the criteria for acute respiratory distress syndrome (ARDS) (**Figure 26.2**).

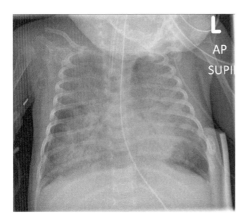

Figure 26.1 Chest X-ray after acute deterioration.

Age	Exclude patients with perinatal lung disease		
Timing	Within 7 days of known insult		
Origin of oedema	Respiratory failure not fully explained by cardiac failure of fluid overload		
Chest imaging	Chest imaging findings of new infiltrate(s) consistent with acute pulmonary parenchymal disease		
Severity	Mild	Moderate	Severe
OI*	4–8	8–16	≥16
OSI**	5–7.5	7.5–12.3	≥12.3
Special populations	Not explained by cyanotic heart disease, chronic lung disease and/or left ventricular dysfunction		

Figure 26.2 Criteria for paediatric ARDS definition.
Oxygenation index (OI) and oxygen saturation index (OSI) formulas:
$$OI = MAP \times F_iO_2 \times 100 / PO_2$$
$$OSI = MAP \times F_iO_2 \times 100 / SpO_2$$
MAP: mean airway pressure (in cmH₂O);
F_iO_2 : fraction of inspired oxygen (0.21–1.0); PO_2 : partial pressure of oxygen (in mmHg); SpO2: oxygen saturation (in %). Pre-ductal PO_2 and SpO_2 should be used.

ARDS is caused by a heterogeneous group of diseases eventually leading to diffuse inflammatory damage involving the alveoli and pulmonary capillaries. The increased capillary permeability leads to alveoli filling with proteinaceous fluid and cellular debris leading to hypoxaemia from ventilation perfusion mismatch and reduced lung compliance.

Mechanical ventilation is critical in this setting to support oxygenation and ventilation but it may promote lung damage, a phenomenon known as ventilator-induced lung injury (VILI). Several mechanisms of VILI have been described including inspiratory and/or expiratory stress inducing overdistension (volutrauma), alveoli that repetitively open and close during tidal breathing (atelectrauma) and ventilator induced pressure damage (barotrauma) among others.

It is important to recognise ARDS early as mortality is high (33% in severe cases), and this mortality can be reduced by a targeted management strategy. 'Open lung' ventilation strategy is suggested for ARDS: target SpO₂ ≥85% (90% if pulmonary hypertension), pH ≥7.2, low tidal volumes (<6ml/kg) and peak plateau pressure (<30 cmH₂O), PEEP 10–14cmH₂O, inhaled nitric oxide if documented pulmonary hypertension or right ventricle dysfunction.

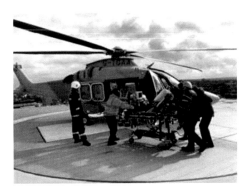

Figure 3.1 The Children's Air Ambulance preparing for a retrieval. (A black and white version of this figure will appear in some formats.)

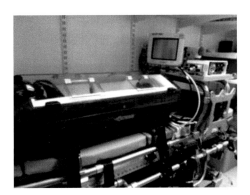

Figure 3.2 Baby pod secured to air stretcher. (A black and white version of this figure will appear in some formats.)

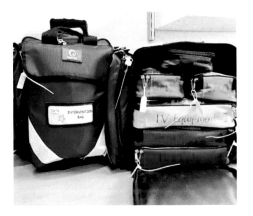

Figure 3.3 Flight bags with colour-coded grab sections. (A black and white version of this figure will appear in some formats.)

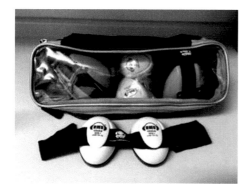

Figure 3.4 A selection of in-flight patient ear defenders. (A black and white version of this figure will appear in some formats.)

(a)

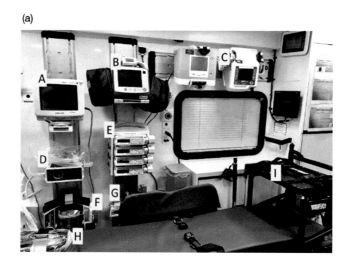

(b)

Equipment wall with electrical appliances safely secured and charging.

A Cardiac monitor
B Defibrillator
C Non invasive ventilators
D Ventilator
E Intravenous infusion pumps
F Suction
G Nitric oxide bracket
H Stretcher with leads
I Equipment bridge

Figure 4.1 (a) STRS bespoke ambulance interior; (b) Ambulance equipment wall checklist. (A black and white version of this figure will appear in some formats.)

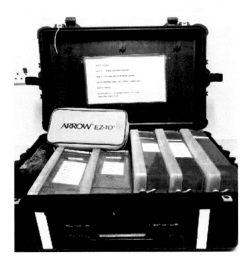

Figure 4.2 Ambulance kit box. (A black and white version of this figure will appear in some formats.)

(a)

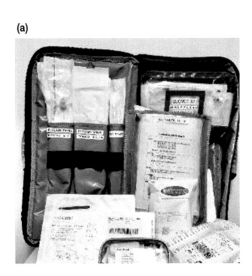

Figure 4.3 (a) Central venous access and chest drain kit. (b) Central venous access and chest drain box contents. (A black and white version of this figure will appear in some formats.)

(b)

Pleural catheters, straight soft radio-opaque
10Fr x 200mm, 12Fr x 250mm, 16Fr x 450mm
Portex seldinger chest drain 12Fr x 300mm; 18Fr
Heimlich drainage valve
Triple lumen CVP catheter set: 5Fr x 5cm, x 8cm, x 15cm
General procedure pack
Sterile gloves Size 6-8 x 2 each
Y connectors, straight connectors, luer lock connector
Straight mosquito forceps x 2
Surgical blade size 10, size 15
Sterile scissors, suture needle holder
Lignocaine
Biopatches
Silk sutures 2.0 x 2

Figure 4.3 (*cont.*)

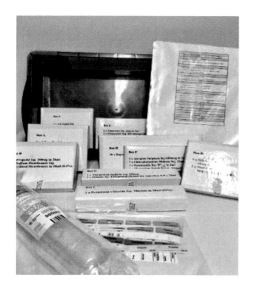

Figure 4.4 Nurse drug fridge pack and controlled drug box. (A black and white version of this figure will appear in some formats.)

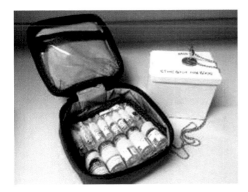

Figure 4.5 Nurse drug fridge pack and controlled drug box. (A black and white version of this figure will appear in some formats.)

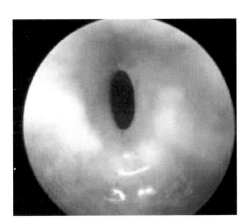

Figure 6.1 Tight grade 3 subglottic stenosis. (A black and white version of this figure will appear in some formats.)

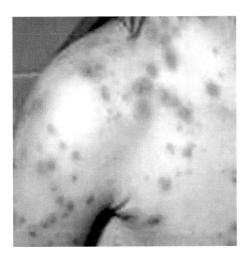

Figure 23.1 Initial presentation of rash. (A black and white version of this figure will appear in some formats.)

SEPSIS SCREENING TOOL TELEPHONE TRIAGE — UNDER 5

01 START CHART IF ANY OF THE FOLLOWING ARE REPORTED:
- ☐ Abnormal temperature
- ☐ Appears to be breathing more quickly or slowly than normal
- ☐ Altered mental state – include sleepy, irritable, drowsy or floppy
- ☐ Abnormally pale / bluish skin or abnormally cold hands or feet
- ☐ Reduced wet nappies or reduced urine output

RISK FACTORS FOR SEPSIS INCLUDE:
- ☐ Impaired immunity (e.g. diabetes, steroids, chemotherapy)   ☐ Indwelling lines / broken skin
- ☐ Recent trauma / surgery / invasive procedure

→ **NO** SEPSIS UNLIKELY, CONSIDER OTHER DIAGNOSIS

YES

02 COULD THIS BE DUE TO AN INFECTION?

LIKELY SOURCE: ☐ Brain   ☐ Surgical   ☐ Other
☐ Respiratory   ☐ Urine   ☐ Skin / joint / wound   ☐ Indwelling device

→ **NO** SEPSIS UNLIKELY, CONSIDER OTHER DIAGNOSIS

YES

03 ANY RED FLAG PRESENT?
- ☐ No response to social cues
- ☐ Doesn't wake when roused / won't stay awake
- ☐ Weak, high-pitched or continuous cry
- ☐ Grunting or bleating noises with every breath
- ☐ Finding it much harder to breathe than normal
- ☐ Very fast breathing / 'pauses' in breathing
- ☐ Skin that's very pale, mottled, ashen or blue
- ☐ Rash that doesn't fade when pressed firmly
- ☐ Temperature <36°C (check 3 times in 10 min)
- ☐ If under 3 months, temperature ≥ 38°C

YES → **RED FLAG SEPSIS START BUNDLE**

NO

04 ANY AMBER FLAG PRESENT?

IF IMMUNITY IMPAIRED TREAT AS RED FLAG SEPSIS
- ☐ Not responding normally / no smile
- ☐ Parental concern
- ☐ Wakes only with prolonged stimulation
- ☐ Significantly decreased activity
- ☐ Having to work hard to breathe
- ☐ Poor feeding in infants
- ☐ Reduced urine output
- ☐ Leg pain
- ☐ Cold feet or hands

YES → FURTHER INFORMATION AND REVIEW REQUIRED:
- ARRANGE URGENT FACE-TO FACE ASSESSMENT USING CLINICAL JUDGEMENT TO DETERMINE APPROPRIATE CLINICAL ENVIRONMENT

NO AMBER FLAGS : GIVE SAFETY-NETTING ADVICE:
CALL 111 IF CONDITION CHANGES OR DETERIORATES.
SIGNPOST TO AVAILABLE RESOURCES AS APPROPRIATE

CALL 999 IF ANY OF:
- Is breathing very fast
- Has a 'fit' or convulsion
- Looks mottled, bluish or pale
- Has a rash that does not fade when you press it
- Is very lethargic or difficult to wake
- Feels abnormally cold to touch

TELEPHONE TRIAGE BUNDLE:
THIS IS TIME-CRITICAL – IMMEDIATE ACTION REQUIRED: **DIAL 999**
AND ARRANGE BLUE LIGHT TRANSFER
COMMUNICATION: Ensure communication of 'Red Flag Sepsis' to crew
Advise crew to pre-alert as 'Red Flag Sepsis'

THE UK SEPSIS TRUST
UKST 2020 TT3.2 PAGE 1 OF 1

The controlled copy of this document is maintained by The UK Sepsis Trust. Any copies of this document held outside of that area, in whatever format (e.g. paper, email attachment) are considered to have passed out of control and should be checked for currency and validity.

The UK Sepsis Trust registered charity number (England & Wales) 1158843 (Scotland) SC050277. Company registration number 8644039. Sepsis Enterprises Ltd. company number 9583335. VAT reg. number 293133408.

Figure 24.1 Sepsis Trust. Acute Hospital Inpatients: Screening and Action Tool for Under 5s. Used with permission. Similar templates for alternative age bands are also available. (A black and white version of this figure will appear in some formats.)

SEPSIS SCREENING TOOL – THE PAEDIATRIC SEPSIS SIX

UNDER 5

PATIENT DETAILS:

DATE:
NAME:
DESIGNATION:
SIGNATURE:

TIME:

COMPLETE ALL ACTIONS WITHIN ONE HOUR

01 ENSURE SENIOR CLINICIAN ATTENDS
NOT ALL PATIENTS WITH RED FLAGS WILL NEED THE 'SEPSIS 6' URGENTLY. A SENIOR DECISION MAKER MAY SEEK ALTERNATIVE DIAGNOSES / DE-ESCALATE CARE. RECORD DECISIONS BELOW
NAME: GRADE:

TIME

02 OXYGEN IF REQUIRED
START IF O₂ SATURATIONS LESS THAN 92% OR EVIDENCE OF SHOCK

TIME

03 OBTAIN IV / IO ACCESS, TAKE BLOODS
BLOOD CULTURES, BLOOD GLUCOSE, LACTATE, FBC, U&Es, CRP AND CLOTTING, LUMBAR PUNCTURE IF INDICATED

TIME

04 GIVE IV / IO ANTIBIOTICS
MAXIMUM DOSE BROAD SPECTRUM THERAPY
CONSIDER: LOCAL POLICY / ALLERGY STATUS / ANTIVIRALS

TIME

05 CONSIDER IV / IO FLUIDS
IF LACTATE IS ABOVE 2 mmol/L GIVE FLUID BOLUS 20 mL/kg WITHOUT DELAY
IF LACTATE >4 mmol/L CALL PICU. (10ml/kg neonates, REPEAT IF REQUIRED)

TIME

06 CONSIDER INOTROPIC SUPPORT
CONSIDER INOTROPIC SUPPORT IF NORMAL PHYSIOLOGY IS NOT RESTORED AFTER ≥20 mL/kg FLUID (10 mL/kg IN NEONATES), CALL PICU OR A REGIONAL CENTRE URGENTLY

TIME

RED FLAGS AFTER ONE HOUR – ESCALATE TO CONSULTANT NOW

RECORD ADDITIONAL NOTES HERE:
e.g. allergy status, arrival of specialist teams, de-escalation of care, delayed antimicrobial decision making, variance from Sepsis Six

SEPSIS TRUST

UKST 2020 1.3 PAGE 2 OF 2 / UKST. REGISTERED CHARITY 1158843

Figure 24.1 *(Cont.)*

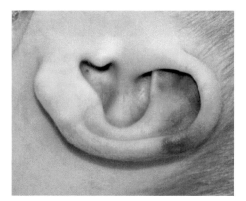

Figure 43.2 Bruising around pinna. (A black and white version of this figure will appear in some formats.)

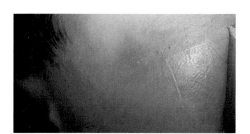

Figure 43.3 Bruising around face. (A black and white version of this figure will appear in some formats.)

Another important and often overlooked contributor to difficulty with ventilation is tube size. This baby had a 3.0 microcuff tube, which is equivalent to a 3.5 uncuffed tube. The difference in resistance between the tubes is based on Poiseuille's equation which describes the relationship between flow, resistance and pressure. Where all other parameters are equal, the resistance to flow is inversely proportional to the radius of the tube to the power of 4 so in this case the difference between $1/3^4$ versus $1/3.5^4$. This means that the resistance to breathing or ventilation is almost twice as difficult with just 0.5mm difference in ETT size, so it is worth considering whether to upsize the ETT, with the weighted risk balance that you will lose the benefits of the cuff, which is reducing the leak and loss of airway pressure at high settings.

2. Should this baby be transferred for extracorporeal membrane oxygenation (ECMO)?

If a patient fails to improve with optimal ventilator management then ECMO should be considered unless the cause of respiratory failure is irreversible. ECMO does not treat the underlying pathology but allows time for the patient to be treated and the lungs to recover without additional VILI.

Indications for a respiratory ECMO are:

a. Oxygenation index (OI) >30–35 on optimal treatment for 4 hours
b. OI >25 on nitric oxide
c. OI >25 with pneumonia, air leak or ARDS (assuming no right to left shunt)
d. Acute hypoxic decompensation unresponsive to any intervention
e. Progressive respiratory failure or pulmonary hypertension with evidence of ventricular dysfunction
f. Pressor resistant hypotension
g. Arterial CO_2 >12kPa for more than 3 hours.

3. Is there anything in the history to exclude this child from ECMO?

Current exclusion criteria for ECMO are:

a. <34 weeks gestation or <2 kg
b. Irreversible cardiopulmonary disease, including pulmonary hypertension in chronic lung disease
c. Lethal congenital abnormalities (including trisomy 13 and 18, but not 21) or other lethal anomaly
d. Established multiorgan dysfunction
e. Uncontrolled bleeding, grade 3/4 intraventricular haemorrhage
f. Mechanical ventilation >14 days
g. Proven necrotising enterocolitis (not absolute)
h. Poor prognosis even with ECMO support (e.g. congenital diaphragmatic hernia never reaching sats >85% and pCO_2 <9kPa).

Increasingly these longstanding exclusion criteria are becoming less absolute. It has recently been shown that paediatric patients with chronic lung disease and pulmonary hypertension do benefit from ECMO if they have pneumonia and adult ECMO services have

Table 26.1. Survival for most common diagnoses requiring respiratory ECMO

Neonatal (up to 28 days old)	Paediatric (29 days to 17 years old)
Meconium aspiration syndrome (MAS) 93%	Asthma 88%
Persistent pulmonary hypertension of newborn 74%	Bronchiolitis 78%
Congenital diaphragmatic hernia (CDH) 50%	Bacterial pneumonia 67%
	Acute respiratory failure 60%
	Pertussis 32%

Table 26.2. Survival for most common diagnoses requiring cardiac ECMO

Neonatal (up to 28 days old)	Paediatric(29 days to 17 years old)
Cardiomyopathy 59%	Myocarditis 76%
Myocarditis 50%	Cardiomyopathy 65%
Congenital heart disease 44%	Cardiogenic shock 61%
Cardiac arrest 41%	Congenital heart disease 54%
Cardiogenic shock 39%	Cardiac arrest 45%

demonstrated that adults with life-threatening bleeding can be placed on ECMO by running the circuits without anticoagulation.

Neonatal diseases requiring respiratory ECMO mostly reflect conditions exclusive to neonates whereas paediatric aetiologies are seen in a small percentage of patients with common diseases (generally infectious) and a progressively worsening picture. On the contrary, cardiac pathologies requiring ECMO are broadly similar across ages but survival rates are better outside the neonatal period. Tables 26.1 and 26.2 show survival rates of both populations and pathologies.

Early transfer to an ECMO centre is better than delaying referral, which potentially leads to further deterioration, making the transfer more difficult or even impossible. Additionally acidosis, end organ injury or cardiac arrest that may arise with delayed referrals increases the risk of neurological complications and death, even if the patient recovers from their initial illness and ECMO as a procedure is 'successful'. Finally, delaying referrals with respiratory disease often leads to cardiovascular compromise because of significant cardiopulmonary interactions associated with worsening lung compliance and greater ventilatory requirements. This results in ECMO centres placing children on veno-arterial (VA) ECMO rather than veno-venous (VV) ECMO. VA ECMO carries a much higher risk and complication profile (see Figure 26.3).

4. The decision was made to transfer the child to the ECMO centre. What investigations and management should be completed prior to transfer?

There should be as little delay as possible when transferring a critically ill child for ECMO due to expected further deterioration. There are certain investigations, however, that need

---

MODALITY OF ECMO

Blood is diverted from the venous system, typically via a cannula in the right atrium, to the ECMO circuit and then returned back to the patient.

Depending on the main goal of therapy we will have:

VENOARTERIAL (VA) ECMO	**VENOVENOUS (W) ECMO**
Return cannula in the arterial side	Return cannula in the venous side
Provides full cardiorespiratory support Preferred modality for cardiovascular diseases	Provides oxygenation and ventilation Preferred modality for respiratory diseases

The access cannula is connected to a pump which sucks blood from the patient and pushes it through an oxygenator, adding oxygen and removing carbon dioxide, before being pushed back to the patient. Patients are anticoagulated (usually with heparin) to prevent thrombosis but this increases the risk of bleeding. The risk of thrombo-ischaemic events is higher on VA ECMO as the emboli can go directly to the brain, whereas on W ECMO they will be directed to the pulmonary vascular bed.

Figure 26.3 Modality of ECMO.

to be completed to ensure there are no current, patient specific contraindications to ECMO and also those needed for transfer/ECMO itself:

1. Echocardiography (echo): Helpful to exclude a cardiac cause of hypoxia and quantify any intracardiac right to left shunt bypassing the lungs and causing desaturation.
2. Cranial ultrasound (CrUSS). In a neonate grade 3–4 intraventricular haemorrhage is a contraindication to ECMO. Findings should be re-discussed with the ECMO centre.
3. Full neurology evaluation is recommended. Major pathology (e.g. seizures or dilated pupils) should be identified.
4. Central venous access. A patient who comes from a PICU setting 'is likely to already have central access; if not, ask the local team to arrange for it but trying to avoid the right side of the neck, which will be necessary for the ECMO cannulation. Although central access is useful, practitioners should not become task-fixated and if it is challenging then it may be better to transfer the patient without ideal access or monitoring.

Transfer of patients requiring ECMO may require the team to tolerate hypoxia, hypercarbia or hypotension that would not be usual for transporting a patient. A risk assessment by a senior clinician must be performed and if mobile ECMO is possible then this may be undertaken. With mobile ECMO, the entire ECMO team comes to the patient and places them on ECMO in the local hospital prior to transfer.

It is also important to note this patient was proned and on HFOV, which is not suitable for transport. After de-proning, a degree of desaturation would be expected and converting to conventional ventilation may prove difficult. Manual bagging with enough pressure to move the chest may be required back to base.

It is important to ensure the patient has been cross-matched for transfusion. If a transfusion is not already in progress, procedures are usually in place to enable blood to be transported on transfer. Local guidelines should be developed. A standard procedure is as follows.

Dispatching hospital:

- Complete a transfer document.
- Place the blood in an appropriate transport box.
- Place all the appropriate documentation in the transport box, retaining a copy of the transfer document.
- Transport box should be sealed (e.g. cable tie).
- Laboratory should telephone the transfusion laboratory of the receiving hospital to confirm dispatch and fax them the transfer document.
- Receiving hospital:
- The blood in the transport box should be sent to the transfusion laboratory as soon as it arrives.
- Transfusion laboratory staff should check the integrity of the transport box, complete the transfer documentation and check the blood is still under correct storage conditions.
- Blood samples must be taken from the patient immediately and sent to the blood transfusion laboratory for testing.
- The laboratory staff must inform the dispatching transfusion laboratory of the fate of the units and return the transit box.

This child was successfully transferred and started on VV ECMO. At the time of cannulation she weighed only 2.1 kg. The course was uneventful. CT head during the ECMO run was normal and after 13 days the patient was successfully decannulated. After a further 12 days the patient was extubated and discharged from PICU 3 days later. She is now well and thriving.

In conclusion, this case highlights:

- The importance of recognising severe ARDS.
- Early referral and transfer for ECMO improves survival and reduces risk of neurological complications.
- Discuss with the ECMO centre about the eligibility of the patient.
- Echo, CrUSS and neurologic investigations need to be done by the referring centre.
- Try to avoid right side of neck for central access.
- With the correct procedure, it is possible to transport the patient's blood from another institution.

Further Reading

Ferreira Cruz F, Ball L, Macedo Rocco PR, et al. Ventilator-induced lung injury during controlled ventilation in patients with acute respiratory distress syndrome: less is probably better. *Expert Rev Respir Med* 2018;;12(5):403–14.

Griffiths MJD, McAuley DF, Perkins GD, et al. Guidelines on the management of acute respiratory distress syndrome. *BMJ Open Respir Res* 2019;6(1):e000420.

Khemani RG, Smith L, Lopez-Fernandez YM, et al. Paediatric acute respiratory distress syndrome incidence and epidemiology

(PARDIE): an international, observational study. *Lancet Respir Med.* 2019;7(2):115–28.

Lillie J, Boot L, Speggiorin S, et al. Factors behind decline of venovenous extracorporeal membrane oxygenation to support neonatal respiratory failure. *Pediatr Crit Care Med* 2020;21(8):e502–4.

Pediatric Acute Lung Injury Consensus Conference Group. Pediatric acute respiratory distress syndrome: consensus recommendations from the Pediatric Acute Lung Injury Consensus Conference. *Pediatr Crit Care Med* 2015;16(5):428–39.

ELSO Guidelines for Neonatal Respiratory Failure 2017. www.elso.org/Portals/0/ ELSOGuidelinesNeonatal RespiratoryFailurev1_4.pdf

Guidance for the emergency transfer of blood and components with patients between hospitals (NHSBT Appropriate use of blood group & National laboratory managers' group of the national blood transfusion committee); www.transfusionguidelines.org/ document-library/documents/transfer-of-blood-appendices-eoe-rtc-v3c-doc/ download-file/Transfer%20of%20Blood% 20Appendices%20EoE%20RTC%20%20V3C .doc.

Cardiac Arrest

Abi Whitehouse and Jon Lillie

A 3-year-old boy with known significant cardiomyopathy presented to his local A&E with a 2-day history of cough and coryza. He had been brought in due to parental concern regarding a reduction in oral intake and lethargy. The referring team described him as being irritable and inconsolable, disorientated but talking. His chest was clear but he had mildly increased work of breathing. Abdominal examination revealed a large liver. The CXR unsurprisingly, showed significant cardiomegaly.

The local team reported that his latest echo showed dilated cardiomyopathy with poor function and he was on lisinopril, digoxin and aspirin usually at home.

The referral and transfer was accepted and the retrieval team headed out to the local hospital to retrieve the child.

On arrival of the retrieval team, the child was asking for water, had mild subcostal recession, saturations were 100% in air and the chest sounded clear. His heart rate was 130bpm, his capillary refill was prolonged at 4–5 seconds peripherally and peripheral pulses were just palpable. He had an audible gallop, significant hepatomegaly and the cardiac apex beat was displaced laterally. Blood sugar was <3mmol/L so the retrieval team increased the maintenance IV fluid infusion rate. While the retrieval team were examining the child, he became agitated, breathless and desaturated to 88% with bilateral crepitations on auscultation. An oxygen facemask was applied, at which point he stopped breathing and had a cardiac arrest.

Questions

1. As the retrieval team, what factors would you consider in team leadership?
2. What would be your approach to ensuring excellent CPR?
3. What are your thoughts about the cause of the cardiac arrest?
4. When would you stop resuscitation?

1. As the retrieval team, what factors would you consider in team leadership?

The retrieval medical lead usually assumes the role of leadership in a cardiac arrest as they are often the most experienced team member in managing paediatric cardiac arrest, which is a rare event. This needs to be a carefully considered decision and it may not always be preferable. In some situations, the local hospital senior nurse or doctor should take on this role, for a number of reasons:

- A local hospital lead is likely to know the patient's previous investigations and management so can start treating potential causes of the cardiac arrest without handover.
- The local hospital lead is likely to know the members of the hospital team best to direct the team during CPR, allocating appropriate tasks.
- The retrieval team may need to perform immediate tasks such as intubation or central access so would be better placed to focus on these (avoid task fixation as team leader).

There is no way to be prescriptive about who should lead every cardiac arrest but consideration of the above factors should take place and brief discussion should occur between team members on who should lead the resuscitation. This may need to change if the team leader is required to perform a task (procedure or talk to family). Crucial to success is that everyone in the team must know who the leader is either by announcement or visual cues (e.g. standing at the end of the bed and not involving themselves in other tasks).

2. What would be your approach to ensuring excellent CPR?

This child has had a cardiorespiratory arrest and should be managed according to the appropriate APLS algorithm.

If not already done, a cardiac arrest call should be put out to ensure appropriate team members are present. If possible, early in the arrest, it is important to quickly familiarise the team with each other and with available personal resources and expertise and to clarify in what role can each team member function at the highest level. Basic universal and national recommendations regarding basic and advanced life support in children should be followed; however, there are some extra points which should be emphasised.

Carbon dioxide trace on intubation or even on mask ventilation, a CO_2 wave form should be seen with chest compressions during cardiac arrest. Basic and advanced life support courses have previously stated that a CO_2 trace is not always seen in cardiac arrest; however, an attenuated reduced rectangular wave form should be seen if the patient is receiving adequate ventilatory breaths and the cardiac compressions are adequate to provide some pulmonary blood flow. If there is no CO_2 trace with chest compressions, then it should be assumed that the endotracheal tube (ETT) is in the wrong place.

The CO_2 trace can also be used to monitor the effectiveness of CPR. If chest compressions or intravascular volume status improve in quality, then more blood is delivered to the lungs which increases the height of the trace. Conversely, after return of circulation, if the CO_2 trace decreases acutely then this is a sign of reduced blood flow to the lungs and ensuing cardiac arrest.

Chest compression effectiveness should be continually monitored via:

- Feeling for the pulse. A pulse should always be palpable during CPR if chest compressions are adequate.
- Saturation trace is usually present, though not numerically accurate, if CPR is effective.
- Arterial line. Although placing an arterial line should not be the focus after a cardiac arrest. If there is one in situ then this can be used to monitor effectiveness of CPR and other resuscitation measures.
- Defibrillator pad accelerometer feedback. Some modern defibrillator pads, for older children, have built in feedback sensors to help improve the rate, depth, recoil and consistency of compressions in paediatric manikin testing.

Other measures to improve chest compression effectiveness include: using steps for shorter team members, using backboards if the bed is soft and rotating team members delivering CPR at each pulse check to prevent tiring.

The child is intubated, requiring suctioning due to large amounts of pink frothy sputum. A venous gas is taken from a cannula and identifies the following:

pH <6.8, pCO_2 7 kPa, pO_2 3 kPa, HCO_3 8 mmol/L, BE −22 mEq/L, Na 130mmol/L, K+ 6.3 mmol/L, Ca 1.0 mmol/L, Hb 90g/L, glucose 5 mmol/L, lactate 14 mmol/L.

3. What are your thoughts about the cause for the cardiac arrest?

The moniker, 'Four Hs and Ts' is useful to ensure that reversible causes of a cardiac arrest are considered and then addressed.

Hypoxia

This is the commonest cause of paediatric cardiac arrest. The rhythm is often pulseless electrical activity (PEA) before asystole.

In this case the patient has severe chronic cardiac impairment that is not likely to be reversible, but their deterioration and cardiac arrest is likely to have been exacerbated by fluid overload, pulmonary oedema and then hypoxia. Intubation with a cuffed ETT, 100% oxygen and a positive end-expiratory pressure of $10–14cmH_20$ would all be recommended.

In other cases, hypoxia may be resolved by simple bag mask ventilation. If, however, the patient had life-threatening asthma with poor compliance and mucus plugs, an ETT, high peak inspiratory pressure ventilation and suctioning may be the key steps necessary to reverse the hypoxia.

Hypovolaemia

This is the second commonest cause for cardiac arrest in children; however; in this child there is nothing to suggest hypovolaemia. The cause for the lower haemoglobin of 90g/L is likely to be due to chronic illness and haemodilution. Additional volume may be detrimental with exacerbation of fluid overload. There is enough evidence with pulmonary oedema, hepatomegaly and the history to avoid giving further fluid and if return of spontaneous circulation (ROSC) is achieved then it would be acceptable to give IV diuretic to try and offload the heart.

Although the primary pathology may not cause hypovolaemia, critically ill children may have suffered a cardiac arrest due to reduced preload which can be caused by increased thoracic pressure, sedation, muscle paralysis or induction of anaesthesia. Small volumes of fluid may improve the situation in these cases. However, if the cause for the cardiac arrest is true hypovolaemia then this group will often need far greater volumes of fluid resuscitation, or blood products if massive haemorrhage is suspected. A child with refractory shock due to Addisonian crisis required 100 ml/kg fluid during CPR, before ROSC was gained.

Hyper/hypokalaemia

The potassium is raised at 6.3 mmol/L but at this level, it is unlikely to have caused the cardiac arrest. Hyperkalaemia is commonly seen during cardiac arrest because potassium becomes extracellular in severe acidosis. A bolus of calcium gluconate to protect the myocardium would be advised but no other management would be required for this.

If serum potassium is >6.5 mmol/L then patients are at risk of cardiac arrest, most likely to be ventricular fibrillation. Patients would usually have a known history or condition that places them at risk of hyperkalaemia, for example, severe renal dysfunction, rhabdomyolysis or tumour lysis syndrome. For management of hyperkalaemia in a cardiac arrest, a calcium bolus can be given followed by an insulin bolus with dextrose, continuing with an insulin–dextrose infusion if necessary. An adrenaline infusion also achieves similar potassium lowering results to insulin–dextrose and may be appropriate in the setting of cardiac arrest with poor cardiac function. Cardiac arrest due to hypokalaemia is much rarer and typically only occurs if K+ is <2mmol/l. IV potassium bolus is required in this situation with frequent re-evaluation of potassium level response.

Hypothermia

There is normally a clear history suggestive of hypothermia, such as submersion in cold water, near drowning or extreme events. The cardiac muscle typically goes into ventricular fibrillation although any rhythm is possible. In profound hypothermia, resuscitation efforts will be futile until the patient is rewarmed>32°C. In this case, aggressive rewarming is indicated which includes multiple different methods:

- Warm IV fluids (38–40°C)
- Heated humidified ventilator gases
- Radiant heaters/warming blanket
- Intravascular temperature control devices, including extracorporeal membrane oxygenation (ECMO), if available
- Bladder irrigation with warm fluids.

Tamponade

Although unlikely, as there is cardiomegaly on CXR –it would be useful to exclude this with an ultrasound. All A&E staff are now trained in point-of-care ultrasound and this training is sufficient to exclude tamponade.

Tamponade should be considered if the patient has had recent cardiac surgery, has an intravascular line in situ where the tip is intra-cardiac (e.g. peripherally inserted central catheter or Hickmann line), cardiomegaly on CXR or has an inflammatory or infective condition that could cause a serositis. Drainage of tamponade should be done by pericardiocentesis or surgical pericardial window.

Thrombosis

Although unlikely in children, if there is an underlying condition which increases the risk of thrombosis or the patient has cardiac defects which increase the risk of stasis, then this should be considered. Post-cardiac surgery, in which an artificial shunt has been placed (e.g. hypoplastic left heart syndrome with gortex shunt), thrombosis in the shunt is immediately life-threatening and should be considered. Cardiology and cardiothorac surgery should be urgently contacted. A heparin bolus is often given in these circumstances to prevent clot propagation but tissue plasminogen activator, which dissolves clots, is not indicated unless there is ROSC.

Tension Pneumothorax

Clinical examination, ultrasound or X-ray may all demonstrate evidence of a pneumothorax. If identified during a cardiac arrest then it should be considered a tension pneumothorax and immediately drained either via thoracostomy (as per trauma) or needle thoracocentesis in the mid-clavicular line, second intercostal space. In practice, a thoracostomy is usually better in a cardiac arrest situation as the needle in the mid-clavicular line becomes dislodged during chest compressions.

Toxins

It may be difficult to determine this but VT or VF in children with no cardiac history should alert the team to consider drugs. Tricyclic antidepressant overdose can cause VF and additional treatment would include giving sodium bicarbonate boluses.

In summary, the 'Four Hs and Ts' are well known but it is important to actively exclude and aggressively treat them if found. Always remember more than one may be present in a child, and all must be treated, (e.g. the child who arrests due to another pathology but becomes hypothermic due to being outside.

After 20 minutes despite effective CPR with good CO_2 trace and oxygenation on the sats trace there is still no return of circulation. The patient remains in PEA.

4. When would you stop resuscitation?

After 20 minutes of cardiac arrest without return of circulation, the patient is most likely to die and if they do survive, the likelihood of significant neurological insult is very high. This cut off of 20 minutes has been used to suggest a point when resuscitation should be stopped for a paediatric population suffering cardiac arrest.

For the individual patient, it may be appropriate to continue resuscitation for longer if remedial measures are still being instituted (or stop earlier than this if the prognosis of their condition is very poor). If the cardiac arrest occurs in hospital, the chance of survival to discharge from hospital is 27%, with 18% having a good neurological outcome if the patient has been receiving CPR for 10 minutes or less. The prognosis can be improved, by offering ECMO from CPR, to 40% and 27% respectively However, even for this modest improvement to be possible, the patient must be in a hospital that offers paediatric ECMO from cardiac arrest and have ECMO instituted rapidly. This is a tiny minority of hospitals in the UK and across the world.

Once the team agree the decision should be made to stop resuscitation, the family should be told that this will be done and supported through this. We would advise the family should be present throughout the resuscitation to appreciate the efforts that have been made to restart the heart. The family should be encouraged to have contact with the child including holding them or their hand. A senior member of the team should explain what has happened and what will now happen.

It is usually advised that all tubes should be left in place as paediatric deaths may often be investigated by the coroner. However, the ETT may be removed to allow the family to see the face if the cardiac arrest occurred before the ETT was placed (i.e. the tube being dislodged cannot be the cause of death) and there was evidence it was in place ($ETCO_2$ or X-ray).

A hot debrief should be performed immediately after the death, in a space away from the patient, with as many members of the team as can stay. This allows for frank discussion and to start to address any concerns or ideas that the team have. It also allows for reflection. If possible a further cold debrief should happen at a later date when emotions have settled. The retrieval team will stay if possible, but they may need to leave if they are needed elsewhere.

Further Reading

Cook TM, Harrop-Griffiths AW, Whitaker DK, et al.. The 'No Trace=Wrong place' campaign. *Br J Anaesth* 2019;122:e68–9.

Lasa JJ, Rogers RS, Localio R, et al. Extracorporeal cardiopulmonary resuscitation (E-CPR) during pediatric in-hospital cardiopulmonary arrest is associated with improved survival to discharge: A report from the American Heart Association's Get With The Guidelines-Resuscitation (GWTG-R) Registry. *Circulation* 2016;133(2):165–76.

A Neurosurgical Emergency

Livia Procopiuc and Alison Pienaar

You have received a call from the paediatric registrar at one of the district general hospitals in the region. A 2-year-old, 11 kg boy was brought in by ambulance 1 hour ago after suffering his first episode of generalised tonic-clonic seizures at home.

The seizures had terminated after administration of 0.5mg/kg buccal midazolam by the paramedic team. The total duration of the seizure was 15 minutes. At the time of the call, the child was maintaining his own airway, displaying no work of breathing, had a respiratory rate of 18 breaths per minute and saturations >95% with a non-rebreather mask. His heart rate was 82 bpm and his blood pressure was 110/64 mmHg. He felt warm and well perfused on examination with a capillary refill time less than 3 seconds, both centrally and peripherally. His temperature was 37.7°C, and he was drowsy but rousable to voice. He had been complaining of diffuse abdominal pain but was not tender nor peritonitic on examination. He had one wet nappy in the ambulance, which was changed after arrival at A&E. A capillary blood gas performed on arrival to A&E showed a mild respiratory acidosis but otherwise normal lactate and glucose levels. A full blood count, biochemistry and CRP had been taken but the results were still outstanding at the time of the call.

In the background medical history, the registrar reported that the child was born prematurely at 29 weeks gestation and had a ventriculo-peritoneal (VP) shunt placed as a neonate for post-haemorrhagic hydrocephalus. He was fed by percutaneous endoscopic gastrostomy (PEG), with significant gastro-oesophageal reflux disease and developmental delay. His mother reported that he had been well until this morning's seizure and had seemed himself.

Questions

1. How would you assess this referral and what investigation and management advice would you give?
2. What are the particular risks of transferring this child?
3. Who needs to perform this transfer? How should it be coordinated?

1. How would you assess this referral and what investigation and management advice would you give?

As always with referrals to a paediatric retrieval service, you need to ask yourself whether the referrer is describing an emergency.

This child is encephalopathic. This may be post ictal but other causes need to be considered especially as this is a new onset seizure.

In any encephalopathic child, the level of the coma may constitute an emergency in itself; however, the potentially rapidly deteriorating emergency would be the concurrent presence of raised intracranial pressure (RICP), and this must be positively excluded in a child who is not normally conscious with a Glasgow Coma Score (GCS) of <15.

This child is encephalopathic (drowsy, rousable to voice=GCS 14, AVPU= V) and has a relative bradycardia and mildly elevated blood pressure in the presence of a VP shunt, with new onset seizures. A malfunctioning VP shunt with or without associated infection and RICP has to be excluded by pre-emptive treatment and urgent CT brain scan.

If confirmed this would warrant urgent transfer to a neurosurgical centre.

With increasing survival of premature neonates, VP shunts inserted for post-haemorrhagic hydrocephalus or neonatal meningitis are not uncommon, and it is important to have a basic understanding of the 'anatomy' of these shunts in order to know how to assess their well-being.

The shunt consists of three parts:

1. The proximal catheter has its tip in the lateral ventricle and exits the skull via a burr hole and continues subcutaneously.
2. A reservoir and valve complex are placed subcutaneously and are palpable on the child's head, usually just behind one of the ears. The valve ensures unidirectional flow and may be adjustable.
3. A distal catheter is tunnelled from the valve onwards, and opens into the peritoneal cavity. This is the long section of the catheter and the portion that usually becomes blocked. Some shunts may end in the pleural cavity (or one of the atria); however, these types are uncommon.

Like all artificially implanted devices, VP shunts are not without the risk of complications with the most common problems being obstruction/blockage and infection.

In both settings the child would present with neurologic symptoms including encephalopathy, seizures and signs of RICP Table 28.1. In the setting of an infected shunt (which is likely blocked) the clinical cardiovascular signs of RICP with relative bradycardia and hypertension may be completely counterbalanced by the septic manifestations of tachycardia and hypotension to produce completely normal heart rate and blood pressure in an unconscious child with a high white cell count and CRP. In children with infected shunts there may be, in addition, abdominal signs associated with peritonitis.

Table 28.1.

In infants and young children	In older children and adolescents
• Tense anterior fontanelle	• Diplopia
• Dilated scalp veins	• Impaired upward gaze
• 'Setting sun' sign	• CN VI palsy
• Irritability	• Headache
• Impaired level of consciousness	• Vomiting
• Vomiting	• Drowsiness or impaired consciousness and coma
• Bradycardia	• Worsened seizure control
• Apnoeic spells	
• Seizures	
• Increasing head circumference	

In this child it would be important to give emergency advice for the management of RICP and then try to establish whether the shunt is blocked and or infected.

Emergency advice for RICP should be structured and succinct:

A: An anaesthetist should be called urgently to attend to manage the airway especially as the level of consciousness falls.

B: Breathing and CO_2 clearance should be supported (by anaesthetic circuit with positive end-expiratory pressure /ventilation) where the respiratory rate is falling due to encephalopathy.

C: Cerebral perfusion pressure must be maintained, assuming the ICP is elevated and over 20 mmHg. The quickest and easiest way to do this, while also actively reducing ICP by osmotherapy, is to administer 3–5 ml/kg of hypertonic saline. Many children's level of consciousness or pupillary reactions will improve in response to this.

D: Seizures must be actively managed and predisposing factors like hyponatraemia, hypoglycaemia and fever all treated.

For CT scan to be performed safely in a child with suspected RICP, the child should be intubated after these initial measures have been instituted.

The shunt can be evaluated by:

- **CT scan**: The newly performed CT should be evaluated with the previous CT to compare ventricular enlargement, and periventricular CSF collections possibly indicating increased ICP.

- **Shunt series (X-rays)**: This consists of a series of antero-posterior and lateral plain X-rays of the skull, chest and abdomen. They may be best performed in a neurosurgical centre and are aimed at detecting catheter disconnections or fractures.

- **Abdominal ultrasound:** If time allows and the child is not clinically unstable, an abdominal ultrasound may be useful, particularly where the patient has associated abdominal symptoms. As the child grows, the intraperitoneal end of the VP shunt can migrate thus leading to catheter blockage. Pseudocysts may form around the end of the catheter which could represent a focus for infection and warrant intervention. The PEG itself may also be associated with complications.

2. What are the particular risks of transferring this child?

In the setting of raised ICP, children may present with Cushing's triad (bradycardia, hypertension and decreased respiratory drive). The relative hypertension and bradycardia might lead to underestimation of the degree of sepsis or septic shock associated with a potential shunt infection, or the underestimation of the severity of the intracranial hypertension. This consideration is especially important when preparing to induce general anaesthesia in these children, and hence a structured assessment and management of these children is vitally important.

During stabilisation and transfer, standard neuroprotective measures should be ensured, with neuromonitoring including examination of the pupils every 15 minutes.

Post anaesthesia and for transfer, the eyelids should not be taped closed.

Common complications during transfer of an intubated, sedated and muscle-relaxed child with a blocked shunt include:

- Child waking up while muscle relaxed with tachycardia, hypertension and dilated responsive pupils

- Onset of seizures while muscle relaxed, identifiable by tachycardia, hypertension and dilated poorly responsive pupils
- Airway secretions mobilised by recurrent movement causing tube obstruction or coughing with rise in CO_2 and accompanying rise in ICP (bradycardia and hypertension)
- Sudden rise in ICP associated with emergency braking of ambulance with profound bradycardia, hypertension and pupillary signs
- Slower relentless rise in ICP to the point that it is unresponsive to hypocarbia induced by short-term hyperventilation, and unresponsive to osmotherapy (repeat boluses of hypertonic saline no longer effective).

Before transfer these scenarios must have been considered and plans made by the team to deal with all in turn.

In the event that the last mentioned becomes the main problem, the shunt reservoir may need to be tapped using a sterile non-touch technique, butterfly needle and syringe with three way tap after cleaning the area of skin over the reservoir.

This is usually undertaken only in extreme circumstances and usually in discussion with the neurosurgical centre; however, the forward journey to the neurosurgical centre must not be interrupted for the tap.

3. Who needs to perform this transfer? How should it be coordinated?

If RICP is suspected clinically or on scan then an urgent transfer should be organised, aiming to depart to the neurosurgical centre within an hour from the end of the CT scan.

This will usually mean the referring hospital will need to perform the transfer. This should be done by the most experienced team that can be assembled and will usually involve liaising with local anaesthetic or pre-hospital teams who have experience in patient transfer and will be able to assist.

It is useful to devise and follow a checklist that can speed up the process to facilitate rapid departure from the local hospital. The following procedure can aid a referring hospital in facilitating this. The retrieval team, although not undertaking the transfer should provide assistance and help co-ordinate the safe transfer to a secure bed or location at the accepting neurosurgical centre.

- Request urgent ambulance transfer by ringing 999 'urgent neurosurgical emergency transfer'
- Emergency airway and breathing equipment + portable suction, IV fluids, drugs and adequate O_2 supply
- Ensure patient and equipment are adequately secured to ambulance trolley
- Ensure smooth journey due to effects on haemodynamics and ICP
- Travel safe – seatbelt on at all times
- Transfer letter with photocopy of relevant notes, results, drugs charts, anaesthetic charts
- Send images across to receiving centre electronically or ensure a copy of all imaging follows the patient
- Document and highlight any safeguarding issues
- Keep parents up to date

- Phone receiving team with ETA and inform them if there are any changes in the patient's condition or you are concerned that the patient is deteriorating further.

Outcome

This child had a *Klebsiella* infected and blocked shunt. He was transferred safely by the local team with difficulties towards the end of the transfer with signs of rising ICP, unresponsive to hypertonic saline. The transferring clinicians did not know the shunt reservoir could be tapped. On arrival at the neurosurgical centre, the child had a heart rate of 42. He was received directly into neurosurgical theatre and the shunt was externalised urgently. Once the shunt infection had been adequately treated he had a new shunt placed and was discharged home 3 weeks later to his baseline health.

Further Reading

Al Holou WN, Wilson TJ, Ali ZS, et al. Gastrostomy tube placement increases the risk of ventriculoperitoneal shunt infection: a multiinstitutional study. *J Neurosurg* 2018;1:1–6.

Barnes NP, Jones, SJ, Hayward RD, et al. Ventriculoperitoneal shunt block: what are the predictive clinical indicators? *Arch Dis Child* 2002;87:198–201.

Chang JJ, Avellino AM. Shunt placement and management. In: Kumar M, Levine J, Schuster J, Kofke A. (eds) *Neurocritical Care Management of the Neurosurgical Patient*, Elsevier 2018:415–27.

Sivaganesan A, Krishnamurthy R, Sahni D, et al. Neuroimaging of ventriculoperitoneal shunt complications in children. *Pediatr Radiol* 2012;42:1029–46.

STRS Guideline: Time Critical Neurosurgical Transfer. www.evelinalondon.nhs.uk/ resources/our-services/hospital/south-thames-retrieval-service/neurosurgical-transfer-mar-2018.pdf.

STRS Guideline: Hypertonic Sodium Chloride. www.evelinalondon.nhs.uk/resources/our-services/hospital/south-thames-retrieval-service/Hypertonic-Saline-2017.pdf

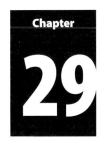

A Fall from Height

Caroline Smith, Sam Fosker and Shelley Riphagen

A 4-year-old child was brought into their local district general hospital in his mother's arms having fallen from a first storey window (around 5 metres in height), and rolled off the porch roof part of the way down. Mum was alerted to the fall by his 5-year-old sister, who was with him when he climbed on the dresser under the window and then fell out of the open window. Mum ran out the house to find the child prone outside the porch, crying and trying to get up on hands and knees. He had some bleeding from his forehead, face, nose and a little from the mouth. She picked him up, called the neighbour for help and took him immediately to the local A&E.

On arrival in the A&E, the child was crying and complaining that his arm hurt. He had multiple visible right-sided and central head and facial lacerations and grazes. At initial triage the observations were as noted in Table 29.1.

A full examination was performed in A&E; he was crying when examined but no longer answering questions. He was refusing to lie flat, preferring lying on his left side. He had several lacerations on the right side of his head and forehead and swelling with bruising down the whole right side of his face. He had fresh blood from his right nostril. There was a small amount of bruising and tenderness down his right chest wall, but his abdomen appeared non-tender. There was bilateral air entry with saturations over 98% with wafting facemask oxygen, as he would not tolerate the facemask. His right upper arm was visibly deformed and swollen, but his other limbs appeared intact. Initial blood tests were sent, seen in Table 29.2 after he had been intubated for CT scan, in view of the mechanism of injury.

CT scan was verbally reported as normal brain imaging with no intracranial or spinal injury, multiple right-sided facial fractures with no obvious damage to bone of the orbit or soft tissue of the eye; multiple right-sided rib fractures with no lung injury, liver laceration with some free fluid in the abdomen; fractured right humerus. The local team were awaiting the formal report, but had made the referral for retrieval of the child to a major trauma centre for ongoing care, as they felt the child was too complex to remain locally.

You have been asked to lead the retrieval of the child.

Questions

1. What advice would you give the local hospital around facial fractures and management of the child's airway?
2. How will you assess the child with regard to the multi-trauma he has sustained and what specific paediatric issues are you aware of in this setting?
3. On arrival the father is shouting at the mother about letting the child out of her sight. How would you approach this as the retrieval team?

Table 29.1.

Heart rate	132 bpm
Respiratory rate	30 breaths per minute
Sats	98% in wafting oxygen
Blood pressure	78/48 mmHg
Temperature	34.8°C
AVPU	A

Table 29.2.

Blood tests		Venous blood gas	
Haemoglobin	133 g/L	pH	7.33
White cell count	8.1 (10^3/mm^3)	pCO$_2$	5.8 kPa
Platelets	324 (10^3/mm^3)	pO$_2$	9.1 kPa
Na	132 mmol/L	Base excess	−2.8 mEq/L
K	4.1 mmol/L	Lactate	2.1 mmol/L
Urea	5.6 mmol/L	Glucose	7.8 mmol/L
Creatinine	36 U/L	HCO$_3^-$	23.4 mmol/L
CRP	<5		

1. What advice would you give the local hospital around facial fractures and management of the child's airway?

Facial fractures are rare in children and the energy transfer required to sustain this injury in childhood is considerable; however, falls are one of the most common causes. In view of the estimated energy transfer and mechanism of injury, it is important to remember that there are likely to be other related injuries (i.e. spine/neurological).

A decision should be made to ensure the safest option for airway management in this child. Although the child was maintaining his airway on admission, there was ongoing bleeding and multiple facial injuries with likely progressive soft tissue swelling over the next few hours. The neurological examination had changed from injury to admission with concerns regarding intracranial injury. In view of both these considerations, and in order to obtain a CT scan of good quality safely, intubation was the safest option. Likely transfer on to a higher level of trauma care could also be facilitated more safely with the child intubated and ventilated, to avoid the possibility of deteriorating airway access during transfer.

It must be remembered that intubation in this setting may be very challenging with unstable jaw, and ongoing bleeding limiting visualisation. A senior anaesthetist should be involved with the consideration of ENT support if available. A full external and internal airway assessment should be made including assessing eyes, facial bones, nose and dentition. A true paediatric maxillofacial emergency that is often missed is the 'white-eye blow out fracture'. Caused by a disruption in the orbital floor, the lack of soft tissue swelling and difficulty in diagnosing it on imaging lends to its 'white-eyed' name and can lead to an underappreciation of the severity of the injury. All transfer clinicians should consider this, as delay in treatment can result in permanent damage to the eye and surrounding structures. Add to this that the oculovagal reflex causes bradycardia, vomiting and headaches, and one can understand how this injury is missed or masked by the signs of a head injury. A thorough eye exam will usually reveal restriction in eye mobility and pain.

Displaced fractures of the mandible and mid-face fractures can cause profuse bleeding intranasally and intra-orally, making visualisation difficult. Mid-face fractures can also result in mobility of the maxilla if a Le Fort fracture is sustained. To combat both mobility of mid-face fractures and profuse bleeding, bite blocks can be used, providing both reduction and pressure simultaneously. To reduce open mandibular fractures quickly, bridle wire can be placed around teeth adjacent to each side of the fracture and wound tight, once again providing stability and haemostasis; although this will require expertise from an adult maxillofacial or trauma surgeon.

The type of mandibular fracture that is most likely to result in an airway issue is a bilateral parasymphyseal fracture. Due to the fact that this area is the point of origin for the mylohyoid, digastric, genius-hyoid and genioglossus muscles, loss of tongue muscle support and mobility of the symphyseal fragment can result. This can, in turn, see the posterior retraction of the tongue, blocking the oropharynx. This is particularly noticeable in a supine patient and often simply sitting the patient forward will clear the airway.

With bleeding ongoing, it is important to identify whether the bleeding site can be seen and if possible controlled. The soft tissues of the oral/nasal cavity may be concealing the bleeding point and when the child is induced this may increase, making the airway even more difficult. Difficult airway equipment, including video laryngoscopy if available, should be immediately accessible. Before commencing anaesthesia, there should be an agreed airway management plan if intubation is not possible.

Although distressing for the child and their family, it must be remembered facial trauma must be managed in an ABC manner before further evaluation by a maxillofacial team. Paediatric mortality is more likely from related airway or neurological sequelae. Once stable, facial fractures should have early assessment by a maxillofacial team due to the potential for serious ongoing functional and aesthetic issues.

To aid this, CT scans must be electronically transferred to the accepting trauma team prior to arrival. Management is generally more conservative in paediatric facial fractures, in order to limit the disturbance to future growth and development. Due to faster healing in children, early fixation and repair may be needed and therefore transfer should be performed as soon as safe.

Although the CT scan does not reveal any bony cervical fractures, the mechanism of injury does not exclude ligamentous injury and transfer should take this into consideration. The child's head and spine should be kept as stable and secure as possible. With an intubated child this can be easily accomplished with head blocks and tapes supporting the head and cervical spine in a neutral position. If not intubated due to less severe injury, the least restrictive option (i.e. towels/blocks to support the head) to obtain the best outcome should be used.

2. How will you assess the child in regard to the multi-trauma he has sustained and what specific paediatric issues are you aware of in this setting?

Much of trauma care in children is extrapolated from adult best practice due to the lack of specific trauma research within the paediatric population. There are, however, some specific considerations when dealing with a paediatric trauma patient that may alter your decisions when treating and transferring these patients.

All critically ill or injured patients should be assessed in a cABCDE manner, with the lower case 'c' (or sometimes 'X') referring to catastrophic haemorrhage. This is more pertinent in a pre-hospital or austere setting due to the immediate nature of treatment needed. Any life-threatening bleeding should be immediately treated with direct pressure, tourniquets or haemostatic dressings prior to airway assessment. If attempted haemostasis has happened in the pre-hospital setting, it is important to remain aware of the risk of clot dislodgement within a hospital and especially transfer setting during moving and handling. Tourniquets should only be removed if definitive care is available.

A: The airway assessment and challenges have been noted above.

B: Rib fractures, as seen in this child, are rare in paediatric patients and signify large transfer of force through the thorax. The likelihood of underlying lung injury is significant. In the presence of a large pneumo/haemothorax, the underlying lung injury may not always be obvious. This injury and resultant oedema may develop over the subsequent hours-to-days impacting gas exchange significantly. Additional to this, children are at much higher risk of cardiovascular collapse due to tension pneumothorax/ haemothorax due to their smaller intrathoracic and circulating blood volume. Any cardiovascular deterioration in a paediatric trauma patient, especially after application of positive pressure ventilation, should result in immediate assessment for tension pneumo/haemothorax.

C: Children presenting with shock after trauma have lost significant amounts of blood. Current advice is for 5 ml/kg boluses of crystalloid only if absolutely necessary (i.e. hypotensive with concern of end organ damage). Blood products should be administered as soon as possible. Although no specific studies on tranexamic acid in the paediatric population are currently available, its administration in a massive haemorrhage setting is thought beneficial. Resuscitation targets should be normalising heart rate and blood pressure at the lower limits of normal for age. In this child, specific attention should be paid to the presence of rib fractures and the liver laceration with free fluid in the abdomen. The risk of haemothorax and haemoperitoneum are significant, especially if attention is not paid to low pressure resuscitation targets. This must be balanced with probable significant head trauma, despite the CT being reported as normal.

D: A specific paediatric Glasgow Coma Score score for non-verbal children has been developed (see Table 29.3), where the assessment of V has been modified for younger children. The child's brain is growing rapidly, with little extra-axial space and much less room for intracranial swelling. This puts children at much higher risk of raised intracranial pressure from any intracranial injury. Spinal cord injury without

Table 29.3. Verbal component of modified Glasgow Coma Score in non-verbal children

	Paediatric response	Score
Best verbal response	Coos and babbles	5
	Irritable cries	4
	Cries to pain	3
	Moans to pain	2
	No response	1

radiological abnormality (SCIWORA) is well documented in a paediatric population and spinal protection should be considered as much a clinical diagnosis as a radiological one. As stated previously with the cervical spine, stabilisation can be difficult in the awake patient and a calm still child is much preferred to an agitated child, where restraint for purposes of spinal protection is attempted. In this child, although the CT scan has been reported as normal, children's head CTs often require review by a paediatric neuroradiologist as it may be difficult to differentiate base of skull fractures, when sutures are not yet fused. The mechanism of injury in this child and significant facial fractures, with blood from the nose should keep base of skull fracture as a significant concern until this can be positively excluded by a paediatric neuroradiologist. The impact of injury with the coup-contrecoup forces that would have been in play also put this child at high risk of cerebral contusion, and the CT brain may be too early or crude to pick this up. For optimal brain protection after trauma, as well as maintaining cerebral perfusion pressure, active temperature and glucose control must also be managed. The objective to maintain adequate cerebral perfusion pressure may be at odds with low pressure resuscitation, to prevent clot disruption.

3. On arrival the father is shouting at the mother about letting the child out of her sight. How would you approach this as the retrieval team?

Your first priority is the safety of the child and ensuring the child is adequately resuscitated and able to be safely transferred. Part of this trauma assessment requires taking a good history regarding mechanism of injury. In some cases with paediatric trauma, this may raise concerns regarding non-accidental injury or neglect. Communication with the family should be within your overall management of the situation and early engagement may help to defuse the situation. A critically ill or injured child is emotionally traumatic for families and will add significantly to the situational stress levels. This can often be worse in a trauma scenario as there may be perceived 'blame' around events. Unfortunately accidents do happen in children even with the best care by parents and caregivers; however, an open mind for the possibility of abuse or neglect should remain in the forefront of consciousness. If there is any professional doubt about the mechanism of injury or the history between parents or witnesses is not corroborated or consistent, then the concerns should be raised and reviewed with your child protection officers.

If parental conflict is detracting from the care of the child, then another professional may be able to deal with the situation while you continue stabilising. If no one else is available, it is essential to explain that the parental conflict is detracting from care and prohibiting stabilisation.

Any concerns raised regarding parental social interactions witnessed should be documented 'verbatim' and escalated through the right channels. Always remember other children within the household who may be at risk, as is the case in this scenario. If there are any concerns about their welfare an urgent referral to social care or relevant services can be made. When transferring the child, it is often possible to have one or more relatives accompany the child, especially as the child may need surgery relatively urgently. If you believe the accompanying parent may be disruptive, which is very rare, you may choose to have no relatives accompany you.

Outcome

This child was transferred to the regional paediatric major trauma centre intubated and ventilated. During transfer he became extremely cardiovascularly unstable. Two units of blood had been taken on the transfer in a blood cool box and were used for ongoing resuscitation.

During the repeat trauma assessment at the major trauma centre, the liver laceration was found to have bled significantly, with a large amount of intraperitoneal free fluid.

On review of the CT head, and subsequent MRI brain scan, he was found to have had an extensive base of skull fracture, with cribriform plate disruption, and accompanying significant cerebral oedema. This worsened over the next 2 days requiring repeated doses of hypertonic saline, and neuroprotective measures. The child was eventually discharged well from hospital after 11 days.

Further Reading

Aires CCG, Ramos LVS, De Figueiredo EL, et al. Airway obstruction after bilateral mandibular parasymphyseal fracture: A case report. *CraniofacTrauma Reconstr Open J* 2020 March.

Braun TL, Xue AS, Maricevich RS. Differences in the management of pediatric facial trauma. *Semin Plast Surg.* 2017; 31(2): 118–22.

Krausz AA, El-Naaj IA, Barak M. Maxillofacial trauma patients: coping with difficult airway. *World J Emerg Surg* 2009;27(4):21.

Mukherjee CG, Mukherjee U. Maxillofacial trauma in children. *Int J Clin Pediatr Dent.* 2012; 5(3): 231–6.

The Royal Children's Hospital Melbourne Paediatric Trauma Manual. Online. www.rch .org.au/trauma-service/manual.

Chapter 30

Brain against the Clock

Tanmay Toteja and Sam Fosker

An 8-month-old baby was brought to a district general hospital A&E with reported right-sided abnormal movements thought to be seizures. She had not been feeding well for the previous 2 days and seemed generally lethargic. The arm movements, described as jerking in the whole right arm, had been noticed by the parents for the first time that day. When the movements did not stop after a few minutes, they called an ambulance.

On arrival of the ambulance team she had been seizing for 20 minutes. She was given buccal midazolam but continued to seize en route to hospital. A dose of rectal diazepam was repeated 5 minutes later but the seizures continued.

After arrival in A&E, the jerking of the right arm initially progressed to involve the right leg and then to involve all four limbs.

Her observations were noted as follows: HR 180/min, sinus rhythm; RR 40/min; SpO$_2$ 86% in air; BP 90/60.

The paediatric resuscitation team were in attendance on arrival of the baby and sited an IV cannula, administered a phenytoin loading dose 20mg/kg and sent baseline laboratory blood tests and blood gas.

The limb twitching continued despite the phenytoin and she began having apnoeic episodes and desaturating into the 70s. Due to this and the continuing seizures the anaesthetic team decided to intubate her. This was done without issue. She was given a dose of ceftriaxone 80mg/kg and CT head was arranged in view of the focal nature and new onset of the seizures.

While awaiting the CT scan, the referring team referred her to the retrieval service. At the time of referral she was intubated with a size 4.0 microcuff tube, 10 cm at the lips. Ventilation was easily achieved. She was not clinically seizing, although the peri-intubation muscle relation made that evaluation more difficult. She was warm and well perfused with capillary refill time <2 seconds. Heart rate had been noted to be extremely variable between 80 and 140bpm. Blood pressure was 90/60. She was also noted to be anisocoric with right pupil 6mm, non-reactive and left pupil 3mm and reactive.

The local hospital was not able to continue her care in light of the need for ongoing ventilation.

The CT report was returned, as follows:

Hyperdense area suggestive of right sided intracranial bleed causing midline shift. Images have been transferred to local neurosurgical hospital. Urgent discussion needed

Questions

1. Should the above information trigger a time-critical neurosurgical transfer? And what management advice would you give to the local hospital?
2. What physiological targets should be identified and maintained during transfer?
3. How do the CT findings affect the roles of the retrieval service and local team?

1. Should the above information trigger a time-critical neurosurgical transfer? And what management advice would you give to the local hospital?

The first and most important aspect of any referral is to recognise and determine the presence or not of an emergency. In this case, the emergency is encephalopathy with status epilepticus and raised intracranial pressure (RICP), which is immediately brain- and potentially life-threatening and requires immediate medical management even without the subsequent CT report .

The immediate and emergency management of RICP should be approached in the same manner as all other emergencies.

A: A competent operator must be assigned to actively manage the airway, assuming that with deepening encephalopathy or progressive RICP, it will be seriously compromised.

B: Breathing must be supported (positive end-expiratory pressure or hand ventilation) in an effort to reduce pCO_2 and thus reduce ICP, prior to intubation and invasive ventilation being established.

C: The potential for cardiac arrest with progressive coning must be anticipated. Hypertonic saline, used to reduce cerebral oedema, acts also as volume expansion to preserve cerebral perfusion pressure. If this is inadequate a pressor may be required

D: Short-term hyperventilation must be followed by induced osmotic diuresis to reduce intracranial swelling. Response can be evaluated by change in pupils.

EFG: There should be no other confounding cause for cerebral swelling or additional brain injury. Sodium, glucose and temperature must be actively addressed and normalised.

The indications for a time-critical neurosurgical transfer are common to children and adults and some are noted below:

- Extradural haematoma
- Acute subdural haematoma with mass effect
- Obstructive hydrocephalus-intracranial haemorrhage, blocked ventriculo-peritoneal shunt
- Acute ischaemic stroke requiring urgent thrombolysis
- Subarachnoid haemorrhage
- Malignant middle cerebral artery infarction
- Penetrating brain injury
- Compound skull fracture
- Uncontrollable bleeding from skull base fracture
- Clinical suspicion of any of the above but no means to perform CT head.

The presence of unequal pupils alongside the presentation of focal seizures is concerning for RICP and even if there was no facility for immediate CT scan, this child would fit the clinical picture of RICP. However, as CT is possible in most UK DGHs, this investigation should be expedited to best identify underlying pathology. Some differential diagnostic causes of the CT findings are shown in the list below and whilst the child is in the CT scanner it is important all these differentials have been investigated and treated.

- Intracranial bleed
- Intracranial space-occupying lesion
- Non-accidental injury.
- Sepsis with meningitis
- Stroke.

In these circumstances, time is of the essence, and it is important to discuss logistics early in the referral. The most expeditious retrieval is usually that delivered by the local team, but the organisational logistics can affect speed of retrieval. The local team should prepare a team and equipment to undertake the transfer immediately after referral to the regional neurosurgical referral centre. There should be facility to undertake a three-way conference call with the retrieval service, attending consultant in the local hospital and the neurosurgeon, if there are any problems with logistics.

The delay in waiting for the paediatric retrieval service to travel to the referral hospital is known to cause more harm than the relative risk of the direct transfer by the non-specialist hospital transfer team. An organised, networked, protocol-delivered solution for neurosurgical transfers with clear instructions for referral and management in these circumstances is of paramount importance.

The anaesthetic team at the local hospital should be responsible for continuing resuscitation, airway support and respiratory support. They should identify competent and senior team members to undertake transfer to the specialist paediatric neurosurgical centre. The retrieval service should help facilitate the transfer and secure an intensive care bed where necessary. This will likely be a highly stressful time for the referring team and organisational logistics will likely detract from clinical care.

Responsibilities of Paediatric Team

Consultant should be present
Referral to STRS and neurosurgical team and co-ordinate ongoing treatment
Contact emergency ambulance service via 999 stating 'Paediatric neurosurgical critical care transfer'
Support anaesthetic team: nurse or doctor in transfer team.

Responsibilities of Anaesthetic Team

Continue resuscitation
Optimise respiratory support
Allocate and mobilise team: ODA/consultant/ICU outreach nurse
Identify and check portable monitor and ventilator
Monitor child closely and transfer **asap**.

Responsibilities of Retrieval Team and receiving PICU
Secure bed on PICU and facilitate neurosurgical referral
Troubleshoot transfer logistics
Advise DGH on patient management
Encourage swift transfer.

Responsibilities of Neurosurgical Team
Diagnosis: identify 'time critical lesion'
Feedback to local DGH within 30 minutes of referral
Liaise with receiving PICU
Inform DGH to what site in receiving hospital the child should be taken.

2. What physiological targets should be identified and maintained during transfer?

Urgent neurosurgical transfer is to be completed from diagnosis to operating table within 4 hours of presentation/injury as indicated in the NICE timeline Table 30.1.

An audit of transfers of patients with head injuries who were transferred from local hospitals to a specialist neurosurgical centre showed a 6% incidence of hypoxia and a 15% incidence of hypotension during the transfer. Each type of brain injury may require specific physiological targets; however, active neuroprotective measures should be maintained in the absence of other guidance from the neurosurgical team.

This involves actively targeting normal values for oxygenation, carbon dioxide, sodium, glucose and temperature. Cerebral perfusion pressure should be ensured. For this reason, assuming ICP is at least 20 mmHg, mean arterial pressure must be kept adequate for age. Although there is no good evidence for neuroprotection in non-traumatic RICP, there is clear evidence that cerebral hypoperfusion (blood pressure), hypoglycaemia (glucose), cerebral swelling (carbon dioxide and sodium) and hypoxia (oxygenation) are all, in their own right, known associations with poorer neurological outcome in other settings.

Mean cerebral perfusion targets can be achieved by an easily remembered set of mean blood pressure targets (Table 30.2). Mean arterial pressure may need to be managed with judicious volume resuscitation including hypertonic saline and vasopressors (which require central venous or intra-osseous access – avoid the jugular veins if possible.)

Table 30.1. Timeline for neurosurgical emergency

Time (min)	Actions required
0	Infant or child identified with suspected mass lesion
0–60	CT scan should be performed within 60 min
60–120	Provisional written radiology report should be available within 60 min of scan being performed.
0–240	If mass lesion identified, prepare to move child to nearest neurosurgical centre within a **maximum** of 60 min from end of scan. Neurosurgery within 4 h if required.

Table 30.2. Blood pressure targets

Age (years)	Mean arterial pressure target (mmHg)
<1	50
1–5	60
5–12	70
>12	80

Table 30.3. Causes acute RICP

Causes of sudden rise in ICP
Airway secretions causing rise in pCO_2
Coughing
Sudden vehicle braking
Seizures
Waking up

Table 30.4. Emergency management RICP

	Emergency management of intracranial hypertensive crisis
A & B	Increase ventilation rate and depth to clear CO_2[en]. Increase sedation then suction airway to ensure clear of secretions.
C	Give hypertonic saline 3 ml/kg as bolus. Request steady journey.
D	Check pupils. Stop seizure with benzodiazepine bolus Ensure adequate background sedation Ensure no painful/ uncomfortable stimuli eg Full bladder, pressure area, vibration.

During transfer, and related to a number of potential factors (Table 30.3), the child may experience a sudden intracranial hypertensive crisis, noted by change in heart rate and blood pressure and pupillary size and responsiveness.

This requires emergency intervention which should have been discussed and prepared prior to transfer (Table 30.4).

During transfer of a sedated and muscle-relaxed child, the only reliable sign of neurologic deterioration may be pupillary changes. Eyelids must not be taped closed, and pupils must be examined for size and responsiveness and documented every 15 minutes.

3. How do the CT findings affect the roles of the retrieval service and local team?

The transfer team should be prepared for transfer as soon as the decision to transfer is taken. Ideally the same team should be involved in the initial resuscitation, management and preparation of the patient. If this is not possible, they should receive a formal handover from the resuscitation team. Good verbal and written communications are vital. This is especially important at the time of referral and when a patient is handed over at the end of the transfer. The national guideline recommends the use of a checklist before departure. All notes (or photocopies) and blood results should accompany the patient. The relevant duty consultant (anesthetist/intensivist/stroke physician/acute care emergency physician/ neuro-surgeon) in the receiving hospital should be made aware of the planned transfer. The transfer team should be told where to go in the receiving hospital. They should be equipped with a mobile telephone to enable contact with the neurosurgical unit and their base hospital en route in case of clinical deterioration.

This kind of transfer does not require any super-specialised equipment. The same equipment used to transfer adults will apply here. Full monitoring as would be in place for a complex surgical case is required.

Neurosurgical transfer guidelines and checklists are readily available from the majority of retrieval services. The local team should be aware of where to find these, and use them to smooth transfer.

Further Reading

Chmayssani M, Vespa PM. Prehospital triage and emergency room care in TBI. *Emergency Med* 2013;4:172. doi:10.4172/2165-7548 .1000172.

Dinsmore J. Traumatic brain injury: an evidence-based review of management. *ContEd Anaesth Crit Care & Pain* 2013;13 (6):189–95

NICE Pathway. Head injury overview. http:// pathways.nice.org.uk/pathways/head-injury NICE

Nathanson MH, Andrzejowski J, Dinsmore J, et al. Guidelines for safe transfer of the brain-injured patient: trauma and stroke, 2019 Guidelines from the Association of Anaesthetists and the Neuro Anaesthesia and Critical Care Society. *Anaesthesia* 2020;75:234–46.

STRS Guideline: Time Critical Neurosurgical Transfer. www.evelinalondon.nhs.uk/ resources/our-services/hospital/south-thames-retrieval-service/neurosurgical-transfer-mar-2018.pdf.

Statement on Provision of Emergency Paediatric Neurosurgical Services; Joint Statement from the Society of British Neurological Surgeons (SBNS) and the Royal College of Anaesthetists (RCoA) Regarding the Provision of Emergency Paediatric Neurosurgical Services.

When Vomit Turns to Blood

Anna Canet Tarres and Shelley Riphagen

A previously fit and well 8-year-old presented with a non-specific week's history of worsening general condition, small blood-tinged vomits as well as vague abdominal pain and difficulty eating and drinking. She had attended her GP who had prescribed a proton pump inhibitor for reflux. This made no significant difference to the child's symptoms. In the week preceding presentation, she had fainted three times while walking upstairs. The morning of presentation, she was noted by her mother to be grey and lethargic and was brought into A&E, where she vomited 250ml of coffee ground blood.

On arrival in A&E she was awake and talking but clearly cold and pale as well as tachycardic. She was given 10ml/kg of crystalloid while blood tests were sent together with a crossmatch because of her striking pallor.

Considering the haematemesis, she was referred to and accepted by a tertiary paediatric surgical service with in-house hepatology. A concurrent referral was made to the retrieval service because of the concerning clinical condition of the child. While awaiting the retrieval team, the child admitted to her mother she had been playing with fridge magnets – moving them inside her cheek using another on the outside of her cheek and had accidentally swallowed one. Shortly afterwards she vomited again. The vomitus contained fresh blood and she became even more tachycardic.

Due to the observations and blood results in Table 31.1, the retrieval team were activated immediately with an estimated time of arrival 25 minutes later

On arrival of the retrieval team, the child was exceptionally pale despite having a blood transfusion in progress and proceeded to vomit over 1000 ml of fresh blood during attempted nasogastric tube insertion by the referring team. She was not jaundiced.

Then while the retrieval team was taking a brief handover, the child stopped responding and had a cardiac arrest with pulseless electrical activity (PEA). She was immediately intubated and resuscitated with 180ml/kg of blood and crystalloid.

Despite ongoing efforts to achieve stabilisation, the child continued to lose very large amounts of fresh blood via the nasogastric tube and proceeded to have a second PEA arrest, evaluated as secondary to profound hypovolaemic, haemorrhagic shock. She was resuscitated once again from this with rapid transfusion of packed red blood cells (RBCs) and plasma, but could not be stabilised for transfer.

Questions

1. In the setting of massive uncontrolled upper gastro-intestinal bleeding in a child, what are the likely causes and viable clinical options to control bleeding?

2. If bleeding control is not achieved, what courses of action can be taken in a setting where there is no on-site paediatric surgical specialist?
3. In view of the massive haemorrhage and the history given, what resources would be required at a tertiary centre to save this child's life?

1. In the setting of massive uncontrolled upper gastro-intestinal bleeding in a child, what are the likely causes and viable clinical options to control bleeding?

Upper gastro-intestinal haemorrhage is defined as coffee ground or fresh blood coming from gastro-intestinal tract proximal to the ligament of Treitz (duodenal-jejunal flexure). In the paediatric age group, it is most often associated with stress ulcers or erosions, but in older children it may also be caused by duodenal ulcer, esophagitis/Mallory–Weiss tears, and oesophageal varices (see Table 31.2). Clinical history is essential to determine if there is

Table 31.1.

Observations		Investigations	
Heart rate	130 breaths per minute	Haemoglobin	51 g/L
Respiratory rate	42 bpm	White cell count	33.2 (10^3/mm^3)
Sats	100%	Platelets	391 (10^3/mm^3)
Blood pressure	115/45 mmHg	CRP	15 mg/L
Glasgow coma score	15	Urea	7.6 mmol/L

Table 31.2.

	Infants	2–5 years	Older
Oesophagus		Oesophagitis Oesophageal varices Mallory–Weiss syndrome	Oesophagitis Mallory–Weiss syndrome Oesophageal varices
Stomach	Gastritis from stress	Gastritis Gastric ulcer Gastric varices	Dieulafoy lesion Portal hypertensive gastropathy Haemobilia
Duodenum		Duodenitis Duodenal ulcer	
Variable location	Vitamin K deficiency Sepsis Trauma (nasogastric tubes) Cow's milk protein allergy	Caustic ingestions Foreign bodies NSAIDs use	Polyps Crohn's disease Telangiectasia Aortoenteric fistula Coagulation disorder Caustic ingestion Foreign bodies NSAIDs use

any background disease (mainly hepatopathies and vasculopathies) that can potentially lead to one of these conditions.

In the setting of haemorrhagic shock, rapid assessment, stabilisation and resuscitation are the priorities before any diagnostic test.

It is essential to:

• Identify shock
• Initiate a major haemorrhage protocol or 'code Red' and to
• Try to identify and control the source of bleeding.

Uncontrolled ongoing internal bleeding can be potentially life threatening and difficult to maintain resuscitation, depending on the aetiology and rate of haemorrhage.

A nasogastric tube placed in this child revealed ongoing large volume losses of fresh blood that proved difficult to keep up with by replacement transfusion.

In this clinical situation, major bleeding leads to two physiological insults that contribute to reduced oxygen delivery and progress of shock: decreased RBC mass which decreases blood oxygen content, and hypovolemia which decreases cardiac output and organ perfusion. Both volume resuscitation and replacement of RBCs are equally important in resuscitation. On presentation, this child had compensated shock which quickly deteriorated to decompensated shock and cardiac arrest, likely due to large circulating blood volume loss of between 25% and 40% (see Table 31.3).

The management of this child is challenging and needs clear thinking, a systematic approach, excellent teamwork and leadership, with all able to contribute to establishing the best management.

Airway and breathing: As part of early resuscitation of shock, to improve oxygen delivery to organs, a 100% oxygen face mask at 15L/min should be placed, even if saturations are normal. This will give some time to try and establish source and rate of haemorrhage and plan further resuscitation.

Table 31.3. Haemorrhage classification

Organ system	Class			
	I	II	III	IV
Blood volume loss	**<15%**	**15–25%**	**30–39%**	**>40%**
Cardiovascular				
heart rate	Normal	Tachycardia	++ Tachycardia	+++Tachycardia
blood pressure	Normal	Normal	Hypotension	++Hypotension
Respiratory	Normal	Tachypnoea	++ Tachypnoea	+++ Tachypnoea
Renal				
urine output	Normal	Oliguria	Oliguria	Anuria
ph	Normal	Normal	Metabolic acidosis	Significant acidosis
Neurology	Anxious	Irritable	Irritable/lethargy	Lethargy
Skin	Warm, pink	Cool, mottled	Cool, pallor	Cold, cyanotic

All necessary equipment for intubation must be prepared, in the event of progression of shock. If the vomiting is significant, intubation with a cuffed endotracheal tube may afford better airway protection.

Circulation: At least two large bore cannulas should be in situ to ensure adequate vascular access. These are usually of larger internal diameter than those of a paediatric central line. As soon as shock has been identified, crystalloid can be given (20ml/kg). In this case, however, it was important (and easily visible) to establish haemorrhagic shock as the mechanism, in which case blood products are ideal resuscitation volume. This requires early consideration of cross-matching, and identification of a 'haemorrhagic emergency' or 'code red' situation to obtain maximum support from the blood bank and haematology. Other considerations of haemorrhagic shock in children are the same as for trauma with low pressure resuscitation targets and consideration and management of dilutional coagulopathy.

In this case, the child had clearly been losing blood (admission Hb 5.4 g/L) before admission. The district general hospital cross-matched and ordered blood immediately, on noticing the extreme pallor on admission. A full cross-match can take 45 minutes or more, and thus in this case, with ongoing active bleeding, O negative blood was initially used.

In critically ill children with haemorrhagic shock, the latest recommendations suggest that red blood cells, plasma and platelets should be transfused empirically in ratios between 2:1:1 to 1:1:1 (which represents the approximate physiologic composition) until the bleeding is no longer life-threatening.

Other major problems associated with large volume blood product transfusion include:

- Significant hypocalcaemia (ionised calcium <0.6mmol/litre), induced by blood product citrate binding to circulating serum calcium and acidosis (pH<7.3). This reduces the activation of coagulation on platelet cell surfaces and disrupts haemostasis, and therefore calcium needs to be monitored and replaced as needed.
- Another important factor regarding massive haemorrhage is maintaining the temperature above 35°C. For each 1°C decrease in temperature, coagulation factor activity decreases by 10% reducing the chance of stopping the bleeding significantly. This is especially important during retrieval, when it is easy to lose heat and therefore needs close monitoring. Apart from keeping the patient warm, heating the fluids prior to their administration should be considered using a blood warmer.
- Depending on the age of transfused RBCs, potassium may be very high in red cell packs with ongoing surveillance of potassium levels needed, especially in the presence of acidosis. A request to a blood bank for the freshest blood available may go some way to alleviate this.

Other Treatments

- Consider starting a proton pump inhibitor, for example pantoprazole, to manage gastritis or oesophagitis.
- If there are clinical signs of hepatopathy (jaundice, hepatomegaly) or the clinical history suggests oesophageal varices, starting octreotide should also be considered.
- Despite weak evidence in the paediatric population, tranexamic acid use should be considered if the initial treatment does not prove effective to stop the bleeding. The recommended dose is: load with 15mg/kg then infusion of 2mg/kg/h for 8 hours.
- There is no evidence to support the use of factor VII; however, it has been used at a last resort when conventional methods have failed.

2. If bleeding control is not achieved, what courses of action can be taken in a setting where there is no on-site paediatric surgical specialist?

In the case of uncontrolled massive upper gastro-intestinal bleeding after all the previously described measures have been exhausted, more invasive procedures should be considered.

If surgery is not an option, a Sengstaken–Blakemore tube must be placed to try to stop the bleeding.

The original Sengstaken–Blakemore tube has three lumens (gastric balloon port, gastric aspiration port and oesophageal balloon port) as seen in Figure 31.1. The Minnesota tube is similar but has four ports (extra oesophageal aspiration port).

The tube should be sized as per Table 31.4 and inserted through one of the nostrils, to sufficient length. Check the tip is in the stomach by aspiration and pH. Firstly, fill the gastric balloon with air (100–150 ml) and then slowly apply traction. Ideally a CXR should be performed at that point to confirm position. Secondly, inflate the oesophageal balloon to a pressure of 35–40 mmHg with a sphygmomanometer attached to a three-way tap. With traction pressure, stick the catheter to the cheek with tape.

Table 31.4.

Patient weight	Sengstaken tube size
10–25 kg	Paediatric, size 14 FG WSP
25–30 kg	Paediatric, size 16 FG WSP
30–45 kg	Adolescent, size 18 FG WSP

Figure 31.1 Sengstaken-Blakemore tube.

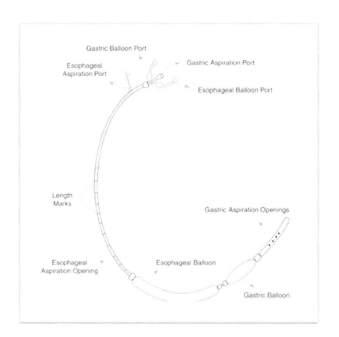

3. In view of the massive haemorrhage and the history given, what resources would be required at a tertiary centre to save this child's life?

When identifying the most appropriate destination for the child, it is important to try and understand the likely pathology and thus the resources that may be required. A massive gastro-intestinal bleed of unknown aetiology will more than likely need paediatric intensive care, paediatric surgery and both diagnostic and interventional radiology.

Although extremely rare, a possible cause of the massive, catastrophic and ongoing bleed after a foreign body ingestion is an aorto-oesophageal fistula. Interventional radiology may be needed.

In the case of this child, cardiac and thoracic surgeons should also be available at the receiving centre.

It is important to consider other diagnoses, such as a possible hepatopathy previously not diagnosed – this would require liver expertise at the receiving centre.

The retrieval team will have detailed knowledge of the services available to children at various tertiary institutions in their region.

Outcome

This young girl had a massive aorto-oesphageal fistula due to oesophageal erosion following a retained lower oesophageal button battery. At the local hospital the adult surgical team, part of the team that saved her life, performed a laparotomy. They opened the stomach to the duodenum but could not find the source of bleeding, which appeared to be coming

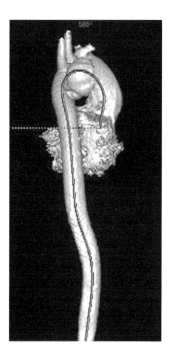

Figure 31.2 CT angiogram.

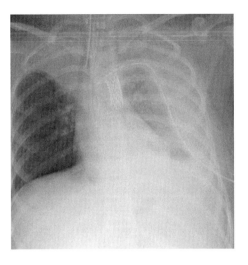

Figure 31.3 Chest radiograph showing covered aortic stents in place.

from the thoracic oesophagus. They passed an adult Sengstaken tube back up the oesophagus and inflated both balloons. Up until the point of bleeding control she had 18 units of blood products to keep her alive. This allowed her to be safely transferred to the tertiary paediatric unit. Here she underwent CT angiogram, shown in Figure 31.2, and then aortic covered stent placement by the interventional cardiology team. This completely stopped all bleeding (see Figure 31.3).

Following this, she underwent oesophagoduodenoscopy the following day. There was a very large, ragged, inflamed defect in the oesophagus, through which the aortic stents could be seen, and it was the opinion of the surgical team that the stomach and duodenum were beyond salvage.

With the help of the adult hospital oesophageal cancer team of surgeons, she underwent total oesophagectomy, gastrectomy and duodenectomy with a cervical oesophagostomy.

She was discharged from PICU 3 weeks later and returned after 1 year to have a colonic interposition to restore oesophago-intestinal continuity and remains well with no neurologic deficit to this day.

Bilious Vomiting and Distended Abdomen?

Let's Find a Surgeon

Xabier Freire-Gomez and Alison Pienaar

A 14-day-old, 4.3 kg term baby presented to his local A&E with an 18-hour history of bilious vomiting and being unsettled. There had been no urine output or bowel motion in the past 8 hours. He was born at term via spontaneous vaginal delivery, with normal antenatal scans, and was discharged home following birth with on demand breastfeeding and no risk factors for sepsis. Further medical history was limited due to language differences with parents who spoke limited English.

On arrival to the A&E, he was triaged as being acutely unwell. He was mottled and lethargic. Abdominal distension was noted. He was apyrexial. Heart rate was 200bpm, blood pressure 50/25 mmHg and capillary refill time centrally was 6 seconds. IV access was established along with initial blood samples (including blood culture) and a 20 mL/kg bolus of 0.9% saline was administered along with a dose of IV cefotaxime and metronidazole. A nasogastric tube was placed and 50 ml of bilious gastric aspirates obtained. Mobile abdominal X-ray was obtained.

Severe hyperkalaemia was noted on the initial venous gas (potassium 8.8 mmol/L) initially managed with salbutamol nebulizers. Initial observations and blood test results are seen in Tables 32.1 and 32.2.

Questions

1. What differential diagnoses would you be considering in this patient, and what management would you institute?
2. How would you manage haemodynamic support and electrolyte abnormalities in this specific patient?
3. How would you overcome the communication difficulties with this patient's parents?

---

1. What differential diagnoses would you be considering in this patient, and what management would you institute?

Surgical Abdomen

Causes for acute abdomen, outlined in Table 32.3, vary with age. Most frequent causes of acute abdomen in paediatrics across all ages are primarily intestinal, for example appendicitis, intussusception and volvulus. In the neonatal period congenital malformations should be considered (e.g. duodenal atresia, Hirschsprung's disease, microcolon). Conditions affecting other intra-abdominal organs can also frequently present with acute abdomen, such as acute hepatitis, pancreatitis or pyelonephritis. The past medical history of the

Table 32.1.

Blood tests		Venous blood gas	
Haemoglobin	156 g/L	pH	7.14
White cell count	3.8 (10^3/mm^3)	pCO$_2$	9.6
Platelets	135 (10^3/mm^3)	HCO$_3^-$	18.5 mm/L
CRP	12 mg/L	Base excess	−5.3 mEq/L
Procalcitonin	34.3	Lactate	11.3 mm/L
Creatinine	34 U/L	Glucose	3.9 mm/L
INR	1.3	Na	134 mm/L
APTT	1.3 secs	K	8.8 mm/L

Table 32.2.

Temperature	36.3° C
Heart rate	200 bpm
Respiration rate	32 breaths per minute
Sats	98–100% (no pre—post ductal gradient)
Blood pressure	50/25 mmHg (no upper-lower limb gradient)
AVPU	Pain
CRT	6secs

patient could give important hints to other causes of intra-abdominal pathology (e.g. obstruction secondary to adhesion in patients with previous laparotomy, or perforation in patients with recent interventions, such as gastric or jejunal feeding device insertions).

However, several conditions that present with a clinical picture suggestive of an acute abdomen might have an extra-abdominal aetiology (e.g. basal pneumonia). This is of paramount importance when it comes to initial stabilisation and resource allocation.

Extra-abdominal Considerations

Cardiac Conditions

In children, both congenital and acquired cardiac conditions represent a subset of situations that merit careful medical management and a high degree of suspicion to achieve a successful outcome. Transfer to a cardiac centre should be preferred in these situations.

- **Congenital cardiac defects:** Specifically in newborns, duct dependent congenital cardiac defects can present, around the time the ductus arteriosus closes and pulmonary vascular resistances drop. An acute abdomen secondary to gut hypoperfusion may arise (cardiogenic necrotising enterocolitis). Conditions such as coarctation of the aorta, interrupted aortic arch or hypoplastic left heart syndrome and its variants may manifest in this way. As an urgent paediatric Echo may not always be available on presentation, it is essential to systematically assess the baby for other signs of congenital cardiac defects,

Table 32.3.

Age group	Diagnosis	Diagnostic clue
Newborns <1month	Intestinal atresia	Double bubble and absent distal gas on plain abdomen X-ray
	Volvulus	Coffee-bean sign on abdomen X-ray
	Meconium ileus	Nil bowel output
Infants <2years	Intussusception	Intermittent pale/pain spells
	Meckel's diverticulum	Bright fresh blood in stools
	Hirschsprung	Progressive constipation
	Incarcerated inguinal hernia	Swollen painful mass
Children 2–10 years	Appendicitis	Progressive right iliac fossa pain, loss of appetite
	Schoenlein Henoch purpura	Abdominal pain with rash and haematuria
	Lobar pneumonia	Respiratory prodromes, lobar consolidation on CXR
Teenagers >10 years	Ovarian torsion	Hypochondrial pain, intermittent at times
	Pancreatitis/ cholecystitis	Jaundice, chyluria, deteriorates with feeding
	Burkitt lymphoma	Systemic symptoms
	Inflammatory bowel disease	Profuse bloody/slimy diarrhoea
	Ectopic pregnancy	Absent period

such as pressure gradient across upper and lower limbs, pre-post ductal saturation difference. In these cases, starting prostaglandin may be life-saving.

- **Acute myocarditis/cardiomyopathy:** Gut perfusion tends to be compromised early on in the context of severe cardiac failure. Tachycardia, hypotension and poor peripheral perfusion are features common to any cause of shock. Other evidence of cardiogenic shock needs to be actively sought before embarking on aggressive fluid resuscitation. In this regard CXR can be a helpful tool to assess cardiomegaly and signs of pulmonary oedema. Hepatomegaly should also be frequently assessed during resuscitation as a sign of fluid overload. It is important to recognise that acute hepatic capsular distension associated with rapid progression of cardiac failure can be exquisitely painful and mimic other right sided abdominal pathologies.

Lobar pneumonia: More frequent in infants and children, lobar pneumonia, often in conjunction with empyema, can present with acute abdomen, referred abdominal pain and vomiting. Again, thorough examination, CXR and point of care chest ultrasound could be helpful.

Abdominal malignancies: Abdominal malignancies often present as abdominal masses rather than as acute abdomen per se. Nonetheless, certain aetiologies, such a Burkitt lymphoma presenting with intussusception, or rapidly growing tumours, for example, hepatoblastoma or neuroblastoma, can sometimes present with obstructive symptoms, tender abdomen and vomiting. History of insidious onset, weight loss, lethargy and general examination findings, such as generalized lymphadenopathy and hepatosplenomegaly, may be clinical clues. If a malignancy is suspected, arranging a transfer to a centre with paediatric oncology services would facilitate further management.

In our case, cardiopulmonary examination including four limb blood pressure, abdominal and CXRs provided enough information to preliminary rule out a primary pulmonary or cardiac condition.

2. How would you manage haemodynamic support and electrolyte abnormalities in this specific patient?

It is most important to recognise and declare that the child was shocked no matter the point in the care pathway you become involved. This newborn presented with tachycardia, hypotension, poor peripheral perfusion and severe acidosis with raised lactate. At presentation to A&E, having ruled out with a sufficient degree of certainty, primary cardiac causes, our working diagnosis should centre on managing septic and hypovolaemic shock.

Antibiotics

Appropriate broad-spectrum antibiotics should be administered as soon as possible. Given the patient is a neonate with suspected abdominal source of sepsis, the agent selected should provide appropriate cover for enteric gram positive, negative and anaerobic organisms as well as for central nervous system infection.

Fluid Resuscitation

Initial fluid resuscitation with isotonic crystalloids (e.g. 0.9% normal saline) up to 60 ml/kg is standard practice for possible septic shock (Surviving Sepsis Campaign guidance). However, patients with abdominal sepsis often require high volume fluid resuscitation. This is attributable to:

- **Intraperitoneal third space losses:** ischaemic bowel becomes inflamed and extremely permeable. This leads to a high volume of fluid lost from the intravascular compartment into the peritoneal cavity. Such losses are difficult to quantify, but an increasing abdominal diameter or a point-of-care ultrasound can give us some information about the degree of intraperitoneal fluid accumulated. If haemodynamic instability persists, assume third space losses and assess haemodynamic response to further fluid boluses.
- **Increased gastric losses:** Our patient had a recent history of copious bilious vomiting and further 250 ml of bilious aspirates was measured on arrival to PICU. These accumulated losses need regular ml by ml replacement to avoid further hypovolemia.

Inotropes and the Cardiovascular System

Shock in neonates and young infants leads to early myocardial impairment. Early addition (consider after 40 mL/kg of fluid without resolution of shock) of inotropic support is beneficial. Dopamine and adrenaline could be considered as first-line choice agents in this case, infused either peripherally (diluted) or centrally. When considering establishing central venous access, bear in mind that an acute abdomen is, until proven contrary, a **surgical emergency**. Definitive surgery should not be delayed achieving central venous access. Have a low threshold for siting an intra-osseous needle for resuscitation. Intubation and ventilation should be considered in children with fluid refractory shock.

Ventilation

Children with abdominal emergencies may require intubation as part of their resuscitation and stabilisation for transfer. Indications for intubation and ventilation may include:

- **Respiratory support**

  Progressive abdominal distension with ongoing fluid resuscitation and associated raised intra-abdominal pressure may cause progressive respiratory embarrassment. Neonates/young infants, in particular, may tolerate this poorly.

- **Cardiovascular support**

  In patients with fluid refractory shock requiring inotropic support, intubation and ventilation for cardiovascular support should be considered: reduce oxygen consumption and reduce left ventricular afterload.

- **Analgesia**

  Patients may have significant discomfort and should receive appropriate analgesia. Requirement for moderate/high dose of opiates may require intubation to ameliorate side effects such as hypoventilation.

- **Access**

  In some cases, in children requiring high volume resuscitation and inotropic support, central venous access may be urgently required. Intubation may facilitate gaining vascular access. These patients often have other indications for intubation.

Overall the threshold to intubate and ventilate patients in this setting is low. It is, however, not without risk. Induction of anaesthesia is associated with significant risk in context of partially resuscitated/ongoing shock.

Non-invasive ventilation may be associated with worsening abdominal distension and would not be favoured in this setting.

When selecting an endotracheal tube keep in mind the potential need for high mean airway pressures to achieve adequate ventilation. A tube of adequate diameter/primary cuffed endotracheal tube should be considered.

Electrolytes

Severe electrolyte derangements can negatively affect haemodynamic stability. This newborn presented with a severe hyperkalaemia (potassium 8.8 mmol/L). The aetiology for hyperkalaemia in this case is likely multifactorial (Table 32.4).

Initial management of hyperkalaemia is aimed at redistribution of potassium ions from the intravascular to the intracellular space and protecting the myocardium against the effects of hyperkalaemia (Table 32.5).

Table 32.4.

Potential causes of hyperkalaemia

Tissue necrosis	Ischaemic bowel
Renal Failure	Shock with acute kidney injury, anuric
Acidosis	Redistribution of hydrogen/ potassium ions

Table 32.5.

Management of hyperkalaemia

Stop any exogenous potassium administration	
Remove potassium from maintenance fluids, avoid blood transfusion	
Redistribution	
Salbutamol	Nebulised/IV
Insulin/ dextrose	Infusion – attention to blood glucose, risk of hypoglycaemia
Protect myocardium	
Calcium gluconate	IV, continuous ECG monitoring, defibrillator available
Source control	
Urgent laparotomy to remove necrotic bowel	
Removal	
Haemofiltration	May be required for acute severe hyperkalaemia

Source Control

Source control is fundamental to resuscitation. Definitive surgery should be undertaken as soon as possible. Ongoing resuscitation will be required during surgery. Delay in surgical intervention may negatively impact on long-term outcome by increasing requirement for bowel resection.

3. How would you overcome the communication difficulties with this patient's parents?

Communication barriers are a commonly encountered challenge in the retrieval setting. In paediatrics, patients are often non-verbal, either because of their early age or because comorbidities, such as neurodevelopmental delay. Often their severe clinical condition or certain medical interventions, such as sedation, can also limit communication. In these situations, parents or carers will be our primary source of information regarding the recent and past medical history.

However, in our globalized society, carers may not be fluent in the local language, posing a challenge for the medical team both to establish a relevant medical history as well as update the carers about the medical plans and patient status and then to take informed consent. This situation also adds extra emotional distress to the family in an already upsetting situation. Do not forget to ask about the carer's mother tongue and which other languages they are confident with.

In this case, mum had no English skills and dad's spoken English was significantly limited, yet fluent enough to provide the team with basic information to focus the case.

There are several resources available which can be useful in these situations:

- Language interpreters: most health facilities will have a language interpreter service available, on site or via phone call. Parents/carers may be accompanied by relatives who could serve as an interpreter in an emergency if no other interpreter can be found.
- Hospital staff: find out whether any of the hospital staff working on that shift might be fluent in the carer's language. This is often the case for the most globalised languages.
- On-line translating services: in some settings, such as during the ambulance transfer, language interpreter services will not be available. Ask carers whether they have any translation mobile phone application they are familiar with or search online for translator services. These tend to be useful for brief updates and simple questions.

Remember also, prior to departure, to facilitate written details of the destination hospital and ward. If the patient being transferred is likely to require emergency surgery always endeavour to have at least one parent with parental responsibility (i.e. able to provide consent for procedure) accompanying the patient.

Summary

Our patient received a total of 70 ml/kg fluid resuscitation, and was intubated by the local team prior to transfer given his progressive lethargy, hypoventilation and severe shock. Haemodynamic parameters (HR 160, BP 80/50, CR 2s) and venous gas significantly improved (pH 7.38, pCO_2 5.0, Lac 1.2, BE -2.3, K 6.8) before being transferred uneventfully to a tertiary PICU for further management.

Urgent exploratory laparotomy revealed gut malrotation with extensive small bowel injury. Our patient underwent a second surgery 24 hours after admission where ischaemic bowel was removed. He was successfully discharged from PICU on day 7 post-admission on total parenteral nutrition and IV antibiotics. He is currently fed enterally and thriving.

Further Reading

Attias O, Bar-Joseph G. Abdominal compartment syndrome in children. In: Wheeler D., Wong H., Shanley T. (eds) *Pediatric Critical Care Medicine.*: London: Springer, 2014:39–55. doi:10.1007/978-1-4471-6416-6_4.

Beck R, Halberthal M, Zonis Z, et al. Abdominal compartment syndrome in children. *Pediatr CritCare Med,* 2001;2(1):51–6, doi:10.1097/00130478-200101000-00011.

Lee HC, Pickard SS, Sridhar S, Dutta S. Intestinal malrotation and catastrophic volvulus in infancy. *J Emerg Med* 2012; 43(1), e49–e51, doi:10.1016/j.jemermed.2011.06.135.

Chapter 33

What Can't Go Down, Must Come Up

Emily Cadman and Alison Pienaar

A previously fit and well 15-year-old boy (weight 65 kg) presented at 15:30 to the A&E in a district general hospital (DGH), with no paediatric surgical service, with abdominal pain and vomiting. The pain and vomiting started the previous night, and the vomitus had 'turned green' that morning. He had no appetite and was struggling to tolerate plain water.

He presented with his mother. She confirmed that he was fully vaccinated, that there were no sick family contacts and no recent foreign travel. She recounted that he had mild hypoxic ischaemic encephalopathy at birth but had no residual neurological problems and was in mainstream education.

On examination his chest was clear and central capillary refill time was normal. His abdomen was tender with guarding present in the central and lower abdomen. No masses were felt and bowel sounds were scanty. As he was very tachycardic for age, and despite a normal blood pressure, he was given an initial fluid resuscitation bolus of 1L 0.9%NaCl, started on appropriate antibiotics (co-amoxiclav, metronidazole and gentamicin) and given morphine for analgesia.

Following review by the adult general surgeons a nasogastric tube was inserted and 1.5L of bilious fluid was drained. He was sent for abdominal and CXRs. The abdominal X-ray was consistent with small bowel obstruction. He was diagnosed by the surgeons as having an acute surgical abdomen, cause as yet unknown, and it was felt he required paediatric surgical input. It was at this point that the referral call was made to the paediatric emergency transport team to help with transfer to a paediatric surgical team.

At the time of the referral call he had been reassessed after initial resuscitation and management. Initially his heart rate improved slightly, and blood pressure was easily recordable, but his capillary refill time was increasing and over time the tachycardia worsened (shown in Table 33.1), his pulses became weaker and he became cool to the touch. Initial blood tests are shown below in Table 33.2.

Questions

1. Is this a clinical emergency and if so what?
2. What risk factors might lead you to suspect bowel obstruction from a patient's history?
3. As the retrieval team, how would you optimise this patient prior to transfer?
4. What factors would influence your decision to intubate and ventilate this child for transfer?
5. What is the role of the surgeon in the acute management?

Table 33.1.

	On arrival	After the 1st bolus	After 2nd & 3rd bolus
Heart rate (bpm)	155	120	140
Respiratory rate (breaths per minute)	45	40	44
Saturations	98%	97%	97%
Temperature (°C)	37.1		
Blood pressure (mmHg)	Unable to get a BP	110/78	90/63
Capillary refill time (secs)	<3	4	4 Pale
AVPU	A	A	V

Table 33.2.

Blood tests		Blood gas (capillary)	
Na	135 mmmol/L	pH	7.28
K	4.7 mmmol/L	PO$_2$	12.5 kPa
Urea	7.0 mmmol/L	PCO$_2$	4.6 kPa
Creatinine	135 U/L	HCO$_3^-$	16.4 mmmol/L
Capillary refill time	8 secs	Base excess	−9.4 mEq/L
Haemoglobin	20.3 g/L	Lactate	7.6 mmmol/L
White cell count	25.4 (10^3/mm^3)	Glucose	11.2 mmmol/L
Platelets	247 (10^3/mm^3)		
Amylase	37 U/L		

1. Is this a clinical emergency and if so what?

The referrer identified the reason for the call being the need for paediatric surgical input into the care of a boy with what appeared to be an acute surgical abdomen. This is a common occurrence for transport teams and it is very important for the individual taking the call to identify if the case presented represents an emergency and if so, what.

In this case, the child presented shocked with tachycardia out of keeping with his temperature or pain level. At first, his blood pressure was in the normal range. Although the local team treated shock with a fluid bolus of 20ml/kg, they did not openly recognise they were dealing with a shocked child.

It is very often the case with children with acute abdominal presentations that the pain associated with the intra-abdominal crisis keeps the child's blood pressure normal early on, and the disproportionate tachycardia may be the only sign of shock initially. Recognition and labelling this as shock secondary to an intra-abdominal event is extremely important in ensuring that the child is resuscitated properly and that ongoing re-evaluation aims at maintaining resuscitation until a surgical solution is secured.

2. What risk factors might lead you to suspect bowel obstruction from a patient's history?

In this child, there were no hints or risk factors in the history that pointed to an underlying cause of his bowel obstruction. The internal hernia found later during surgery was unknown and felt to be congenital. In some cases, the following may provide a clue:

- **Previous abdominal/pelvic surgery:** The most common cause of small bowel obstruction (adults and children combined) in the developed world is adhesions from previous surgery (accounts for 65–75% of cases) Following abdominal surgery 5% of children will develop adhesions that go on to cause obstruction.
- **Ex-prematurity with necrotising enterocolitis**
- **Any hernias or suggestive lumps on examination:** Obstruction is more common in inguinal hernias and less common in umbilical hernias. Umbilical hernias are often bigger (with a wide neck) and so can look more alarming and cause more parental anxiety, but they are less likely to obstruct. Internal hernias are rare, with an incidence of 0.2–2%, and they rarely cause small bowel obstruction.
- **Intermittent crying, pallor or 'looking lifeless':** Intussusception is the most common cause of bowel obstruction in infants and young children. Redcurrant jelly stool is a late sign and is only reported in 10% of cases.
- **History of foreign body ingestion:**- More common in younger children or children with learning or behavioural difficulties.
- **Symptoms suggestive of tumours:** Intra- or extraluminal.

3. As the retrieval team, how would you optimise this patient prior to transfer?

This child had ongoing features of shock and needed further resuscitation. He was persistently tachycardiac, hypotensive for age and had a markedly raised serum lactate. In patients presenting with abdominal sepsis, ischaemic bowel may contribute to the raised serum lactate; however, ischaemic bowel is likely to be associated with shock and appropriate resuscitation is imperative.

Surviving Sepsis Campaign guidelines for management of sepsis should be instituted.

After initial resuscitation with 40ml/kg of fluid, the addition of inotropic support to ongoing fluid resuscitation should be considered. With only peripheral access, dilute dopamine or adrenaline can be started while central venous access is secured.

Intra-abdominal sepsis often results in excessive third space fluid losses (within intestinal lumen, into the peritoneal cavity, by gut losses). This child had high volume nasogastric losses. Ongoing fluid resuscitation well beyond 60mL/kg is frequently required. It is important to re-assess response to volume resuscitation with every bolus by re-evaluating heart rate, peripheral warmth and perfusion, blood pressure, liver size, urine output and gases.

Patients with significant intra-abdominal pathology leading to gross abdominal distension may develop abdominal compartment syndrome with impaired venous return from the lower body, further compromising haemodynamic stability and intra-abdominal organ perfusion.

Table 33.3.

Parameter	Comment
Heart rate, blood pressure, capillary refill time	Monitor trend against age related norms
Lactate	Rising lactate may represent poor systemic perfusion and/or progressive bowel ischaemia
Urine output	Insert urine catheter, regularly review output
Lactate	Rising lactate may represent poor systemic perfusion and/or progressive bowel ischaemia
Central venous saturation	Monitor central venous saturation if patient has an internal jugular central venous line
Haemoglobin (Hb)	Anticipate fall with haemodilution, consider transfusion if Hb low and persistently shocked

The response to ongoing resuscitation can be assessed via the parameters outlined in Table 33.3. These should be viewed as a whole as other pathologies may be impacting on the individual values.

4. What factors would influence your decision to intubate and ventilate this child for transfer?

Intubation and ventilation should be considered for the following reasons:

- Refractory shock
  - ○ In fluid and inotrope refractory shock, intubation and ventilation is indicated. Severe sepsis can be associated with myocardial dysfunction. Positive pressure ventilation will provide cardiovascular support and reduce myocardial oxygen demand.
  - ○ High volume fluid resuscitation may be associated with third space losses of fluid. This may manifest progressive abdominal distension with associated respiratory embarrassment. Ventilation may be required to maintain adequate tissue oxygenation and reduce respiratory workload.

- Central venous access
  - ○ In children where percutaneous central venous access under local anaesthetic may not be tolerated, intubation and ventilation may be required to undertake line insertion safely and comfortably for the child.

- Analgesia
  - ○ This child had significant discomfort which would be aggravated by travel in an ambulance. Opioids will provide good analgesia, but at higher doses the risk of hypoventilation may require mechanical ventilation to enable safe transfer.

- Source control
  - ○ Achieving source control is an essential component in the management of septic shock. The patient is likely to require a laparotomy, and transfer intubated and

ventilated with adequate vascular access in place ensures that these procedures do not delay the child getting to theatre for definitive management.

As this child has ongoing and progressive shock, haemodynamic instability around the time of induction should be anticipated and should inform discussion with parents regarding intubation risks. Abdominal compartment syndrome and mechanical ventilation will reduce right ventricular preload, particularly if high mean airway pressures are required.

For this reason, when anaesthetising and intubating a child with an acute abdomen and associated shock, the following precautions should be taken.

- Prior to intubation:
  o Administer further fluid resuscitation boluses with more on standby via good vascular access
  o Commence inotropic support (via peripheral cannula/intra-osseous needle if central venous access is not available) even if the blood pressure, before induction, is good. It can always be stopped later.

- Intubation:
  o Select induction agents with stable cardiovascular profile, e.g. ketamine, low dose fentanyl
  o Have resuscitation drugs prepared, additional resuscitation fluid and intra-osseous needle should be available. Designate personnel to specific tasks in advance in the case of decompensation.
  o Insert a large bore nasogastric tube and actively aspirate gastric contents prior to and during induction and intubation.
  o Adequately pre-oxygenate the patient.
  o Anticipate requirement for high mean airway pressure ventilation if there is significant abdominal distension. Site an adequately sized cuffed endotracheal tube, to ensure high ventilatory pressures can be achieved if required.
  o Post intubation sedation/analgesia should be selected considering haemodynamic status and pain control.

5. What is the role of the surgeon in the acute management?

In any case of acute abdomen, don't forget to involve local surgeons early on and ensure your patient has an urgent surgical review. In DGHs, the general surgeons may not operate on younger children, but they should still assess the patient and liaise with the paediatric surgeons at the tertiary centre.

The surgeon, and the radiologist, may be able to guide you, while you are concentrating on the resuscitation, on the differential diagnosis of the acute abdomen and the investigations that may need to be performed urgently.

Most surgical departments have a service agreement to operate on children over a certain age/weight, especially in extremis. Surgical treatment and/or decompression of raised intra-abdominal pressure may be crucial to the management of your patient in cases of abdominal sepsis. Delay in surgical intervention may result in loss of viable bowel. Surgical intervention at the DGH with postoperative transfer to a specialist paediatric intensive care unit may be more appropriate. If this is looking likely, early engagement (especially if this is due to the child being in extremis) with the surgical team is imperative to ensure there are no delays in proceeding to theatre.

Outcome

The patient was intubated and ventilated at the DGH. He was transferred to his local paediatric tertiary centre for PICU care and paediatric surgical management, where he was taken to theatre for an emergency laparotomy. At laparotomy he was found to have a midgut internal hernia through the foramen of Winslow and out through the lesser omentum. He had an ischaemic small bowel but no evidence of necrosis. The hernia was reduced, small serosal tears in the bowel were repaired and the abdomen was able to be closed primarily. He was kept nil by mouth for several days, with an nasogastric tube on free drainage and started on total parenteral nutrition. He was successfully extubated the day after surgery. The following day he stepped down to the ward from PICU and was discharged home 10 days after first presenting at his local A&E.

Further Reading

Beck R, Halberthal M, Zonis Z, et al. Abdominal compartment syndrome in children. *Paediatr Crit Care Med* 2001;2(1):51–6.

Carlotti A, Carvalho W. Abdominal compartment syndrome: A review. *Paediatric Critical Care Medicine* 2009;10(1):115–120.

Crisp S, Rainbow J. *Emergencies in Paediatrics and Neonatology* OUP, 2013.

Hryhorczuk A, Lee E, Eisenberg R. Bowel obstructions in older children *Amer J Roentgentol* 2013;201:201–8.

Jarvis A, Freedman S, Helman A. Paediatric gastroenteritis, constipation and bowel obstruction. *Emergency Medicine Cases* January 2012. https://emergencymedicinecases.com/episode-19-part-2-pediatric-gastroenteritis-acute-constipation-bowel-obstruction.

Menzies D, Ellis H. Intestinal obstruction from adhesions-how big is the problem? *Ann R Coll Surg Engl* 1990;72(1): 60–3.

Pearson E, Rollins M, Vogler S et al. Decompressive laparotomy for abdominal compartment syndrome in children: before it is too late. *J Paediatr Surg* 2010;45:1324–9.

Roil F, del Favero A. Ondansetron clinical pharmacokinetics. *Clin Pharmacokinet* 1995 29(2):95–109.

Shiozaki H, Sakurai S, Sudo K, et al. Pre-operative diagnosis and successful surgery of a strangulated internal hernia through a defect in the falciform ligament: a case report. *J Med Case Rep* 2012;6:206.

Chapter 34

Not All Burns Can Be Seen

Alex Williams and Ariane Annicq

A 5-month-old baby, weighing 5 kg, had been brought into A&E following a fire at a beauty parlour that was precipitated by an acetone explosion. He was an ex-premature baby, born at 31 weeks gestational age, and ventilated for a short time post delivery. No further medical history was available at the time of admission to A&E because both his parents were in the fire and were admitted as patients to A&E with severe burns requiring intubation and ventilation. At the time of referral, the baby had been in A&E for 50 minutes. He was self-ventilating in air, saturating 100%, with a respiratory rate of 45. He was alert, active, distressed, crying and tachycardic. No blood pressure had been performed. Pupils were equal and reactive to light.

The local team had assessed his injuries. The back of his head was swollen and both ears were burnt. He had burns on the right side of his face to the middle of his chin. He had blisters around his mouth, and his neck and lips were swollen. They had estimated the burns as 15% of his body surface area. Local first aid had been performed.

Questions

1. Does this child need intubation at this point? Explain your reasoning.
2. What key points should you consider prior to intubation in a burns patient and how will you secure the endotracheal tube?
3. What ventilation strategies are advised?
4. What are the additional key points to consider before transferring of a burned child to a specialist paediatric burns centre?

1. Does this child need intubation? Explain your reasoning.

Although this patient appears well, with no respiratory compromise, he should be intubated and ventilated without delay. A careful airway and breathing assessment is of greatest priority in burns patients. Consider the following points and compare them with the patient's clinical status above.

- Up to 20% of patients with burns will have an inhalational burn. Risk factors for associated inhalation injury include the size of the burn, type, presence of particulate matter (soot), magnitude of the exposure and individual host factors, such as underlying lung disease and inability to flee the incident.

- Children under 4 year old (with the youngest more affected) have several risk factors that increase both the chance of inhalational injury and death. These include smaller airways, less well-developed broncho-pulmonary tree, a high skin surface area to body

weight and large total body water percentage, (leading to proportionally more fluid resuscitation and chance of pulmonary oedema).
- Inhalational injury nearly doubles the mortality rate of burns patients and has a significant impact on morbidity.

Inhalational injury can be divided into three groups: supraglottic, subglottic and systemic toxicity. The injuries to the subglottic airway and the systemic toxicity will be further discussed in question 3.

The supraglottic injury is typically a thermal insult, whereas the lower airways are protected by the glottis (unless large quantities of steam have been inhaled). This heat injury can cause significant swelling of the tongue, epiglottis and aryepiglottic folds, potentially complicating intubation attempts. This swelling can take between 2 and 4 hours post injury to develop. For this reason, it is advised to **intubate early** if there is any suspicion of inhalational component to the burn.

The following factors should be triggers to intubate:
- Burns involving the face or entire neck circumference; stridor, singed nasal hair, carbonaceous debris in/around mouth or nose and in sputum
- Exposure to flame, smoke or chemicals, duration of exposure, exposure in an enclosed space
- Reduced or falling level of consciousness
- Large burn (>25%) expecting higher fluid resuscitation volumes and inflammatory response causing generalised oedema
- Electrical burns.

2. What key points should you consider prior to intubation in a burns patient and how will you secure the endotracheal tube?

Think carefully when selecting and securing the endotracheal tube (ETT). A cuffed tube should be used, since it can ensure adequate ventilation at all stages of potential tracheal and/or pulmonary oedema and also reduces the chance of the ETT moving. As the airway swelling evolves, the ETT can be pushed out and potentially displaced. Using either tape or a marker pen, place a mark on the tube at the appropriate length, once position has been confirmed on X-ray. This will be a visual indicator if the ETT does begin to slip. Do not cut the ETT at any stage. Any adhesive dressing or tape to the burnt area is clearly contraindicated in this scenario. The simplest solution to securing the ETT is to use soft ties, with a protective, non-adherent dermal pad underneath, to prevent further trauma to burnt skin underneath the ties. The use of sutures/wires/dental fixation to anchor ETTs is inadvisable at this stage and is not normal practice in a tertiary burns centre.

3. What ventilation strategies are advised?

The subglottic inhalational injury is most often a chemical injury. Noxious substances released by burning materials strip the airway mucosa, leading to sloughing, destroying cilia and depleting surfactant. An inflammatory cascade is triggered, which results in oedema in the lower airways, bronchoconstriction with bronchospasm and pulmonary vasodilation, creating a ventilation/perfusion mismatch, leading to systemic hypoxia. Already constricted airways can become blocked by mucous plugs and casts, and subsequent overventilation of unaffected areas of lung can lead to pneumothorax. Eventually the patient may develop acute respiratory distress syndrome (ARDS) and/or a secondary bacterial infection due to the factors outlined above.

Acute ventilation management should aim to keep oxygen saturations >92% without causing additional ventilator-induced lung injury. If the lung involvement progresses to ARDS, ventilation should be managed in this manner.

In burns patients, other relevant causes for respiratory failure should be considered including:

- Chest wall trauma
- Burns eschar (can restrict chest wall movement)
- Systemic effects of inhalational injury.

The systemic effects of the inhalational injury stem from altered respiratory physiology affecting oxygenation and carbon dioxide clearance. The inflammatory process initiated in response to damaged lung tissue can lead to a systemic inflammatory response. Carbon monoxide and/or cyanide poisoning from the fire should also be considered.

Careful evaluation of simple blood gas helps to get a more accurate assessment of these toxins:

Carbon monoxide (CO) poisoning:

Diagnosis: On pulse oximeter SpO_2 95–100%; however, on arterial blood gas a low PaO_2 + high carboxyhemoglobin (COHb) level (normal 0–5%)
Management: CO should clear with FiO_2 of 100% in 3–4 hours. If COHb level > 20% hyperbaric oxygen therapy will clear CO faster.

Cyanide poisoning (aerosolisation of upholstery and fabrics)

Diagnosis: High anion gap metabolic acidosis (esp. if lactate >10 mmol/L) despite 100% O_2 & adequate fluid resuscitation in first 2 hours of presentation; difference between arterial and venous oxygen saturation (i.e. oxygen extraction ratio) is less than 10%
Treatment: Hydroxycobalamin (Cyanokit) 70 mg/kg IV or 50% sodium thiosulphate 0.5 ml/kg over 10 minutes.

Discuss both these scenarios with burns centre and a consultant toxicologist.

4. What are the additional key points to consider before transferring of a burned child to a specialist paediatric burns centre?

Further stabilisation should follow the conventional systematic approach.

Following **Airway** and **Breathing**, **Circulation** should be carefully assessed and managed. The patient has significant burns and requires fluid replacement.

C: Initial fluid resuscitation should be based on clinical presentation: if clinical signs of shock give fluid bolus 20 ml/kg and titrate further to cardiovascular response.

The Lund and Browder chart can be used to calculate the burn percentage. Further fluid replacement is based on the Parkland formula and is preferably with a balanced crystalloid such as Hartmann's solution (if normal serum potassium).

> **Burns replacement fluid calculation using Parkland formula**
> **4 ml × weight (kg) × % total burn surface area**
> (i.e. 4 × 5 ×15 = 300 ml in 24 hours)
> **50% of volume in first 8 hours** =150 ml in 8 hours
> **50% of volume in next 16 hours**=150 ml in next 16 hours

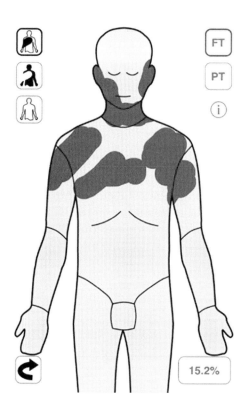

Figure 34.1 Mersey Burns smartphone application (www.merseyburns.com).

Remember that this is a first estimate of fluid replacement requirement and must be re-evaluated every hour to check that volume replacement is not falling behind or becoming excessive.

Re-evaluation is based on clinical appearance: is the child warm and well perfused to fingers and toes?, Are the heart rate, blood pressure and urine output all normalised, when other contributory factors (pain and temperature) have been accounted for?

Background maintenance fluids should also be run at 2 ml/kg/hr for this weight patient.

Ongoing clinical assessment and monitoring of urine output to verify whether this is adequate or excessive. (Aim urine output>0.5 ml/kg/h.)

There are many charts and apps available (eg. Mersey Burns smartphone application (www.merseyburns.com) Figures 34.1 and 34.2) that combine burn percentage calculation and the Parkland formula to rapidly guide management.

Adequate IV access is crucial. At the very least, two large bore cannulas should be inserted and secured with sutures to prevent displacement from burnt skin. Central IV access would be a sensible consideration especially if the distance of travel is more than 1 hour. Inotropic support should be prepared and ready to administer if required.

The patient should be catheterised early, before oedema develops and to allow accurate monitoring of urine output.

Baseline bloods should include a creatinine kinase to assess rhabdomyolysis. If elevated, titrate fluids to increase urine output to >2 ml/kg/hr. In this case, a bolus of hypertonic saline in nephroprotective.

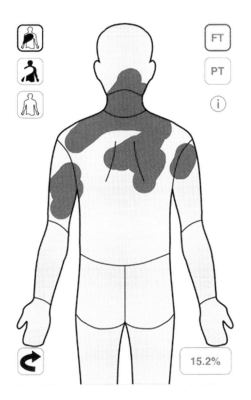

Figure 34.2 Mersey Burns smartphone application (www.merseyburns.com).

If the patient continues to be hypotensive, be suspicious of associated trauma or blast injuries. Perform an extensive secondary survey prior to departure.

Pain control is of paramount importance in burn victims. Since the patient is intubated and ventilated, a morphine infusion should be commenced. Sedation requirements may well be higher than average. IV ketamine is recommended for painful and stimulating procedures.

Hypothermia is a real risk in these patients and will delay further treatment at a burns centre. Normothermia must be restored. Temperature should be constantly monitored with an appropriate probe and every effort should be made to guard against hypothermia.

Further Management

Around the world, burns care is centred around specialist burns centres. These cover much larger geographical areas and smaller surrounding hospitals will feed into them. The burns centres will provide tertiary care and expert opinion on burns patients and associated follow-up.

England and Wales is divided into four burn care networks. These are further divided (in descending order of severity managed) into centres, units and facilities. Any child intubated for burns or if total burn surface area is >20% requires a specialist burn centre. These are listed below:

- London and South East England Burn network

  o St Andrew's Burn centre, Broomfield Hospital, Chelmsford

- Northern Burn Care operational delivery network

  o Alder Hey Hospital (Liverpool)
  o Royal Manchester Children's Hospital
  o Royal Victoria Infirmary (Newcastle)

- Midlands Burn Care operational delivery network

  o Birmingham Children's Hospital

- South West UK Burn care network

  o Bristol Royal Hospital for Children.

Bearing this in mind, and considering the different structures of burns care around the world, the child might need to travel a great distance before arriving at the destination. This is an important factor to think about for your stabilisation and preparation for transport.

Because of the distance, this child had to be transferred, helicopter transfer may be preferable. Transferring a child in a helicopter adds extra complicating factors such as noise, lower temperatures at altitude, limited access and vibration. Vibration in particular will make securing of IV access and pain control in this setting even more crucial.

Finally, social services will need to be alerted. Safeguarding documents should be completed with a detailed body map and medical report.

Further Reading

Dries DJ, Endorf FW. Inhalation injury: Epidemiology, pathology, treatment strategies. *Scand J Trauma Resusc Emerg Med*, 2013;21,31. DOI: 10.1186/1757-7241-21-31.

Foncerrada G, Culnan DM, Capek KD, et al. Inhalation injury in the burned patient. *Ann Plastic Surg*, 2018;80(3):S98–105. DOI: 10.1097/SAP.0000000000001377.

Mersey Burns smartphone application (merseyburns.com).

Walker PF, Buehner MF, Wood LA, et al. Diagnosis and management of inhalation injury: An updated review. *Crit Care*, 2015;19, 351. DOI: 10.1186/s13054-015-1077-4.

With thanks to St Andrew's Children's Burns Unit at Broomfield Hospital, Chelmsford.

Chapter 35

Drowning and Organ Donation

Emma Prower and Joanne Perkins

An 11-month-old girl was brought into the A&E. She had been left in the bath with her older sister for what the parents reported was approximately 10 minutes. When their father returned to the bathroom, he found the baby submerged, blue and making no respiratory effort.

He took the child downstairs and started CPR causing the baby to vomit. He also called the ambulance service, who arrived shortly afterwards to find the baby asystolic. CPR was continued by the ambulance staff and the baby regained palpable cardiac output after one cycle of CPR and one dose of adrenaline but failed to regain consciousness. She was transferred intubated to the local hospital.

On arrival in the A&E she was cold and mottled and given 20 ml/kg of warm IV fluid for hypotension. Her initial arterial blood gas showed: pH 6.7, pO_2 13, pCO_2 11, lactate 18, BE -25, HCO_3 11, K 4, Na 133, Glucose 12. On examination the baby was noted to have fixed dilated pupils, no purposeful movements on painful stimulation and gasping respiration. CT head was performed and was consistent with hypoxic brain injury with reduced grey-white matter differentiation.

Following transfer to the PICU, a further MRI was performed after 48 hours which showed severe hypoxic ischaemic insult with cortical, deep grey matter and brainstem involvement. EEG showed severe encephalopathy and brainstem testing confirmed absent reflexes and apnoea.

Questions?

1. What are the specific concerns when managing a child with return of spontaneous circulation after drowning?
2. What are good and bad prognosticators when considering the outcome after drowning?
3. When should organ donation be considered?
4. What are the clinical and logistic considerations regarding paediatric organ donation?

1. What are the specific concerns when managing a child with return of spontaneous circulation after drowning?

Resuscitation after cardiac arrest due to drowning is associated with predictable clinical sequelae including the development of acute respiratory distress syndrome, various degrees of multiorgan dysfunction and most importantly hypoxic ischaemic brain injury.

The main aim of management is to re-optimise all organ perfusion and achieve reasonable oxygenation and ventilation without further injuring the lungs. The main aim of neuro-protection is to avoid additional cerebral insult by further hypoxia or hypoperfusion.

As with all clinical emergencies, it is important to evaluate and manage this situation with a well-structured, systematic approach.

An accurate history of the situation that led to drowning is important to ensure head or neck trauma is considered, and to consider safe-guarding issues in younger children.

- Protection of airway and C-spine:
  - Assume cervical injury until proven otherwise and ensure care when rolling and transferring
  - High flow oxygen and intubation with cuffed endotracheal tube.

- Protective lung ventilation:
  - Target tidal volumes 6–8 ml/kg, limit peak inspiratory pressure to 30 cm H_2O
  - Permissive hypercapnia (balanced with the need for neuroprotection)
  - Permissive hypoxia (sats 90–94%)
  - Optimisation of PEEP to improve oxygenation (may need 10–15 cm H_2O) without compromising cardiac output
  - Send bronchoalveolar lavage specimen and treat with antibiotics if infection is a concern.

- Circulatory support:
  - Central/intra-osseous and arterial access
  - Restrict maintenance fluids to 50% maintenance (0.9% saline +/- glucose)
  - Ensure age appropriate mean arterial pressure (MAP) and maintenance of cerebral perfusion pressure (CPP).

    - Assuming intracranial pressure (ICP) is at least 20 cmH_2O, CPP=MAP−ICP
      Initially use hypertonic saline, inotropes or vasopressors if needed to achieve this, targeting Na >145 mmol/L
  - Treat arrhythmias by optimising electrolytes, normalising temperature to low normal range (35–36°C) and keeping inotropes to a minimum
  - Actively manage hypothermia.

    If cardiovascularly stable: slowly re-warm by 0.5 degrees per hour to a target of 35°C using:
    - warm IV fluids (38–40°C)
    - heated humidified ventilator gases
    - radiant heaters/warming blankets
    - IV temperature control devices.

    If unstable: aggressively re-warm using bladder irrigation, continuous veno-venous haemofiltration or cardiopulmonary bypass /ECMO if it is available and severe neurologic insult has not been confirmed.

- Neuroprotection:
  - 30 degree head up
  - Normoglycaemia
  - 2.7% saline (2–5 ml/kg) for a target sodium of 140–150 mmol/L
  - Ventilate to normocapnia ETCO$_2$ 4–5 kPa (if possible)
  - Slow re-warming if possible

    o Seizure control with phenytoin if needed.

- Examine and document fully any bruising or other signs of injury or abuse:
  - o Follow usual child protection procedures if there is any concern about neglect or abuse
  - o Ensure the parents are cared for as well as the child, no matter the circumstances.

2. What are good and bad prognosticators when considering the outcome after drowning?

A full history of a drowning incident may be difficult. On most occasions with children, the exact lead up to the event is unwitnessed. Rarely under certain conditions (very cold water) despite a long period of submersion and prolonged cardiac arrest there may be a more favourable outcome; however, this is not usually the case in indoor drowning events. Retrospective analysis of data displayed in **Table 35.1** showed the following indicators to be good and bad prognosticators post drowning.

3. When should organ donation be considered?

Your first priority is to stabilise the child and institute neuroprotective measures. Reassessment should be continuous. Following prolonged cardiac arrest with hypoxic ischaemic brain injury, cerebral oedema is at its worst between 24 and 72 hours. After this time, oedema starts to reduce. In a child who appears to be severely brain injured, there is an ideal period in which to obtain further neuroimaging and undertake full neurologic examination for prognostication in the 24–72 hours post insult.

    In this case there were numerous poor prognostic factors present:

- Situational factors: Age <3 yrs, submersion time potentially >5 mins, likely no or ineffective CPR at scene with asystole on arrival of paramedics
- Examination findings: Fixed dilated pupils with GCS <5
- Investigation findings: Evidence of prolonged period of hypoxaemia from initial blood gas (high lactate, low pH) and initial early CT head showing reduction in grey white matter differentiation.

In the event that further more definitive neuro-imaging (MRI) and investigations (EEG) demonstrate extensive irreparable brain injury, which is corroborated by clinical examination and absent brainstem activity, a redirection of care should ensue. It is important at this time to break the news to parents empathetically with family support on hand, and to

Table 35.1.

Good	Bad
Short submersion time	Submersion >5 mins
GCS >5 at scene or after resuscitation	No CPR >10 mins, asystole at scene
Cardiac output and spontaneous respiration in A&E	Resuscitation >30 mins
	Age <3 yrs
	Multi-organ dysfunction

involve the organ donation team, referred to as Senior Nurses in Organ Donation (SNODs) in the UK, so that they are aware of the child and the clinical condition and can support the PICU consultant and team in discussions with the parents regarding the concept of brain death and the prognosis of a child in this condition. The parents must first be brought to an understanding that the child is dead (brain death) before any discussions regarding next steps, including the opportunity for the family for organ donation, are discussed.

SNODs are valuable assets to the PICU team at this point in the child and family's care as they are able to dedicate themselves to the care of the family, while the PICU nursing and medical staff ensure the child's clinical condition remains optimised until a decision has been made by the family.

4.   What are the clinical and logistic considerations regarding paediatric organ donation?

Organ donation is a process that includes both the discussions and decision to donate organs and then the process itself, optimising physiology and organ condition.

As discussed earlier, discussions with the organ donation team should take place at the earliest opportunity as forewarning to the SNOD team and to give the parents access to expertise regarding available options. In the UK this can be done via referral to the National Organ Retrieval Service (NORS) who will then pass the information to the available local team. After referral to the organ donation team the process usually includes:

- Confirmation of the history and diagnosis of the patient to allow the organ donation team to assess the patient's suitability to be an organ donor **before** approaching the family
- Patients who are potential donors (according to UK NICE Guideline 135) show:
  - The absence of one or more cranial reflexes **and** a GCS of 4 or less that is not explained by sedation

- The intention to withdraw life sustaining treatment with a life threatening or life limiting condition which will, or is expected to, result in circulatory death.
- A member of the organ donation team should always be present when organ donation is first discussed with the families. Once it has been decided that a child may be an organ donor, optimisation of physiology for organ recovery is important. An outline of this is shown in Figure 35.1 but may differ between localities.

Max and Keira's Law (a new opt-out system for organ donation) was enacted in England in spring 2020. The new law means that all adults over 18 will be considered potential donors unless they opt-out or are excluded. Organ donation within the paediatric population is not included in this law; however, the organ donation statistics and situation for children is worse than adults and all front line clinical teams should have knowledge regarding paediatric organ donation.

- Children wait 2.5 times longer than adults for transplantation.
- Children die on the transplant list waiting for suitably sized organs.
- Donations in children have been static whilst adults have increased 20%.
- There is an evolving role of hepatocyte transplantation for inborn errors of metabolism and as a bridge to recovery or transplantation.

Donor Optimisation Care Bundle – Paediatric (37 wks CGA - 15 yrs)

Patient Name_____   Date of Birth_____

Unit Number_____   Date _____

Cardiovascular	Y	N/A
1. Monitor cardiovascular state aim for normal parameters[1]	☐	◼
2. Measure CVP (4 – 10 mmHg) (if suitable access available)	☐	☐
3. Review intravascular fluid status and correct hypovolaemia with isotonic Fluid boluses (10mls/kg aliquot)	☐	◼
4. Measure central venous oxygen saturation (maintain >70%)	☐	◼
5. Measure cardiac output if appropriate (non-invasive monitoring is appropriate if availiable)	☐	☐
6. Commence vasopressin where vasopressor required, wean or stop catecholamine pressors as able	☐	☐
7. Commence dopamine / noradrenaline to maintain MAP as required	☐	☐
8. Introduce adrenaline / dobutamine if echo indicates poor cardiac function	☐	☐
9. Consider esmolol / labetalol in cases of persistent hypertension in the absence of vasopressors.	☐	☐

Respiratory
(>1 month old - pH > 7.25 PaO$_2$ ≥ 10 kPa)
(37wk CGA - <1 month old pH >7.2 PaO2 >8kPa)

	Y	N/A
1. Perform lung recruitment manoeuvres (following apnoea tests, disconnections, suctions, de-saturations).	☐	◼
2. Review ventilation, ensure lung protective strategy (Tidal volumes 6– 8ml/kg (< 1month old 4-6mls/kg) and optimum PEEP (5 – 10 cm H$_2$O), PIP <30cmH$_2$O)	☐	◼
3. Maintain regular chest physio incl. suctioning as per unit protocol	☐	◼
4. Maintain 30 – 45 degrees head of bed elevation	☐	◼
5. If appropriate use a cuffed endotracheal tube and ensure it is adequately inflated (consider changing to cuffed tube if indicated)	☐	☐
6. Patient positioning (side, back, side) as per unit protocol	☐	◼
7. Where available, and in the context of lung donation, perform bronchoscopy, bronchial lavage and - toilet for therapeutic purposes	☐	☐

Fluids and metabolic management	Y	N/A
1. Review fluid administration. IV crystalloid maintenance fluid (or NG water where appropriate) to maintain Na$^+$ < 150 mmol/l	☐	◼
2. Maintain urine output between 1.0 – 2.0ml/kg/hr (if > 4ml/kg/hr, consider Diabetes insipidus and treat promptly with vasopressin and/or DDAVP.)	☐	◼
3. Administer methylprednisolone	☐	◼
4. Start insulin infusion if necessary to maintain blood sugar (4 –12 mmol/l)	☐	◼
5. Continue NG feeding as appropriate, ensure prescribed gastric protection as unit policy	☐	☐
6. Correct electrolyte abnormalities (maintain Na, K, Ca, Phos, and Mg within normal ranges)	☐	◼

Thrombo-embolic prevention	Y	N/A
1. Ensure prevention measures in place as per unit policy	☐	☐

Lines, Monitoring and Investigations (if not already completed)	Y	N/A
1. Insert arterial line	☐	◼
2. Continue hourly observations as per critical care policy	☐	◼
3. Perform CXR (post recruitment procedure where possible)	☐	◼
4. Perform a 12-lead ECG	☐	◼
5. Send Troponin level in all cardiac arrest cases (and follow-up sample where patient in PICU > 24 hours)	☐	☐
6. Where available, perform an echocardiogram	☐	☐

Other	Y	N/A
1. Maintain normothermia using active warming /cooling where required	☐	◼
2. Review and stop all unnecessary medications	☐	◼
3. Consideration for blood sampling volumes [2]	☐	◼
4. Family considerations and support throughout	☐	◼

Paediatric Donor Optimisation Care Bundle 2016

Figure 35.1 Paediatric donor optimisation bundle. Used with permission.

As a complicating factor in this type of situation is the need to refer the child to the coroner. If organ donation is a possibility, permission to proceed down this route needs to be obtained from the relevant coroner. In many cases this comes with conditions and in some cases restrictions, which may be negotiable with more clinical information provided to the coroner.

Further Reading

Drowning Guidelines. www.evelinalondon.nhs .uk/resources/our-services/hospital/south-thames-retrieval-service/drowning-mar-2018 .pdf.

Integrated Care Plan for Paediatric Organ Donation. www.odt.nhs.uk/deceased-donation/best-practice-guidance/paediatric-care/.

Diagnosis of Death by Neurological Criteria
https://nhsbtdbe.blob.core.windows.net/ umbraco-assets-corp/4759/form-for-the-diagnosis-of-death-using-neurological-criteria-under-2-months-abbreviated-v1.pdf.

https://nhsbtdbe.blob.core.windows.net/ umbraco-assets-corp/4756/form-for-the-diagnosis-of-death-using-neurological-criteria-2-months-to-18-years-abbreviated-v1.pdf.

Donation after Cardiac Death
https://nhsbtdbe.blob.core.windows.net/ umbraco-assets-corp/1360/donation-after-circulatory-death-dcd_consensus_2010.pdf.

Organ Donation and Babies with an Ante-natal Diagnosis of a Life-Limiting Condition
https://nhsbtdbe.blob.core.windows.net/ umbraco-assets-corp/11786/inf1299-july-2018.pdf.

Ethical Issues in Paediatric Organ Donation: UK Position Paper
www.aomrc.org.uk/wp-content/uploads/2016/ 04/Paediatric_organ_donation_position_ 0615-2.pdf.

The Cold Shocked Child

Sam Fosker and Shelley Riphagen

An 11-month-old, 8.7 kg baby was brought in to hospital urgently by ambulance in shock.

He had been seen that morning by his GP due to increased agitation overnight and was given antibiotics for a diagnosis of otitis media. After his parents returned home with him, they noted discoloration of his abdomen near his percutaneous endoscopic gastrostomy (PEG) site and he became increasingly floppy and pale. The parents became increasingly alarmed, and called the ambulance.

He had a history of complicated tracheoesophageal fistula repair as an infant and had had multiple gastric operations. He was usually fed through a PEG. This had been changed as usual at home by the community nurse on the day prior to this presentation.

On arrival of the ambulance to the local A&E, the child was triaged as an emergency. He was pale, grey and grunting with a firm tense abdomen and para-umbilical discolouration.

His oxygen saturations were 100% in 30% nasal cannula oxygen. His heart rate was 180 bpm and blood pressure was 73/40mmHg after receiving a volume bolus of 20 ml/kg crystalloid administered by the ambulance crew. Shortly after arrival into the A&E, the child had a generalised tonic clonic seizure, treated with weight-specific benzodiazepines. Immediately thereafter the child had a pulseless electrical activity (PEA) cardiac arrest. CPR was started and after 2 minutes and one dose of adrenaline, the child had return of circulation. A referral call was made to have the child transferred to intensive care with the presumed diagnosis of septic shock. The retrieval team were dispatched immediately.

After return of cardiac output the child was intubated with a size 4.0 microcuff tube. Oxygenation and ventilation were difficult. Saturations were 98% with FiO_2 0.7. High pressures were required to move the chest. Heart rate remained elevated at 185bpm and blood pressure 67/38mmHg.

Venous blood gas was as follows: pH 6.8; pCO_2 12 KPa; BE: -17; lactate 8 mmol/L. Haematocrit on the gas was 15 with Hb 53 g/L.

CXR showed bilateral lower zone whiteout suggestive of pleural effusions.

As ventilation was difficult and high ventilatory pressures were thought to be adding to cardiovascular compromise, a decision was made to proceed to chest drain insertion.

The retrieval team arrived at the child's bedside 70 minutes after the referral call. They took handover, noting the extreme pallor and very poorly palpable peripheral pulses.

The combined team made a plan for urgent chest drain insertion, with the retrieval team taking the lead with their critical care expertise.

On insertion of the left chest drain by blunt dissection, 200 ml of fresh blood emptied immediately under pressure into the chest drain bottle and the child experienced a second PEA cardiac arrest. Return of cardiac output was achieved by volume resuscitation with blood. Fresh blood continued emptying from the left chest drain. Before the right chest drain was inserted, precaution was taken to volume resuscitate the child with more blood. A 'code red' or major haemorrhage protocol was declared. Fresh blood emptied into the right chest drain with rapid bleeding from both.

Questions

1. What is your differential diagnosis for this presentation?
2. What are the complications of PEG insertion/change?
3. How are you going to resuscitate and stabilise the child for transfer? How will you manage ongoing blood loss?
4. On your arrival who should be in charge of the situation within the A&E?

1. What is your differential diagnosis for this child's presentation?

The child was shocked. What was the possible cause of the shock? The abdomen was grossly distended with some peri-umbilical discolouration.

The causes of shock that were considered were:

Abdominal – perforation, malrotation and trauma

Pancreatitis

Sepsis – intra-abdominal or pleural/ respiratory.

The commonest causes of shock in children are septic and cardiogenic shock. This child had a short preceding history, not suggestive of cardiogenic shock. The fact that the gastrostomy tube had been changed the day before must not be overlooked and may have been the cause of a septic shower or gastro-intestinal or abdominal trauma.

The presence of fresh blood in both chest drains made diagnosis of sepsis highly unlikely, and intra-abdominal trauma had to be most likely. This became a major haemorrhage scenario. Trauma in a child of this age is suspicious with no corroborative history. There was no other evidence of injury to the child beside the 'bruising'/ discoloration of the abdominal wall. The parents reported no trauma. They independently repeated the story as outlined above.

Without further imaging or blood test results, it may not be possible to achieve a definitive diagnosis. Nevertheless it is possible to continue managing the clinical emergency and maintain resuscitation. In these situations, careful assessment allows identification of emergencies that need intervention, without knowing the underlying cause. Although haemorrhagic shock was likely, sepsis needed to be treated.

Ongoing large volume blood loss must be managed as for major haemorrhage with blood product replacement at a ratio of 1:1:1 of red cells, platelets and plasma with lower pressure targets. Tranexamic acid must be given in addition. Maintaining pressure on bleeding points is essential, however, in intrathoracic and intra-abdominal bleeding, this is not possible.

2. What are the complications of PEG insertion/change?

PEG complications are frequent, reported in 0.5–22% of all percutaneous insertions. They can be split into major and minor complications. Major complications generally occur at the time or within a few days of insertion or following revision or replacement of the PEG. These include:

- Haemorrhage
- Peritonitis from gastric/bowel perforation
- Dislocation of the PEG tube.

Minor complications tend to manifest a few days post insertion or in the case of dislodgement, in a well-formed tract at any point during its use. Minor complications include:

- Peristomal erythema and infection
- Minor granulomas
- Limited leakage
- Buried bumper syndrome (internal flange embedded abdominal wall).

Parents should be counselled about PEG safety and specific complications and be alert to changes in the child's clinical condition in the days around PEG interventions. Longer-term PEG tubes are often changed in the community and parents should be aware what to look for in the first few days post change.

3. How are you going to resuscitate and stabilise the child for transfer? How will you manage ongoing blood loss?

In this situation, the possibility of undertaking surgery locally should be explored. Many district general hospital adult surgeons would not be prepared to undertake surgical exploration in a young child with a complex surgical background especially where the exact aetiology of the surgical emergency is unclear. In these cases, the child will need urgent transfer to a paediatric surgical centre with resuscitation maintained for the transfer. The paediatric surgical team at the receiving centre should be placed on standby with a theatre kept open for emergency admission.

The child had ongoing large volume blood loss from both chest drains. Before transfer the child must be resuscitated as well as possible and active resuscitation must be ongoing. The approach should be systematic to ensure a full assessment is completed even if the underlying diagnosis is unclear.

A: The child had an age appropriate size 4.0 microcuff tube. Correct tube placement was assured by end tidal CO_2 monitoring and CXR. The cuffed tube meant that respiratory compromise by increased abdominal distension could be managed with increased ventilation pressures.

B: Chest drains had been inserted with release of large tension haemothoraces bilaterally. This suggested an arterial source of bleeding. While it is possible to attach a Heimlich (flutter) valve to pneumothorax for transfer, this is not possible for fluid collections. Chest drain bottles must be secured for transfer and 5–15 minute checks in place for volume loss into the bottles. This allows volume-for-volume fluid replacement. In the case of haemothoraces, the underlying lung may also be injured. Ventilation targets should achieve adequate oxygenation and ventilation with lowest peak pressure.

C: The child remained shocked despite fluid boluses and the dose of adrenaline. In the case of blood loss, the main focus should be restoration of intravascular volume with resuscitation targets lowered to achieve 'low pressure' resuscitation. Vasopressors may be counter-productive in the first instance. Large bore vascular access will be required to maintain resuscitation. If this cannot be achieved (which is likely), central venous access or reliable intra-osseous access should be obtained.

The child's total blood volume is estimated to be around 75 ml/kg. For this child this equated to approximately 650 ml. Blood loss of 200 ml from the first chest drain represented ~30% total blood volume, with further blood loss from the other chest drain and possible concealed blood loss in the tense abdomen.

Research on massive blood loss in the paediatric population is minimal and much of the advice is adapted from the adult population. The diagnosis of major haemorrhage in adults is based on the volume and speed of blood loss. Blood loss causing shock in children, must be escalated to a 'major haemorrhage' protocol.

Treatment should follow the APLS guidelines, with tranexamic acid and early use of blood products, aiming to keep a balanced ratio of Packed Red Cells to Frozen Fresh Plasma. Attention should be paid to temperature management and electrolyte balance with derangements of calcium and potassium likely to compromise clinical condition further if untreated. A blood warmer should be requested as soon as major haemorrhage protocol is activated.

Major haemorrhage and large volume transfusions are associated with a significant risk of complications which can be categorised as follows:

- Transfusion reactions
- Immunological complications
- Metabolic derangements
- Hypothermia
- Miscellaneous

D: You must ensure the child is adequately sedated and muscle relaxed for the journey. When resuscitating an acutely unwell child, this can sometimes be overlooked. Ensuring clear documentation of drug administration and timing, and establishing maintenance sedation infusions early will aid this aspect of care.

Identifying the 'window of opportunity' to transfer is often exceedingly difficult in these circumstances and requires team work and team risk-benefit evaluation. There may not be a perfect time. The risk balance of remaining or moving must be evaluated. There must be enough personnel during transfer to ensure safety and ensure CPR and ongoing resuscitation can be achieved in transit.

All aspects of the transfer must be considered including that moving the child may disrupt newly formed clot. Resources for ongoing resuscitation during transfer with large volume blood product requirement must be in place, with the correct procedures followed with regard to moving blood products. In this child's case, transfer out to a paediatric specialist centre was the only option considered acceptable. Transfer had to occur as soon as possible.

4. On your arrival who should be in charge of the situation within the A&E?

The local team may look to the transfer team to take charge of the situation on arrival. The safety of the child is of paramount importance and in order to achieve this, the retrieval team will need to achieve the following in the most efficient manner possible.

- Comprehensive, systematic and succinct handover from local team
- Thorough assessment and formulate plan for stabilisation for transfer
- Support of further interventions necessary prior to transfer
- Communication with receiving centre to facilitate pre-admission patient registration can be achieved to allow the child to proceed direct to theatre if necessary.

One of the members of the local team may be able to continue being in charge of the situation whilst the retrieval team assesses the child. If resources allow, it may be possible to take one of the local team on the retrieval to provide additional senior support.

Whoever is in charge, it is vitally important that adequate numbers of personnel are retained around the child to help with ongoing resuscitation and stabilisation until ready for transfer. In this situation, the local team must remain actively involved in teamwork to achieve optimal stabilisation time. The local team will also have easy access to additional local resources required.

Outcome

This child was safely transferred to a paediatric specialist centre where he underwent emergency laparotomy, because of suspicion of a complication associated with the PEG change in view of the timing, the abdominal distension, the abdominal wall discoloration and the bilateral haemothoraces, without any other history or evidence of trauma. During transfer and surgery, he needed a total of 22 units of packed cells, plasma and platelets for over 3000 ml blood loss.

At laparotomy, the child was found to have a posterior gastric perforation with the PEG tube displaced through the posterior gastric wall. There was evidence of injury to the pancreas. The splenic artery had been digested/injured and had bled retroperitoneally until the collection ruptured into both thoracic cavities.

After a prolonged stay in paediatric intensive care, the child made a full recovery with no neurologic sequelae. This is a rare but described complication of PEG insertion.

Further Reading

Blain S, Paterson N. Paediatric massive transfusion. *BJA Education*. Volume 16, Issue 8, August 2016, Pages 269–75, .doi.org/10.1093/bjaed/mkv051

Cyrany J, Rejchrt S, Kopacova M, Bures J. Buried bumper syndrome: A complication of percutaneous endoscopic gastrostomy *World J Gastroenterol* 2016;22(2):618–27.

Diab Y, Wong E, Luban N. Massive transfusion in children and neonates. *Br J Haematol* 2013; 161: 15–26.

Macchini F, Zanini A, Farris G, et al. Infant percutaneous endoscopic gastrostomy: Risks or benefits? *Clin Endosc* 2018;51(3):260–5, doi:10.5946/ce.2017.137.

Encephalopathy

Fiona Bickell and Shelley Riphagen

A 9-year-old girl had been admitted to A&E with drowsiness and reduced responsiveness. She had not been eating or drinking properly for the past day or so and the parents were concerned.

Up until 10 days previously, she had been completely fit and well, but at the beginning of the illness had been febrile with a sore throat. She had seen the family GP, who had diagnosed tonsillitis, and she had been given a course of oral amoxicillin. Although her temperature had settled on the antibiotics, she had remained very lethargic with general malaise and had been kept off school at home. By the day of presentation, she was so weak that she could not walk unaided. That morning her parents noted she had slurred speech. Her dad had taken her back to the GP, supporting her walking to such an extent that she was almost carried in. While waiting to be seen in the general practice waiting room, she became acutely agitated and incontinent of urine. An ambulance was called and she was transferred to the nearby hospital emergency department. There was no other significant history of illness, allergies or medication use, and she had all her childhood immunisations to date.

On arrival in A&E she was breathing normally with no work of breathing or added sounds. Oxygen saturations were normal. Cardiovascular examination was normal with heart rate 115bpm and blood pressure 102/55 and brisk capillary refill.

Her neurological examination was concerning. Although she had some spontaneous eye opening and would open eyes to command, she could not follow motor instructions, though she could move all limbs spontaneously and withdraw from pain. The only sounds she was making were incoherent words. Pupils were equal and reactive to light. Her Glasgow Coma Score was calculated at 11/15.

At this point the child was referred to the retrieval service for further management advice.

Questions

1. Based on your assessment of the situation, what would your evaluation and management strategy be for this child?
2. Based on progress described during this case, what would be your management suggestions for transfer of this child?
3. The parents are very concerned and want to accompany the child during transfer. They have asked what to expect for recovery.

1. Based on your assessment of the situation, what would your evaluation and management strategy be for this child?

There is an apparently vague history of general malaise following what sounded like an insignificant infection that cleared within a few days. However, the child has presented encephalopathic. Depending on the disturbance of level of consciousness and deterioration of neurological functioning, encephalopathy in itself may warrant emergency management.

Of paramount importance in the encephalopathic child is to establish the presence or absence of raised intracranial pressure (RICP) as an immediate life-threatening emergency. In encephalopathic children, psychiatric disturbances, seizures and movement disorders may all also require emergency intervention on their own merit and the clinical team should maintain vigilance for these clinical manifestations.

At the time of this child's presentation, she had a significantly reduced level of consciousness, but not to such a level as to put airway safety or breathing at risk. Acceptable advice may be to admit the child to the paediatric ward for investigation and observation, in consultation with the neurology team. Prior to this course of action, it is necessary to check for the absence of RICP, the speed of deterioration up until now and thus the anticipated course of encephalopathy. If admission to a paediatric ward is determined appropriate, the admitting clinician must ensure that the child is carefully monitored with regular and complete neurological observations undertaken right throughout the day and night, to ensure deterioration is detected early.

Besides the depressed level of consciousness, there are no other signs of RICP in this child; however, she seemed to have deteriorated significantly from the day before admission including the description of what may have been a seizure at the GP surgery (unexplained incontinence in an older child).

With this change in rate of progression, it would be advisable that she is moved to a tertiary neurology centre for further investigation and management.

Prior to transfer, it is essential to ensure some basic investigations have been sent including chemistry for electrolytes, liver and renal function, ammonia and blood glucose, blood and urine for toxicology, and blood culture, full blood count, CRP and erythrocyte sedimentation rate for infection/ inflammation. Throat and rectal swabs for viral PCR and herpes PCR should also be sent. Although the child has a significantly altered level of consciousness, without neuroimaging it is unwise to proceed to lumbar puncture.

2. Based on progress described during this case, what would be your management suggestions for transfer of this child?

It is important as the referring team to establish the need for transfer of this child to a tertiary centre with onsite paediatric neurology and intensive care. When making referral calls or taking referrals, it is of paramount importance to critically analyse the question to be asked/being asked. In this case, the referring team were ostensibly calling for advice, but in reality they were alarmed at the history of sudden change in the child with slurred speech and incontinence. It is more helpful if the referring team are highly specific about the request they are making, and if the request is not evident at first, it is of prime importance that the team taking the referral clarify the key concerns and questions.

The acceleration of disease progression in this child over the previous day puts the child at increased risk of further deterioration, and that disease progress needed to be carefully evaluated. A paediatric neurologist must review the child urgently with the correct neuroimaging and ensure all the correct special investigations were undertaken, including a lumbar puncture after clinical review and results of neuroimaging. Appropriate treatment needed to be instituted to try and arrest the progression and return the child to normal functioning.

The primary questions to be answered prior to transfer were:

1. Did the child need urgent CT head prior to transfer to exclude a brain tumour, as this may change the destination to a neurosurgical centre?
2. Was it safe to transfer the child in the current condition?

The answers to both are most likely yes.

Regarding the need for CT brain, MRI brain would be the definitive neuroimaging of choice in this child; however, that will require 45 minutes of lying still, and it may not be possible without some level of sedation. For this reason, it needs to be done with anaesthetic evaluation and support of the procedure. CT brain can be undertaken in less than a few minutes, and in this child with retained airway protection, it would be safe to do so without anaesthesia prior to transfer, to ensure there is no obvious space-occupying lesion.

Regarding transfer, the answer would depend on anticipated delay to retrieval and further witnessed disease progression or development of obvious seizures. In the current condition, as long as transfer was expedited, and the child remained unchanged, she could be safely transferred unintubated.

While awaiting transfer, appropriate antibiotics and antivirals could be started to treat encephalitis/meningitis as one of the differentials.

The destination in the tertiary institution must be either to PICU for initial evaluation and HDU monitoring, or to a neurology HDU with PICU on site and PICU forewarned of the admission.

3. The parents are very concerned and want to accompany the child during transfer. They have asked what to expect for recovery.

In cases where the likely diagnosis or exact aetiology are still a broad differential, it is unwise to give parents reassurance regarding the progress, course or outcome, no matter how distressed they are.

It is important to be honest about the large differential diagnosis and many unknowns. This child most likely has a post-infectious encephalitis and after MRI brain will need the appropriate CSF and blood tests prior to commencing therapy. This may involve a combination of immune modifying-treatments including steroids, immunoglobulin and plasmapheresis depending on response in addition to the antibiotics and antivirals, already commenced. These can be stopped once all microbiology tests are returned negative.

The outcome of post-infectious or immune-mediated encephalitis depends on the aetiology or trigger, and the progression and extent of neurological involvement. It may involve a long period of treatment and a stuttering response to therapy by the child.

It can be a very difficult and distressing time for parents and family, with a child who may be entirely different to the child they know. It is better to prepare them for a long stay in hospital, with neurological outcome unknown for the present. There is no guarantee at present that the child will not still deteriorate further to difficult to control seizures, or a level of consciousness that requires intensive care support. Facilitation of plasmapheresis may be necessary in PICU. The only comfort you can give is that the child will be in a safe, monitored environment with the appropriate expertise in house for direction of treatment, and that they will be kept fully informed of plans and progress.

Adolescent Psychosis and Seizures

Infection, Ingestion or Encephalitis?

Sasha Herring and Marilyn McDougall

A 15-year-old girl, previously fit and well, presented with a 5-day history of headache. Two days previously, she had attended school, but the morning before presentation she was confused and disorientated to time and place.

On arrival in A&E she was described as being 'psychotic', due to her confusion and incomprehensible speech. She was admitted to the paediatric ward and reviewed by the psychiatric team. After further questioning, it was found that her brother had been recently presented to A&E with a psychiatric problem for which he was discharged. The family were not known to social services.

Later that evening she had an episode of being unable to talk and became very agitated. At this time, she was also noted to be febrile. A CT of her head was performed. The radiologist's report queried 'features of immune/infective encephalitis with subtle sulcal effacement and no focal intracranial abnormality. The cerebellar tonsils are seen to be low-lying which may represent early crowding at the foramen magnum'.

A referral was made to the paediatric neurology team at a nearby tertiary centre, who advised on management and accepted the child for admission to the paediatric neurology ward. Whilst awaiting transfer, she had a number of tonic clonic seizures which were managed with benzodiazepines and subsequently was loaded with phenytoin.

Because of the seizures, the referring hospital referred the transfer to the paediatric retrieval team, requesting an urgent PICU transfer. She was continuing to have further seizures with ongoing decerebrate posturing, and a Glasgow Coma Score (GCS) 10 (E = 4, V = 4, M = 2) was documented. The team at the referring hospital were planning to intubate and ventilate her prior to transfer. Her observations at the time of referral are shown in Table 38.1 and blood results in Table 38.2.

Questions?

1. What are the urgent management priorities at the referring hospital prior to transfer?
2. What is the differential diagnosis?
3. What investigations and additional management should be considered at the referring hospital and how should these be communicated between referring and retrieval teams?
4. What are your priorities for managing this patient during transfer?

Table 38.1.

Heart rate	120–130 bpm
Respiratory rate	38 breaths per minute
Sats	100%
Blood pressure	118/72 mmHg
Temperature	38.1°C

Table 38.2.

Blood results				Venous gas	
Haemoglobin	115 g/L	Na	132 mmol/L	pH	7.49
White cell count	10.1 (10^3/mm^3)	K	3.4 mmol/L	pO$_2$	9.4 kPa
Neutrophils	6.3 (10^3/mm^3)	Creatinine	83 U/L	pCO$_2$	3.5 kPa
Lymphocytes	2.4	Urea	3.2 mmol/L	Lactate	4.0 mmol/L
Plts	106	APTT	28.8		
		PT	16.5		

1. What are the urgent management priorities at the referring hospital for this patient prior to transfer?

The combination of sulcal effacement and the low lying cerebral tonsils on the CT scan indicate cerebral swelling which may be associated with increasing raised intracranial pressure (RICP).

This child has an encephalopathy with RICP and the emergency management should be directed to address this urgently in a systematic and stepwise manner.

Priorities for managing this emergency include supporting and then securing the airway and controlling ventilation and carbon dioxide clearance to prevent further cerebral swelling and injury to the brain. Smooth induction of anaesthesia and good control of pCO$_2$ and blood pressure are essential to prevent any acute spikes in the intracranial pressure.

Optimal ventilation with careful management of end tidal carbon dioxide (3.5–4.5kPa) and target oxygen saturations >92% are recommended to prevent secondary cerebral injury and optimise cerebral blood flow. In addition, use of a short-acting, bolus muscle relaxant is advised to enable assessment of ongoing seizure activity, after induction. Appropriate systolic blood pressure must be maintained in order to provide adequate cerebral perfusion pressure using fluid boluses and inotropic support if required. Age and weight-based parameter tools give a systolic blood pressure range from 95–126 (10th–90th centile), therefore it would be appropriate to target a systolic blood pressure greater than 100 mmHg for this patient. In addition, blood glucose should be strictly maintained within the normal range and pyrexia treated to optimise cerebral metabolic status in a fragile brain. The low sodium should be corrected with hypertonic saline bolus and kept at the upper limits of the normal range. The patient should be positioned with her head in the midline and elevated by 30° and carefully observed for ongoing seizure activity. Although there is no good evidence for neuroprotection in non-traumatic RICP, we do know that attention to this detail ensures no secondary injury occurs.

The patient's pupils should be assessed frequently (before and after any intervention and at 15 minutes intervals). Pupillary dilation could indicate further brain swelling causing uncal herniation which may respond to osmotic therapy such as 3–5 ml/kg bolus of hypertonic saline. Bilateral pupil dilatation may indicate awareness under sedation and would be an indication for increased sedation. Divergent or abnormal pupillary responses may indicate seizures which require anti-convulsant therapy in a muscle-relaxed patient.

2. What is the differential diagnosis?

Sudden onset of encephalopathy is rare and the differential diagnoses need to be carefully considered to ensure that the appropriate therapy is initiated promptly and that the patient is transferred to the appropriate centre. The differential possibilities, though not exclusive, would at least include the following:

- Infective – meningitis and encephalitis
- Autoimmune encephalitis
- Space occupying lesion
- Toxins – ingestion/poisoning
- Metabolic causes
- Psychosis.

Infective Cause: Meningitis and Encephalitis

The history and investigations are strongly suggestive of an infective cause (pyrexia, white cell count, CT result). A contrast CT would be helpful for eliminating meningitis but in the absence of this she needs triple therapy including broad spectrum antibiotic (cephalosporin), antiviral therapy and macrolide for atypical infections (e.g. mycoplasma) and a plan for further imaging at the tertiary centre.

Autoimmune Encephalitis

Autoimmune CNS disorders should be suspected in the encephalopathic child who has seizures, movement disorder, neuropsychiatric or cognitive dysfunction on a background of being previously fit and well. A child who presents with a viral or pyrexial prodrome, or a child with a history of autoimmunity in the individual or family should have an auto-immune work up.

MRI and magnetic resonance angiography should be performed as soon as possible, and further imaging of the lower abdomen to exclude tumours, in particular ovarian teratoma in young girls, which is associated with anti-N-methyl-D-aspartate receptor (NDMA) encephalitis.

The first line treatment for autoimmune encephalopathy is high dose IV steroids followed by intravenous immunoglobulin (IVIG), which cannot be commenced until infective and life-threatening metabolic causes are excluded. If infection cannot be excluded, IVIG may be considered prior to steroid therapy. This will be decided with the paediatric neurology team. In some very unwell children treatment with plasma exchange may be considered prior to both steroids and IVIG.

Anti-NMDA encephalitis is the most common cause of non-infectious encephalitis in children and adolescents.

The presentation is predictable and evolves in stages beginning with a prodrome of fever and viral-type symptoms, then the onset of psychiatric and behavioural changes, which is consistent with the presentation of this case. Diagnosis of NDMA disorder is confirmed by detection of antibodies in the serum or cerebrospinal fluid.

Approximately 80% of NDMA disorders occur in women and may include tumours, most commonly teratoma (ovarian or testicular), but also lymphoma, small cell lung carcinoma and neuroblastomas. In children, the association with tumours is less strong: the presence of teratoma has been demonstrated in approximately 9% of girls under the age of 14 years who experience autoimmune encephalitis.

Space-Occupying Lesion

Cerebral imaging will assist with elimination of a space-occupying lesion or abscess as a differential diagnosis, and it is essential in order to make sure the patient is transferred to the appropriate tertiary centre. In a child without seizures requiring a CT scan for abnormal neurology, a general anaesthetic/anaesthetic presence for CT may be the safest strategy. In this case, the imaging excluded space occupying lesion as a differential diagnosis.

Toxins: Ingestion/Poisoning

The possibility of drug ingestion should always be considered, especially in adolescent patients, presenting with new neurological symptoms. Urine dipstix should be performed at the local hospital, and blood and urine samples saved for formal toxicology screening. ECG is essential. A careful social history should also be taken to assess the availability of drugs, both recreational and prescription, in the home.

Metabolic Causes

Some rare metabolic conditions present in adolescence – in order to exclude this, blood levels of ammonia, glucose and sodium need to be sent.

Psychosis

It is possible for adolescents to present with psychiatric illnesses at this age. A careful family history should be taken, including possible recreational drug availability in the home. Although rare, pseudo seizures may also be considered in this gender and age range.

3. What investigations and additional management should be considered at the referring hospital and how should these be communicated between referring and retrieval teams?

It is worth remembering that at this stage of the child's illness, the imaging may be reported as normal. Normal imaging does not exclude many of the causes considered (e.g.

encephalitis, meningitis). Baseline investigations that should be performed at the local hospital include a full septic screen, procalcitonin, herpes simplex virus PCR and saved serum for antibody screening and drug screening for toxicology.

Immunotherapy treatment for autoimmune disorders cannot be commenced until infective and life-threatening metabolic causes are excluded.

A lumbar puncture should not be performed at the referring hospital. It should not be undertaken at all until the PICU and neurology team are satisfied that there is no risk to the patient from RICP or coagulopathy. Antibiotics and antiviral therapy should however not be delayed. CSF studies are necessary for microscopy and infective investigations, as well as oligoclonal bands and IgG index plus antibody studies when it is safe to do them.

Finally, in this age group a pregnancy test should be performed to eliminate the possibility of pre-eclampsia, and prior to administration of anti-convulsants due to potential teratogenic effects on the developing foetus.

The retrieval team will lead the transfer but it is also important that they are aware of all communication that has occurred prior to them being called. If a child has been planned for a standard ambulance transfer and then requires a full retrieval team due to deterioration, it is important to ensure there is a record of prior correspondence and communication of what has been said to the parents. When communicating between teams, they should ensure they are aware of which results have been requested so they can ensure all results are transported or sent over. It is of equal importance they are aware of which investigations have not been sent or are awaited. This is highlighted in this case due to the need for many investigations and also to reduce delay if the child needs immunotherapy. Once the child is transferred both teams should have contact information for each other to ensure further communication can occur if needed.

4. What are your priorities for managing this patient during transfer?

A secure airway should be maintained as a priority, and the child should be ventilated as described above. Similarly, cardiovascular targets should be maintained as discussed previously.

This case highlights the need for a low threshold for intubation and ventilation in patients with neurological pathology when considering transfer. The child was safe whilst having her CT but soon deteriorated and would not have been safe if she had developed seizures and a decreased GCS on transfer. Contingency plans should always be discussed amongst the retrieval team and plans made for worsening clinical state.

Use of short-acting muscle relaxant is recommended in order to balance the need to be able to recognize seizures with the need to manage RICP. Spikes in intracranial pressure should be minimized by ensuring adequate sedation and administering muscle relaxants prior to noxious stimuli such as suctioning and movement in order to prevent coughing. A high degree of suspicion for evolving increases in intracranial pressure should be maintained throughout the transfer, monitoring for decreased heart rate, hypertension and pupillary changes, or signs of seizure activity. Additional bolus doses of hypertonic saline can be given as first line of management for RICP, whilst also increasing levels of sedation. Seizures should be managed with benzodiazepines (bolus or infusion) and levetiracetam may be useful if seizures are resistant to benzodiazepines.

Outcome

This child was difficult to manage in PICU with psychosis and seizures. Her intracranial hypertension subsided during treatment. She was found to have an ovarian teratoma identified on abdominal MRI, but not seen initially on abdominal ultrasound. She had NMDA receptor antibodies documented and improved slowly over 6 months after plasma exchange, steroid therapy and resection of the teratoma.

Further Reading

Armangue T, Petit-Pedrol M, Dalmau J. Autoimmune encephalitis in children. *J Child Neurol* 2012;27(11):1460–9.

Evelina Children's Hospitaldrug calculator. www.evelinalondon.nhs.uk/resources/our-services/hospital/south-thames-retrieval-service/Drug-calculators/age-based-calculator.pdf.

Ramanathan S, Mohammad SS, Brilot F, Dale RC. Autoimmune encephalitis: recent updates and emerging challenges. *J Clin Neurosci* 2014; 21(5):722–30, doi: 10.1016/j.jocn.2013.07.017.

Chapter 39

The Collapsed Neonate

Ain Satar and Shelley Riphagen

You have been referred a 12-day-old neonate who was brought into her local A&E by her parents an hour ago. The parents have reported a 2-day history of tachypnoea and poor feeding. They feel she is increasingly lethargic and not herself. On admission, the referring registrar reported that she was tachypnoeic (respiration rate 70 breaths per minute) with mild subcostal recession and had been started on wafting oxygen as her initial saturations were 88% in air. She was tachycardic (heart rate 190 bpm) and mottled and felt cool peripherally with mildly prolonged capillary refill time. She was not pyrexial and was neurologically appropriate with a flat fontanelle. Her abdomen was soft with a 2-cm liver palpable.

The registrar felt she had weak femoral pulses with a higher right arm non-invasive blood pressure reading compared to her other limbs and was concerned she might have coarctation of the aorta because of the discrepancy between pre-ductal (right arm) and post-ductal systolic blood pressure (legs) of over 20 mmHg. The referral was to request urgent transfer to a cardiac centre for definitive evaluation and diagnosis.

Besides the history above, the baby was born at 39 weeks via lower segment C-section at 4.06 kg. There was no history of Group B streptococcal colonisation or other infectious concerns in her mother. The referring registrar reported that there had been documented polyhydramnios at initial antenatal scans, which had subsequently resolved. Although mum and baby were discharged on day 2 post section, she needed a 1 day readmission on day 4 for jaundice, which subsided with phototherapy and the baby had been well since then until 2 days ago.

Based on her initial clinical examination, the registrar had given her one 10 ml/kg 0.9% sodium chloride fluid bolus and 50 mg/kg IV ceftriaxone to treat possible sepsis. They were planning to start prostin; however, this needed to be couriered from a nearby Trust hospital as nothing was available locally. CXR has been done and can be seen in Figure 39.1.

Questions

1. How do you approach diagnosis in this group of babies?
2. The referring hospital is 3-hours drive from the nearest cardiac surgical centre. Helicopter transfer is available. What would be your considerations for this mode of transfer in this setting?
3. What are your other considerations when undertaking neonatal transfer?

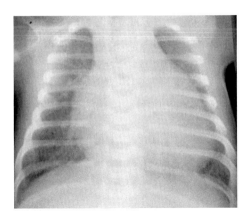

Figure 39.1 Admission chest radiograph.

1. How do you approach diagnosis in this group of babies?

The first and most important point at the time of referral is to evaluate whether this is an emergency presentation, and if so what the emergency is.

A neonate who has any cardiorespiratory compromise should be taken seriously as this can rapidly deteriorate into a 'collapsed neonate'.

Neonatal collapse usually has a non-specific presentation, which may include a history of the baby being off feeds, lethargic and sleepier than usual but little else. On clinical examination, the baby may display any of these concerning signs including hypothermia, respiratory distress, poor pulses, tachycardia and low blood pressure.

Most neonatal collapse will present with three main emergency presentations: respiratory distress, shock or encephalopathy, or a combination of the three. There are five or six common diagnostic groups into which the aetiology can be separated.

Sepsis is by far the commonest accounting for up to 50% of cases and including both vertically and horizontally transmitted infections. All sources of sepsis must be adequately covered in management including broad spectrum antibiotic cover with good CNS penetration and aciclovir for disseminated herpes.

Congenital cardiac lesions account for up to 20–25% of neonatal collapse with shock and include cardiac anatomical defects impairing systemic blood flow (like coarctation, critical aortic stenosis etc), or associated with such severe cyanosis that myocardial hypoxia and cardiogenic shock ensue (like transposition of great arteries or total anomalous pulmonary venous drainage). IV prostaglandin, which will partly restore fetal type circulation by reopening the ductus arteriosus, may be lifesaving in these situations and should be started if there is even a concern that the baby could have a congenital heart lesion, and before definitive ECHO evidence is obtained.

Even in the cases where the clinical diagnosis appears clear but no definitive diagnosis has been obtained, all possible causes of neonatal collapse must have been considered and treatment in place until a definitive diagnosis can be secured.

Other important differentials to consider would include metabolic conditions associated with 'energy deficiency' or 'metabolic intoxication' to the point of cellular dysfunction, which could be implicated in shock. Trauma is an unusual cause of neonatal collapse, but unfortunately must remain a consideration with deterioration occurring due to intracranial or intra-abdominal bleeding.

A thorough history, clinical assessment and basic investigations, with these differentials in mind, will help narrow down the possible diagnosis.

Management of the collapsed neonate should include supporting ventilation to the point of intubation, management of shock, with the addition of prostaglandin, stopping all feeds and ensuring a secure supply of IV dextrose and broad spectrum, CNS-penetrating antibiotics and antivirals.

2. The referring hospital is 3-hours drive from the nearest cardiac surgical centre. Helicopter transfer is available. What would be your considerations for this mode of transfer in this setting?

The decision to intubate and ventilate a neonate is dependent on the presence or likely development of shock and the condition of the baby on presentation.

In babies with congenital heart lesions who are not shocked, there may be a concern that the commencement of low dose prostaglandin at 5–10 ng/kg/min will cause apnoeas; however, at this low dose this is less likely. Prostaglandin-related apnoea also usually becomes evident within the first hour of starting the infusion. If there are no apnoeic episodes in this time and the baby is in good condition, then it is more than likely safe to transfer the baby self-ventilating.

Airway and Breathing

A secure airway is preferable considering the clinical picture, resources and mode of transfer. Assessment and decision need to be made based on apnoeas, rate of prostin, clinical stability, impact on transfer efficiency, team experience and travel time. Apnoea during the flight or loading and unloading could cause severe clinical deterioration with significant challenges to facilitate an emergency airway management procedure. A further complication of air travel is excessive vibration, which impedes consistent and accurate assessment of respiratory effort, rate and saturations. Gel-filled or air-foam mattresses can reduce the effects of vibration on both neonate and equipment.

If there is high suspicion or confirmed cardiac cause, ventilate in enough oxygen to achieve target saturations of 75–85%. This may not always be achievable. Ensure the ventilator used is connected to an air and oxygen source, not just oxygen.

It would be ideal to have both pre and post-ductal monitoring of saturations but this may be a challenge during air transfer. Pre-ductal saturations, the measurement most reflective of cerebral perfusion, should be prioritised. Visual rather than audio alarms of the monitoring equipment should be used where possible, as noise levels are high during air transfers.

Circulation and Access

It is of critical importance to ensure prostaglandin E2/dinoprostone (Prostin) is available and to commence it early when a duct dependent congenital heart lesion is suspected. The dose of Prostin depends on the assessed clinical state. Apnoea is common in the first hour of starting Prostin and with increasing dose in critically ill or premature neonates. Higher doses of >20 nanograms/kg/min, if required, are generally only commenced in discussion with consultant intensivist or cardiologist.

Hypotension may occur with high doses of Prostin. Adequate, reliable, easily reachable and visible IV access, monitoring and preparation to include availability of emergency intra-osseous access, fluid boluses and inotropes are crucial. This cohort of patients can be very sensitive to fluid boluses necessitating cautious fluid resuscitation and continued assessment of heart failure.

Optimisation of systemic blood pressure and, if feasible, haemoglobin concentration may improve oxygen delivery.

Disability and Neurology

If the neonate is intubated and ventilated, ensure adequate sedation with morphine infusion. Muscle relaxant should be considered to reduce risk of endotracheal tube dislodgement during transfer as well as reducing metabolic demand.

The importance of temperature regulation in a neonate is well documented. A reliable method of monitoring neonatal temperature during transfer should be used. Altitude affects environmental temperature and can increase demand on the transport incubator/babypod. Hyperthermia is a known side effect of Prostin and should be managed to reduce energy consumption. Depending on flight conditions and weather, transwarmer mattresses or incubator covers can be used to warm up or avoid overheating from strong sunlight.

Glycaemic Control

Neonates with sepsis, heart disease, metabolic condition or intracranial bleed are all at high risk of hypoglycaemia. Careful management with adequate continuous glucose infusion and regular monitoring is important.

Communication and Clinical Preparedness

A neonate who is likely to need cardiac specialist management and intervention needs to be transferred to an appropriate PICU.

Effective communication between team members and reliable air to ground links should be well established. A clear plan anticipating and preparing for potential complications is important in any retrieval, more so in a neonatal helicopter transfer.

A typical helicopter transfer involves at least four loading and unloading events with the inability to immediately stop during the journey. It is important to minimise any adverse events by optimising management prior to transfer and accounting for the effects of the flight environment as well as physiological effects on the pathology of the neonate.

3. What are your other considerations when undertaking neonatal transfer?

A holistic approach towards the family is required with the management of any paediatric patient. In our region, a specialist neonatal transport team usually undertakes neonatal transfers unless a cardiac condition is suspected or confirmed. There are a few specific considerations for a neonatal transfer as discussed briefly below.

The mother's health and wellbeing as well as her fitness to travel post-partum with her infant should be considered. Discussions with parents will need to be had early on for a helicopter transfer as individual passengers and equipment weight impacts flight planning and activation. Expressed breast milk, if available, should be transported in an appropriate container with the infant.

Maternal pain management must be optimised prior to travel with help from the local team to ensure smooth air transfer. Motion sickness is more likely with helicopter transfers and parents should be informed of this. Occasionally, a mother may still be an in-patient and if appropriate, the local team should make every effort to transfer her care to be closer to her infant.

Siblings health and safety in an emergency may not be at the forefront of parents' minds. Older siblings' care needs to be arranged and if they themselves are unwell, they will need to be seen locally. Similarly, if the neonate is one of twins, every effort should be made to support parents in managing the logistics of both children's care.

This is a stressful and worrying time for a new parent; kindness and compassion from the team will make a huge difference.

Further Reading

Browning Carmo KA, Barr P, West M, et al. Transporting newborn infants with suspected duct dependent congenital heart disease on low-dose prostaglandin E1 without routine mechanical ventilation air air *Arch Dis Child Fetal Neonatal Ed* 2007;92(2):F117–19.

Dijkema EJ, Leiner T, Grotenhuis HB. Diagnosis, imaging and clinical management of aortic coarctation *Heart* 2017;103(15):1148–55.

Doshi AR, Chikkabyrappa S. Coarctation of aorta in children. *Cureus.* 2018;10(12):e3690.

Singh S, Hakim FA, Sharma A, et al. Hypoplasia, pseudocoarctation and coarctation of the aorta– a systematic review. *Heart Lung Circ* 2015;24:110–18.

Skeoch CH, Jackson L, Wilson AM, et al. Fit to fly: practical challenges in neonatal transfers by air *Arch Dis Child Fetal Neonatal Ed* 2005;90:F456–60.

Suradi H, Hijazi ZM. Current management of coarctation of the aorta. *Glob Cardiol Sci Pract.* 2015;2015(4):44, doi:10.5339/gcsp .2015.44.

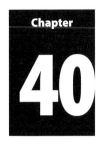
A Floppy Breathless Child

Sam Fosker and Shelley Riphagen

Initial Call

A 2-year-old girl with known spinal muscular atrophy (SMA) was referred with a 3-day history of worsening tachypnoea and increasing lethargy. She was no longer tolerating feeds and had visible mild intercostal and subcostal recession. Initially the child had improved on high flow nasal cannula (HFNC); however, oxygen requirements gradually increased to FiO_2 of 0.64 in 3 L/kg HFNC by the time of referral.

The child had been started on appropriate antibiotics and had received regular chest physiotherapy with moderate effect. She was only tolerating lying on her left hand side with oxygen saturations of 92–96% with the optiflow. She was alert but lethargic, answering questions in single words. Her physiological observations are noted in Table 40.1. There was no reported growth on blood cultures and nasopharyngeal aspirates were negative.

The referring team was unsure of her baseline, and it was difficult to elicit further information from her mother, who was inconsolably upset regarding the possibility of the child requiring transfer to PICU. The only additional relevant information was that the child had been reviewed by the tertiary respiratory team 2 months previously and was being considered for home non-invasive respiratory support. Her investigations from blood tests are shown in Table 40.2 and her admission CXR in Figure 40.1.

Questions

1. How will you best manage this patient's airway and breathing for transfer?
2. How might the patient's other medical conditions affect your plan?
3. How are you best going to support the mother?

1. How will you best manage this patient's airway and breathing for transfer?

Children with neuromuscular weakness are not always straightforward to evaluate with respect to respiratory failure. They may not have the power to increase their respiratory work. The only sign of respiratory failure in this group may be increasing tachypnoea, tachycardia and increasing lethargy or falling level of consciousness. They do not have the same reserve as children without muscle weakness.

Table 40.1. Physiologic observations

Heart rate	110 bpm
Blood pressure	113/66 mmHg
Respiratory rate	42 breaths per minute
Oxygen saturations	92%
Level of consciousness	A**V**PU

Table 40.2.

Blood tests		Venous gas	
White cell count	13.3 (10^3/mm^3)	pH	7.32
Haemoglobin	127 g/L	pO$_2$	32 kPa
Plts	493	pCO$_2$	5.9 kPa
Na	139 mmol/L	HCO$_3$	20 mmol/L
K	3.8 mmol/L	Basic excess	1.9 mEq/L
Urea	1.5 mmol/L	Lactate	0.7 mmol/L
Creatinine	18 U/L		

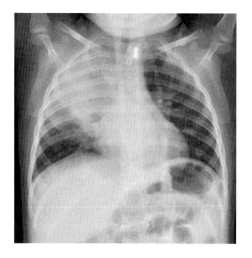

Figure 40.1 Admission chest radiograph.

Safety of the child during transfer is paramount. This requires anticipation of deterioration during the transfer. Factors affecting this evaluation include the current clinical status of the child, your plans for transfer and respiratory support available.

Your transfer ventilator may not allow for all modalities. HFNC is not available without specific equipment.

You must take into consideration how the transfer will affect both the clinical status and your ability to control respiratory support. The main options to consider for this child would be as follows.

Non-invasive Ventilation (NIV)

HFNC (Optiflow, vapotherm, AIRVO 2) The child is currently managing with this support. The humidified HFNC circuit may make it more comfortable for the child. This mode is not available on all transport ventilators. Additionally the stress of transfer and moving may destabilise the child. Not all ambulances carry the air cylinder capability for HFNC.

In this case, an alternative respiratory support modality will need to be started. Be prepared when changing a child from HFNC to another modality as the loss of positive pressure can lead to acute loss of recruited lung and acute desaturation.

Continuous/bilevel positive airway pressure (CPAP/BiPAP) These offer an alternative non-invasive support mode which is more widely available and can be delivered through a variety of different airway interfaces. **Nasal masks** can be sized with the relevant size guide. Aim to use the smallest fit to minimise leak. Nasal masks can be used as full face masks in younger children. **Full face masks** include masks that cover the mouth and nose, up to the forehead and full-head/helmet masks. Again these need to be sized appropriately so always take a variety of sizes on the transfer. Due to the variety of masks and devices available, ensure you take appropriate masks for your ventilator as these may not be available locally. CPAP/BiPAP can be delivered via dedicated devices (e.g. NIPPY/Trilogy) or as a setting on some transport ventilators (e.g. Babypac). Ensure all the correct equipment is taken on transfer as the invasive ventilation circuits are different to those used for NIV. Some teams produce a purpose-made box for NIV with all the equipment you will need. Table 40.3 summarises initial settings to use when setting up NIV.

There are some relative and absolute contraindications to the use of NIV including: airway obstruction, base of skull fracture, undrained pneumothorax, decreased level of consciousness, large amounts of secretions or possibility of vomiting, bowel obstruction, haemodynamic instability, severe hypoxia/hypercarbia, combative/unco-operative patient, recent facial trauma/burns/surgery preventing a good seal with the mask.

Once NIV has been started the settings can be adjusted depending on the clinical status of the child:

Table 40.3.

Mode	Pressure support/ pressure control
Inspiratory positive airway pressure	5–12 cm H_2O (start low if child is anxious and gradually increase)
Expiratory positive airway pressure	4–5 cm H_2O
Insp time in pressure control mode	0.4–0.8 sec depending on spontaneous rate
Backup rate	5 breaths per min below normal patient rate
F_iO_2	As required to maintain saturations >90%
Trigger	Inspiratory and expiratory trigger set to 4 (normal default)
Flow alarms	High alarm 20% max flow recorded at peak pressure Low alarm 20% below min recorded at peak pressure

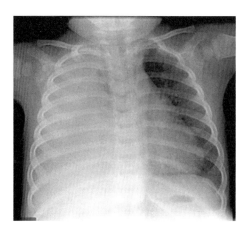

Figure 40.2 Repeat chest radiograph after acute respiratory deterioration.

Increase expiratory positive airway pressure by 2–3 cm H_2O (to a maximum of 10 cm H_2O) to improve oxygenation

Increase inspiratory positive airway pressure by 2–4 cm H_2O (to a maximum of 25 cm H_2O) to improve ventilation.

Children requiring in excess of these pressures, should be re-evaluated carefully for invasive ventilation.

Invasive Ventilation

If non-invasive methods are not suitable or the child deteriorates, the child will need to be intubated. This should be undertaken prior to transfer with careful consideration regarding anaesthesia and muscle relaxation, remembering that some children with myopathies react adversely to anaesthetic agents, and muscle relaxants have a more prolonged and profound effect.

Decision for intubation to facilitate invasive ventilation should be made with the referring team based on response to treatment and the duration of the transfer.

The child had a CXR prior to you arriving at the referring hospital. This is shown in Figure 40.2. How would this affect your plan?

The CXR has worsened markedly from the admission CXR only a few days prior. This is in keeping with the clinical picture. This would change your decision regarding intubation and ventilation as clearly the non-invasive support has not prevented this deterioration. With such significant parenchymal changes and reduction in lung compliance, the child is less likely to tolerate NIV and will have reduced reserve.

Having the child supine and secured to a stretcher will likely worsen their respiratory distress. This child is best managed with intubation and invasive ventilation which will also allow adequate airway toilette and some gentle physiotherapy prior to transfer.

2. How might the patient's other medical conditions affect your plan?

SMA is an autosomal recessive disease characterised by progressive muscle wasting due to degeneration of motor neurons in the spinal cord and brainstem. The defective *SMN1* gene

Table 40.4.

Name (type)	Age of onset	Characteristics
1. Wernig–Hoffmann disease (Infantile)	0–6 months	Quick onset in first few months of life 'floppy baby syndrome'. Very aggressive form known as SMA type 0.
2. Dubowitz (Intermediate)	6–18 months	Children not able to stand or walk, slower progressive deterioration. Can develop scoliosis requiring brace to help support respiration.
3. Kugelberg–Welander	>12 months	Usually able to walk, often requiring support as develops later. Less respiratory involvement and hence life expectancy is near normal.
4. Adult onset	Adulthood	Usually after 3rd decade of life. Mostly affecting proximal muscle groups, person may need wheelchair but other complications rare

results in inadequate production of SMN protein, which is vital for growth and development of motor neurons. There are four types of SMA as noted in Table 40.4.

As well as SMA, children with other neuromuscular disorders (e.g. muscular dystrophies/congenital myopathies) may experience an apparently acute deterioration with any respiratory illness. Muscle wasting and weakness associated with these conditions means children may not be able to generate the required clinical respiratory response and the work of breathing may look falsely reassuring until very late in clinical deterioration. Alongside the respiratory issues, this group of children may have other problems associated with their underlying disease process. These can include unsafe swallow and poor feeding, gastro-oesophageal reflux, excessive secretions, scoliosis and cardiomyopathy. These all need to be taken into account when managing the child (e.g. making the child nil by mouth if aspiration is a risk due to poor swallow).

Understanding of the child's baseline function, may affect the assessment for intubation. Discussion with the family, which may not be possible in this case, or review of relevant letters and investigations within the child's notes will aid decision making.

Some children with myopathies have home NIV already and this can be used for increasing periods to prevent the need of intubation. Their mask will have been properly sized and the child will be used to it, reducing the risk of respiratory deterioration.

Families of children with chronic conditions will often have extensive knowledge around the condition and prognosis. This may make any difficult conversations easier as discussions around long-term ventilation, management of deterioration and end-of-life care planning may have been started previously. Never assume these have happened and identify the family's understanding of the situation and how the disease process may progress.

If the child needs intubation, there is a possibility this may be for a prolonged period. Successful extubation on first attempt may be difficult and early discussion into potential issues will make it easier for the family. The child may have advanced care plans in place and knowing the ceilings of treatment will be important when transferring them to higher level care.

New treatments with SMA and other neuromuscular disorders are continually being developed. Some of these have shown improvement in long-term survival but are also changing parental expectations of care. Always discuss the child's acute presentation with the primary clinical team responsible for their long-term care. They may be able to offer guidance on the disease progression and expected clinical course of the individual child.

3. How are you best going to support the mother?

In this scenario you are told the mother had become inconsolable and wasn't engaging with the referring team. This would make communicating with her and discussing ongoing plans difficult. Ultimately the child's safety and getting them to the relevant care facility is your main priority but involvement with the family and carers should happen at all stages.

This becomes more relevant when considering transfer options as you will often be in a confined space and need to be certain you can perform any needed interventions. If there is any concern that having a parent/carer on the transfer compromises this safety, other options should be sought. These discussions are often difficult and decisions should be made as a team to ensure everyone is in agreement. Other options include:

- Giving the parent details of your destination to arrange their own transport with a family member for support. Depending on local resources, you may be able to assist with this (e.g. booking a taxi).
- If there are concerns the child may deteriorate en route or having the parent close on the transfer may provide benefit, for example as comfort for an awake child, the parent or carer should be encouraged to accompany the transfer.

Taking time to speak to parents and carers is a vital part of any transfer or retrieval. The journey to PICU with an accompanying caregiver provides uninterrupted time to take a good history and understand the child and family. Parents will often have much more detailed insight into the acute state of the child and also their background medical history. Time taken in this setting often pays dividends later. It is an opportunity to ensure crucial information has not been lost in the handover between teams and to begin to establish a working relationship with the parent.

Further Reading

Davidson AC, Banham S, Elliot M, et al. BTS/ICS guideline for the ventilatory management of acute hypercapnic respiratory failure. *Thorax* 2016;71:ii1–ii35.

Farrell PT. Rigid bronchoscopy for foreign body removal: anaesthesia and ventilation. *Ped Anaes* 2004;14(1):84–9

Hull J, Aniapravan R, Chan E, et al. British Thoracic Society guideline for respiratory management of children with neuromuscular weakness. *Thorax* 2012;67:i1–40.

Zhao H, Wang H, Sun F, et al. High-flow nasal cannula oxygen therapy is superior to conventional oxygen therapy but not to noninvasive mechanical ventilation on intubation rate: a systematic review and meta-analysis. *Crit Care* 2017;21(1):184, doi: 10.1186/s13054-017-1760-8.

Fever in the Time of COVID-19 (SARS-CoV2)

Marilyn McDougall

A 9-year-old, previously well girl presented with a 5-day history of lethargy, fever and muscle pain. In addition, she had experienced significant abdominal pain with diarrhoea for 3 days. In the previous 2 days her mother had also noted a painless non-purulent conjunctivitis. This child presented 10 days after the SARS-CoV2 /COVID-19 pandemic had reached peak incidence in London, UK.

At the time of presentation she was febrile (temperature 39°C), tachypnoeic (respiratory rate 22 breaths per minute) and without any other signs of respiratory distress. She was well saturated (98%) in room air, but tachycardic (heart rate 140bpm) and hypotensive (BP 80/ 35). Her peripheries were warm but her pulse volume was reduced. She had been treated with a bolus of 20 ml/kg of normal saline for shock. This had not resulted in any significant change in her clinical condition. A second bolus of 20 ml/kg was in progress at the time of the referral. As the referral was made she had an acute episode of profound hypotension (systolic BP < 60 mmHg) with impalpable pulses as she was being lifted onto a bedpan. She was immediately placed back in a supine position and the retrieval team was called for advice.

Her abdomen was distended without any palpable organomegaly. She had passed urine earlier in the day. There were no focal neurological signs and she appeared to be alert and appropriate.

Of note in her history, her maternal uncle was a doctor who had been working in A&E at the time of the SARS-CoV2 outbreak. He had contracted coronavirus and was still critically unwell when this patient was admitted. Investigations are shown in Tables 41.1 and 41.2.

Questions

1. What is your advice for ongoing management of this patient?
2. What antimicrobial therapy should be given?
3. What clinical conditions/ syndromes have been noted in children during the 2019/2020 SARS-COV2 pandemic that might be relevant for this patient?
4. Would you consider any additional therapy for this patient?

1. What is your advice for ongoing management of this patient?

The patient remains shocked despite 40 ml/kg of fluid boluses. The clinical features presented are suggestive of septic shock. Adequate IV access, ideally at least two large bore (22/20 gauge) cannulae, is essential to provide ongoing therapy. The patient should be

Table 41.1. Initial blood tests

Blood tests		Further blood tests	
Haemoglobin	122 g/L	CRP	278 mg/L
White cell count	$15.6 \times 10^3/mm^3$	Procalcitonin	70 µg/L
Neutrophils	$12.1 \times 10^3/mm^3$	Fibrinogen	4.1 g/L
Lymphocytes	$0.75 \times 10^3/mm^3$	Ferritin	924 µg/L
Platelets	$175 \times 10^3/mm^3$	Troponin	830 µg/L
Na	126 mmol/L	Pro BNP	35,000 nanograms/L
K	4.3 mmol/L		
Creatinine	110 U/L		

Table 41.2. Initial blood gas

pH	7.36
pCO_2	4.6 kPa
pO_2	NA
HCO_3	23 mmol/L
Base excess	−3.mEq/L
Lactate	4.5 mmol/L
Glucose	5.7 mmol/L

carefully examined to exclude features of cardiac failure which may complicate septic shock in children. The elevated cardiac enzymes (troponin T and brain natriuretic peptide [BNP]) are concerning and may indicate myocardial involvement. In children <5 years of age, an enlarged liver and gallop rhythm may be noted. In older patients elevated jugular venous pressure, gallop rhythm and new onset mitral regurgitation murmur may indicate heart failure. An ECG should be performed once the patient's blood pressure and clinical state has stabilised. Any evidence of an abnormal ECG or signs of heart failure would mandate transfer to a PICU with onsite cardiology for an urgent assessment.

In children who remain hypotensive and tachycardic despite appropriate fluid resuscitation (40–60 ml/kg), early initiation of inotrope therapy is indicated. Dopamine 5 mcg/kg was started in this patient after the acute episode of hypotension. The patient remained tachycardic and hypotensive. The dopamine was escalated which resulted in a gradual rise in the BP (98/58) and fall in the heart rate (118 bpm).

If the patient had not responded to dopamine, noradrenaline could have been added to support the blood pressure. This is in keeping with the latest Surviving Sepsis guidelines and an appropriate response to the wide pulse pressure (diastolic BP <½ systolic BP) at the time of presentation. Noradrenaline could be commenced at a low dose 0.05 mcg/kg and escalated to a maximum of 1 mcg/kg depending on the clinical response. Noradrenaline is best administered via central line. Even a single lumen femoral cannula would be appropriate in this setting. Any inotropes, such as adrenaline, noradrenaline or dopamine, which are given via a peripheral cannula should be administered in a dilute formulation to prevent local tissue injury.

The patient remained well saturated without any signs of respiratory failure, therefore no respiratory support apart from face mask oxygen at 10 L/min via non-breath bag for shock management was applied.

2. What antimicrobial therapy should be given?

Surviving Sepsis Campaign guidelines recommend the administration of broad-spectrum antibiotics within 1 hour of recognition of septic shock. This patient has features which would be in keeping with toxic shock (fever, conjunctivitis and diarrhoea) therefore broad spectrum antibiotics which cover both Group A *Streptococcus* and *Staphylococcus* such as ceftriaxone would be appropriate. In addition clindamycin is recommended to inhibit further toxin production by the bacteria.

The lymphopenia may be suggestive of a viral infection or overwhelming infection. However careful monitoring of this patient would be important to ensure that an underlying immune disorder is not missed if the lymphopenia does not resolve.

3. What clinical conditions/ syndromes have been noted in children during the 2019/2020 SARS-COV2 pandemic that may be relevant for this patient?

A new multisystem hyper-inflammatory disorder was identified in children during the COVID-19 pandemic. This is called PIM-TS(**P**aediatric **M**ultisystem **I**nflammatory **S**yndrome – **T**emporally Associated with **S**ARS-CoV-2) in the UK and MIS-C (Multisystem Inflammatory Syndrome in Children) by the Center for Disease Control in the USA and the WHO. The combination of fever, abdominal pain, shock, elevated CRP, procalcitonin (PCT) and lymphopenia are highly suggestive of this diagnosis in the patient. The recent contact with an uncle who has SARS-COV-2 would be an additional risk factor for the diagnosis.

The RCPCH case definition is broad:

1. A child presenting with persistent fever, inflammation (neutrophilia, elevated CRP and lymphopenia) and evidence of single or multiorgan dysfunction (shock, cardiac, respiratory, renal, gastrointestinal or neurological disorder) with additional features. This may include children fulfilling full or partial criteria for Kawasaki disease.
2. Exclusion of any other microbial cause, including bacterial sepsis, staphylococcal or streptococcal shock syndromes, infections associated with myocarditis, such as enterovirus. Waiting for results of these investigations should not delay seeking expert advice.
3. SARS-CoV-2 PCR testing may be positive or negative.

Many features of this overlap with Kawasaki disease. During the 2020 COVID19 pandemic in one region of Italy, paediatricians noted a 30-fold increase in the number of children presenting with Kawasaki disease.

Due to the similarities, and many clinical features of this new condition, which overlap with both Kawasaki disease and toxic shock syndrome, early support from both infectious diseases and cardiologist is recommended. Very close monitoring and anticipation of cardiovascular deterioration and the risk of development of coronary artery aneurysms is essential in the care of this group of patients.

Early experience of this disease supported early escalation of inotrope therapy including milrinone, dopamine and noradrenaline to support the cardiovascular system. Respiratory failure was rarely present in these cases and many children were able to be supported with non-invasive ventilation.

A comprehensive list of the clinical and laboratory features and appropriate initial management and investigations is available on the RCPCH website: www.rcpch.ac.uk/resources/covid-19-guidance-management-children-admitted-hospital.

4. Would you consider any additional therapy for this patient?

The patient would fulfil the criteria for PIMS-TS while further microbiological tests are pending. Due to the risk of coronary artery aneurysms developing, several immunomodulatory and anticoagulation treatment options should be considered with support from paediatric infection and cardiology experts.

IVIG 2 g/kg has been shown to reduce the incidence of coronary aneurysms in Kawasaki disease and is therefore usually recommended for PIMS-TS cases. For refractory cases of Kawasaki disease or PIMS-TS defined as persistent fever and progressive aneurysms despite IVIG therapy, prednisolone may be added.

Low dose aspirin 3–5 mg/kg is recommended to reduce the risk of coronary ischaemia in the presence of coronary artery inflammation.

Finally due to the increased incidence of thrombosis in adults with COVID19 related hyper-inflammatory conditions, thromboprophylaxis is recommended for children admitted to hospital to prevent thrombotic events. The elevated fibrinogen and other inflammatory markers would suggest an increased risk of thrombosis in this cohort of patient.

Further Reading

Riphagen S, Gomez X, Gonzalez-Martinez C, et al. Hyperinflammatory shock in children during COVID-19 pandemic. *The Lancet* 2020;395 (10237):1607–8.

Royal College of Paediatrics and Child Health (RCPCH) Guidance: Paediatric multisystem inflammatory syndrome temporally associated with Covid-19. www.rcpch.ac.uk/resources/covid-19-guidance-management-children-admitted-hospital.

Verdoni L, Mazza A, Gervasoni A, et al. An outbreak of severe Kawasaki-like disease at the Italian Epicenter of the SARS-Cov_2 epidemic: an observational cohort study. *The Lancet* 2020;395(10239):1771–8.

Weiss SL, Peters MJ, Alhazzan W, et al. Surviving sepsis campaign international guidelines for the management of septic shock and sepsis-associated organ dysfunction in children. *Intensive Care Med* 2020;46:10–67, doi.org/10.1007/s00134–019-05878-6.

A Palliative Care Transfer Home

Miriam Fine-Goulden and Jo Laddie

A 6-week old baby, who was intubated and ventilated, had been managed in PICU for a complex congenital heart defect. Second and third opinions had been sought from additional paediatric cardiac centres, including in the United States, and after much consultation and discussion, it had been agreed by the multidisciplinary team, including all the external consultations, that the heart defect was inoperable.

He had been receiving an infusion of prostaglandin E2 (prostin) to maintain ductal patency while the consultation was ongoing. IV access had been challenging towards the end of the 6 weeks, and he had one patent cannula through which the prostaglandin infusion was running. Parents had come to the point where, if there was no medical or surgical solution for their baby, they did not wish their baby to have another IV cannula sited. The palliative care team had been involved with the baby's care as part of the multidisciplinary team, and discussions with the family had taken place to consider his end-of-life care.

With support from the palliative care team regarding their choices in this situation, the parents had decided that they wanted to take their baby home to spend whatever time they had with him at home. The retrieval team had been asked to facilitate the transfer home of this baby, and the subsequent extubation in the home setting, with the support of the palliative care team, and a prior agreed plan of care for the baby. This plan had been made in consultation with the parents. Imagine yourself in this position.

Questions

1. In this setting, is it appropriate to have a discussion about organ donation?
2. What preparation is required when planning this transfer?
3. What do the PICU and retrieval team need to hand over to the children's community nurses or paediatric palliative care team?

1. In this setting, is it appropriate to have a discussion about organ donation?

Absolutely. Paediatric donation following circulatory death (DCD) rather than donation following neurological determination of death (also known as 'donation after brain death', or DBD) would be applicable in this situation. As DCD involves a degree of ischaemic time following cessation of the circulation, the potential for organ donation is more limited than in cases of DBD. In addition, it would require that the baby dies in hospital – in particular in theatres under controlled conditions. For some families, this is a death that they would be prepared to plan for, but others might prefer to plan for a death outside of a hospital environment. The family would need to be aware of this choice when discussing options for end-of-life care including organ donation.

Although this baby would have been ineligible to donate his heart, he may have been eligible to donate other organs. This should be discussed with the Specialist Nurses for Organ Donation (SNODs). Organ donation at this age is uncommon, but there are many babies awaiting transplant of different organs for whom an infant donor is essential. Furthermore, hepatocyte donation can help multiple recipients.

Organ donation laws in England in place from spring 2020 include a newly introduced opt-out system but this does not apply to children under the age of 18 years. (Max and Kiera's Law) Organ Donation (Deemed Consent) Act 2019.

2.   What preparation is required when planning this transfer?

In particular:
- What paperwork needs to be completed prior to transfer?
- What community support needs to be arranged?
- What medications should be prescribed for discharge?
- Is there any special equipment required?

Transferring the Baby Home for Palliative Care

Ideally, the transport team would consist of a doctor or advanced nurse practitioner and a transport nurse who are not only trained in the transfer of the critically ill patient but also know the baby and family and have managed end of life before. The transport should have been arranged electively – preferably in the morning, as this allows for delays and also ensures arrival during working hours, when community services are most likely to be available. Palliative care transfers out of hours and on weekends are much more difficult in terms of logistic support and should be avoided if possible.

The transport team should inform the community team of the expected time of arrival at the home or hospice, call them to inform them of their departure as they leave the unit, and update the team if there are any delays en route.

The PICU and palliative care teams should have had discussions with the family about the transport arrangements. There may be space to take both parents in the ambulance with the baby, but if not, arrangements should be made to transfer the remaining parent home at the same time as the ambulance.

Discussions must have taken place – and been documented appropriately – regarding the potential for the baby to become unstable, deteriorate or die during the journey. One aspect of care that must be clarified is the potential for loss of IV access in the ambulance, and the parents' stated wish for no further attempts at IV cannulation. For this baby, it was therefore agreed that in the event of loss of IV access, the prostaglandin would be given via the oral route.

The baby had been receiving morphine and clonidine for sedation via the enteral route (via nasogastric tube) whilst intubated and ventilated. Clinicians unaccustomed to end-of-life care for children may feel uneasy about using higher than usual doses of sedating medications, which are prescribed to help maintain comfort. If these medications continue to be delivered by the clinical teams to this end, there need not be undue concern that a child's death is being expedited. If any concerns persist, these should be discussed with the palliative care team prior to transfer. Sedative medications may be weaned prior to transfer and extubation, although this may not be feasible depending on the clinical state of the patient. If, however, they are only being used for comfort for an endotracheal tube, they should be discontinued before extubation. Before leaving hospital, the resuscitation status of the child must be clear to all. A plan should be agreed with regards to what to do should a baby extubate during transfer or deteriorate en route. If it is the parent's wishes, it may be possible for the ambulance to stop in a place of safety, and the baby could be taken gently out of the transport pod and placed into their arms. If the baby died in the ambulance, then at an appropriate time, the ambulance would continue to the family home and care of the family would be transferred to the community team.

The time of death is accepted as the time of confirmation of death by a medical practitioner.

What paperwork needs to be completed prior to transfer?

Symptom management plan – this is a comprehensive list of anticipated symptoms that the baby may experience and detailed plans of management that include both comforting measures and pharmacologically appropriate dose regimes. This plan would be prepared by the palliative care team who will provide support once in the community.

There are contact details for the palliative care team involved, for additional guidance and support. A 2-week supply of all the medications listed on the plan may need to be sent with the plan, in addition to all the consumables required (syringes, flushes, etc).

Emergency Care Plan – this will include:
- demographic details of the patient and family
- contact details of all healthcare teams involved with the patient
- diagnosis
- a plan of action in the event of an acute deterioration (e.g. if an ambulance was called to the home or hospice) with specific agreements on levels of escalation and/or intervention and a plan of action in the event of a more gradual deterioration. This should also include a plan for what to do if the patient deteriorates during transfer.
- some details of additional preferences that have been discussed, for example, about organ donation, preferred place of care and death, use of bereavement suite at the hospice. In addition, there should be documentation regarding explanations about confirmation of death, certification of death, post-mortem, etc.
- signatures of palliative care team and parents to reflect care wishes at time of discussion, with the caveat that parents can change their mind about treatment plans at any time.
- Resuscitation status: Do Not Attempt Cardiopulmonary Resuscitation (DNAR) which has been signed by a consultant and dated.

Additional documentation: Nursing Care Plan, medical notes and drug chart

What community support needs to be arranged?
Community Paediatric Palliative Care Team

This family will need the support and care from a children's community nursing team. They should also have the support of a team of paediatric palliative care nurses, with liaison from a palliative care consultant (these may be community based or from a tertiary team).

Children's Hospice

The local children's hospice should be involved in discussions about the baby's discharge at the earliest opportunity as although the parents have chosen to take their baby home, they may change their minds and wish for hospice care at any time. If the baby dies at home, then his parents would also be offered (if available) the use of the bereavement suite at the hospice, which allows them to spend time with their baby after he dies. Referral to a hospice needs to happen whilst the child is alive and requires the consent of the family as information is transferred across sectors. Of note, a family does not have to actually use the hospice at all during their child's life to be able to use it in their death or afterwards. The palliative care team will be able to explain what services hospices offer. Sometimes, hospice staff will come and meet parents prior to discharge.

General Practitioner

It is essential that the local GP is informed of the planned discharge of the baby from the hospital for end-of-life care. It is helpful if the GP comes to review the baby following transfer to facilitate optimal care of the baby and family. The ideal time for the GP to meet the child and family is when the child had arrived safely and been settled in by the transport team, so that if there are any questions, they can be answered immediately. In addition, for a doctor to be able to issue a Medical Certificate of Certification of Death (MCCD – usually referred to as 'death certificate'), following certification of death, he/she must have seen the baby alive in the 14 days preceding death, otherwise the death must be referred to the coroner before it can be registered. It is important that the family knows whom to contact if their baby dies outside normal working hours. The palliative care team will also be able to talk them through care of the body after death. Under certain circumstances, GPs may only meet the child and family via a video conference and do not have to physically see the baby face to face.

What medication should be prescribed and dispensed for discharge?

It is good practice for all medication that has been prescribed for symptom management as well as all regular medication that the baby requires, to be supplied for transfer and for the first 2 weeks in the community. Paediatric hospices do not have drug stores. In addition, medications should be dispensed with all appropriate consumables. After 2 weeks, on-going supplies, if required, will be provided by the GP.

Is there any special equipment required?

In certain situations equipment such as feed pumps, suction, oxygen or syringe drivers may be required, and these need to be sourced prior to transfer. Often, such equipment is available in the ambulance for the transfer home or to the hospice and then not required thereafter. A plan needs to be agreed for safe return of hospital equipment from the community when it is no longer needed.

3. What do the PICU and retrieval team need to hand over to the children's community nurses or paediatric palliative care team?

- Baby's medical notes, nursing care plans, emergency care plan and symptom management plan, contact details of referring team.

- The take home drugs could include controlled drugs such as midazolam or morphine, and these will need to be stored in a locked box within the parents' home.
- Family dynamic – who are the main carers, names of siblings or others who may be present.
- Religious considerations and plans either before death or after.

A member of the community or palliative care team should be present at handover and once everything is handed over. It is the responsibility of the transport team to identify a suitable time to stop ongoing therapy and remove life-sustaining equipment, for example stopping ventilation and removal of the endotracheal tube. This should have been explored when completing the Emergency Care Plan with the palliative care team who will have explained that prolonged periods of ventilation (in general more than 2 hours) are not feasible. There is never a 'right time' and it is so important that the family do not feel 'rushed', but the family should have time for cuddles and photos, time to make themselves comfortable, to have family support present if so desired or religious leaders at hand, before gently asking if they were ready.

It is very important to establish who is present and what they have been told before talking to the present company because occasionally parents have made their decision about palliative care but do not want this decision publicised as their community may not support this action.

Previous discussion at the hospital prior to transfer will guide what therapy is discontinued (e.g. positive pressure ventilation), cessation of IV therapy and removal of IV cannulae, but may also guide what therapy is continued, for example medication, feeds or the use of suction.

There should also be an agreement, prior to transfer, regarding who will remove any life-sustaining treatment and who the family want present in the room at the time. It is often not appropriate for all members of the clinical team to remain in the room. Generally, we would recommend one member of the transfer team and one member of the palliative care team or community nursing team who will be responsible for withdrawal and then subsequent initial symptom management.

It is good practice to agree, prior to withdrawal, a plan for administration of any medications around the time of withdrawal, for example sedative or analgesic medicine may be continued for the purpose of pain relief and sedation (The Rainbows Children's Hospice Guidelines 2016). It is important to note that medications should be available to administer via subcutaneous, buccal or enteral route if the baby becomes distressed. It is important that families have had normal anticipated physiological changes explained in advance, so they understand the rationale for when it is and is not, appropriate to administer medications.

Memory Making with the Family before or after the Death of Their Baby

Care of a dying baby includes trying to find moments of joy and making happy memories. There are many different charities that not only fund memory boxes for families, but also support them after the baby or child has died. Photographs are very important, but also families may wish to be involved helping make hand and footprints, giving a baby bath or hair wash, either before or after their baby has died. Hand over to the community palliative care nurses what the parents' preferences are at the time, although they may change later.

Although the transport team is not able to change the outcome for children at the end of their lives, being able to provide kind and compassionate care to families at this most difficult of times is of tremendous value and is something they will never forget.

Further Reading

Basic Symptom Control in Paediatric Palliative Care, 2016. Together for Short Lives. The Rainbows Children's Hospice Guidelines. www.togetherforshortlives.org.uk/resource/basic-symptom-control-paediatric-palliative-care/.

Max and Kiera's Law. Organ Donation (Deemed Consent) Act 2019. UK Parliament. Effective Spring 2020.

Together for Short Lives. A UK charity for children with life threatening and life limiting conditions. www.togetherfor shortlives.org.uk. This is also a great resource for healthcare professionals caring for these children.

Winston's Wish Charity www.winstonswish.org. Free National Helpline 08088 020 021 Giving hope to grieving children.

Acknowledgement: With thanks to Dr Jo Laddie, Consultant in Paediatric Palliative Medicine, Evelina London Children's Hospital for checking and editing the chapter for accuracy.

A Story that Just Doesn't Add Up

Emma Smith and Shelley Riphagen

A 3-year-old boy who was previously fit and well was reported to have fallen down the stairs at home 4 days previously and had been brought to his local hospital A&E with vomiting.

On the day of the fall he had been taken to a hospital nearby the home, had been reviewed and discharged after being seen in A&E, with written head injury advice. The mother reported that for the following 2 days he was not 'himself' and returned to the referring hospital on the third day after injury with lethargy, fever and vomiting. The referring hospital had no record of exactly what had been done at the first hospital, with only history from mum. For this reason he had had a CT head performed, which was normal, but he had remained in hospital for observation, because of the head injury concern.

On the day of referral, he had developed significant abdominal pain and on examination had a generally tender abdomen with guarding and a low grade temperature. He was reviewed by the local surgical team who felt he had likely appendicitis but had performed abdominal X-rays to exclude other causes (Figure 43.1). Following discussion with the tertiary paediatric surgical team they were concerned about the recent fall, and had asked for him to be transferred to the tertiary hospital for review. He had been accepted by the tertiary surgical team. The transfer was referred to the retrieval team in view of the child's worsening clinical picture.

A second phone call was received prior to the retrieval team leaving. The local team reported that on further examination, they had seen some bruising on his face including both pinna (Figures 43.2 and 43.3), and also on his back, that had not been noticed before. They have given him a 20 ml/kg fluid bolus of 0.9% NaCl because of his heart rate. Observations and blood results at the time of referral are shown in Tables 43.1 and 43.2.

Questions

1. What are your current concerns, both clinical and social, regarding the child's presentation?
2. What are your immediate considerations in regard to transferring this child?
3. You are concerned about the mechanism of injury: how would you approach this with the parents?

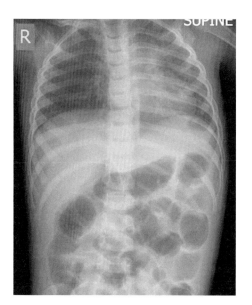

Figure 43.1 Admission abdominal radiograph.

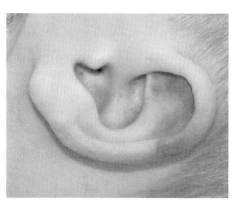

Figure 43.2 Bruising around pinna. (A black and white version of this figure will appear in some formats. For the colour version, please refer to the plate section.)

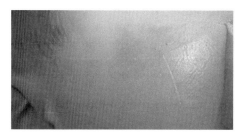

Figure 43.3 Bruising around face. (A black and white version of this figure will appear in some formats. For the colour version, please refer to the plate section.)

1. What are your current clinical concerns, both clinical and social, regarding the child's presentation?

At the time of referral the child was tachycardic despite being afebrile. His blood pressure was preserved and he had a mildly raised CRP. He had a generally tender abdomen, and

Table 43.1.

Blood tests		Venous blood gas)	
Haemoglobin	12.3 g/L	pH	7.34
White cell count	$12.1 \times 10^3/mm^3$	pCO_2	5.8 kPa
Platelets	$300 \times 10^3/mm^3$	pO_2	7.6 kPa
Na	129 mmol/L	Base excess	−1.3 mEq/L
K	5.0 mmol/L	Lactate	1.5 mmol/L
Urea	5.6 mmol/L	Glucose	7.8 mmol/L
Creatinine	36 U/L	HCO_3^-	23.4 mmol/L
CRP	86 mg/L		

Table 43.2.

Heart rate	160 bpm
Respiratory rate	40 breaths per minute
Sats	100% in 4 L/min O_2
Blood pressure	105/57 mmHg
Temperature	36.6°C
AVPU	Alert

Table 43.3.

Gastrointestinal	Genitourinary	Respiratory	Other
Intussusception	Urinary tract infection	Pneumonia	Ovarian torsion
Malrotation and volvulus	Testicular	Empyema	Abdominal malignancy
Appendicitis	torsion		
Meckel's diverticulum			
Pancreatitis			
Inflammatory bowel disease			

there was a history of falling down the stairs. Your immediate concern should be that of an acute abdomen, possibly secondary to trauma. A significant head injury had been excluded by the previous CT head.

Causes of acute abdominal pain are wide and could involve a number of body systems as seen in Table 43.3.

It is important to consider all of these possibilities but in this case your initial concern would be trauma following the fall, in the presence of facial and back bruising.

Paediatric trauma, beyond the regular bumps and bruises, is an area that can cause much worry, particularly because children can't always tell us what the problem is and where it hurts.

When thinking about a child vs an adult in regard to trauma, there are a number of important differences:

- Children have a large head compared to body – therefore are more at risk of cervical shearing injuries
- Neck muscles are weaker, cervical spine injuries occur at a higher spinal level
- Cartilaginous ribs lead to a more compliant chest wall, pulmonary contusion occurs without rib fractures
- Intra-abdominal organs are less protected and so more at risk of solid organ injury
- The bladder is an abdominal rather than pelvic organ and so there is increased risk of bladder injury
- Children, in general, have an absolute smaller blood volume – an insignificant haemorrhage in an adult might be life threatening for a child
- Long bones are more flexible leading to greenstick fractures

Abdominal injuries are something not often seen in paediatrics. A history of trauma might prompt the clinical team to consider it earlier, but it should be high on your differential list as it often goes unrecognised.

Abdominal injuries are a significant cause of morbidity and mortality in abused children, particularly as symptoms are often non-specific, and as reported in a RCPCH review article, mainly occur in pre-school children with limited communication.

A key clue that abdominal trauma might be present is bruising found during careful examination (though up to 80% of cases have no bruising present). Other investigations such as FAST scan, urine dipstick for haematuria or an abdominal ultrasound might also help, particularly if performed by a paediatric radiologist. A CT abdomen is, however, more beneficial, particularly if looking for pancreatic or duodenal injuries, as it can identify small amounts of free intraperitoneal air more accurately.

The commonest missed intra-abdominal pathology is retroperitoneal duodenal injury.

2. What are your immediate considerations in regard to transferring this child?

It is best in this situation to split your thoughts into those that are medical and those regarding the parents.

- The child has an unexplained tachycardia. This could be due to pain but also shock due to inadequate fluid resuscitation and this should be your first priority.
- Fluid resuscitation is important. The gut is a key area where fluid can be lost into the third space and if there is any pathological intraperitoneal process, then further boluses will be needed, often more than you think.
- Fluid can be given in 10 ml/kg aliquots – APLS guidelines suggest 10 ml/kg increments so that you do not give too much volume and disrupt any clot formation as 'the first clot is the best clot'. If you do have any intra-abdominal bleeding concerns then you may also need to give platelets or additional blood products.
- Aim for **Hb>10 g/dl, platelet >100 × 10^9/L** until major bleeding is no longer a risk and **INR/APTT <1.3** and **fibrinogen >1.5**.
- If you have a falling Hb then consider getting blood for transfer. It can be started at the hospital prior to transfer and continued en route, although all efforts should be made to control any bleeding if possible.

- Use small doses of analgesia to relieve both pain and also prevent both hypertension (to prevent clot rupture) and tachycardia – generally aim for a slightly lower systolic BP than higher.
- Be aware of evolving abdominal compartment syndrome which could impede ventilation. You may need to intubate the child prior to transfer and use higher ventilation pressures then you might initially anticipate. This may necessitate a cuffed endotracheal tube.
- Following your assessment it is important to consider if you are transferring to a suitable site. If you have concerns of abdominal injury, is a general surgeon available at the admitting tertiary institution and willing to take over care. You may also need the advice or input of a neurosurgeon.

Parents are usually encouraged to be present for transfer but this has to be balanced with both yours and the child's safety.

If you are concerned about a mechanism of injury then transfer can be an ideal time to both observe the parent interacting with the child but also take the opportunity to obtain a history from that parent and allow the receiving hospital to take a history from the second parent, to see if they corroborate. Any conversations should be documented 'verbatim'.

If you are concerned that the parent/s could become disruptive to the child's care, which is unusual, then they should not travel in the ambulance with you. You will need to explain that they can meet you at the local hospital.

3. You are concerned about the mechanism of injury: how would you approach this with the parents?

Children often injure themselves. They are very mobile, active and have significantly less fear than adults. What is important to always consider, is whether the history you have been given fits with the clinical findings you have in front of you. Paediatricians have extensive training with regards to safeguarding, but in the acute situation it is easy to get distracted with addressing immediate clinical concerns. Whilst it is always important to ensure that the child is stabilised, you must always consider 'does this make sense?' and if in doubt discuss your concerns with colleagues.

In this case, the child had bruising on his ears and back which are not areas that children commonly have bruising from normal play, and would have been difficult to bruise by a fall downstairs without significant bruising elsewhere.

If the concern about non-accidental injury has not been raised previously and you are concerned, then speak to the local team looking after the child and ensure that any concerns that you or they have are handed over to the receiving hospital.

It is particularly important when you have potential concerns of non-accidental injury that you do a careful examination of the child when you first see them. Important areas not to miss are shown in **Figure 43.4**. This includes documenting attempts for IV access that you have seen and any bruising noticed, particularly in unusual areas, identifying the site of bruising, and a description of size, colour and any open trauma.

Impeccable documentation is important as you might be required to use this in later reports and body maps can be useful and are available in all paediatric departments.

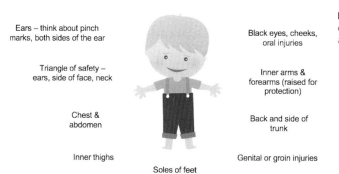

Ears – think about pinch marks, both sides of the ear

Triangle of safety – ears, side of face, neck

Chest & abdomen

Inner thighs

Soles of feet

Black eyes, cheeks, oral injuries

Inner arms & forearms (raised for protection)

Back and side of trunk

Genital or groin injuries

Figure 43.4 Important areas to examine if concerned about non-accidental injury.

Discussion with Referring Team Regarding Your Concerns and What Steps Have Been Taken

It is important that the local hospital team have highlighted their concerns. They must do a social services referral and if there are significant concerns then ask them to contact the police.

Whilst focus should be on the child who is acutely unwell, it is also important to think about other siblings. If there are other children in the family, or in the family home, then the referring team must discuss the case with social services, to ensure that siblings are also in a place of safety as they may require emergency foster placement.

If the referring team are referring to social services and/or the police then ask them to have this discussion with the parents to inform them of this. It is important to be open and honest about this with the parents and explain the reason for the referral.

Outcome

On arrival at the tertiary centre, the patient had evidence of abdominal bruising and imaging showed signs consistent with an abdominal perforation. A discrete line on his abdominal film indicated a retroperitoneal duodenal perforation. A retroperitoneal duodenal perforation does not cause classic 'air under the diaphragm' and instead is seen as highlighting of the Ligament of Treitz, which can be seen as a sharp white line on a plain abdominal X-ray.

The child went to theatre for a laparotomy and was found to have multiple intestinal 'burst' injuries with intestinal serosal bruising and small perforations in multiple sites of the small bowel. These injuries were consistent with direct blunt trauma to the abdomen such as from a punch or a kick. Appropriate child protection measures were instituted and the child made a good recovery.

Further Reading

Browning JG, Wilkinson AG, Beattie T. Imaging paediatric blunt abdominal trauma in the emergency department: ultrasound versus computed tomography. *EmergMed J* 2008;**25**:645–8.

Child Protection Companion. RCPCH. https://pcouk.org/companion.

Child Protection Evidence: Systematic Review on Visceral Injuries. RCPCH. Published November 2018 www.rcpch.ac.uk/sites/default/files/2018-11/child_protection_evidence_-_visceral_injuries.pdf.

Multidrug Overdose
A Practical Guide to Stabilisation and Transfer

Nav Somasinghe and Joanne Perkins

A previously fit and well 13-year-old girl was referred to the paediatric retrieval service for transfer and request for admission to PICU. She had been found collapsed by police approximately 4 hours after she had messaged a friend saying she was suicidal. Her friend raised the alarm to her parents and subsequently to the police. The friend was able to identify her location by her phone for the police. The child had taken a deliberate mixed overdose of her father's antihypertensive medication. She has no history of mental health problems and the current situation was felt to be due to school stressors (potential bullying and academic pressure).

When found by the police, she was too drowsy to give a full history; however, it was assumed she had taken a mixed overdose. The amounts taken (and usual maximum dose) were estimated from the empty boxes found in her bag and included amlodipine 280 mg (10 mg), doxazocin 112 mg (16 mg), perindopril 600 mg (10 mg), trimethoprim 1 g (400 mg), paracetamol 3.5 g (4 g) and methylated spirits (isopropyl alcohol 95%, approx. 150 ml.

On admission to A&E she had been persistently hypotensive with systolic BP 50–70mmHg and drowsy but responsive and answering questions. Full blood count, urea and electrolytes were all within the normal range. An arterial blood gas showed a lactate of 2.3, but all other parameters were within normal range. Her observations at the time of referral are shown in Table 44.1.

Questions

1. How would you approach the multidrug aspect of this overdose, and what is the most potentially significant of the antihypertensive agents taken?
2. What would be your initial management and stabilisation priorities?
3. What would be the key priorities for facilitating a safe transfer of this patient?
4. Should this child have a psychiatric assessment prior to transfer?

1. How would you approach the multi-drug aspect of this overdose, and what is the most potentially significant of the antihypertensive agents taken?

As with all assessments, a structured approach should be taken; however, due to this being a mixed overdose, there will be drug-specific management which will need to be initiated in a timely fashion.

Table 44.1.

Heart rate	100 bpm
Respiratory rate	28 breaths per minute
Sats	95% in air
Blood pressure	85/50 mmhg
Temperature	36.6°C
Glasgow coma score	14/15

It is very important to try and verify what was taken and the quantity. Obtaining this information is not always straightforward, particularly where the child is not able to tell you. You might need to speak to family and parents and explore what drugs or substances they could have had access to at home and the quantities of each. It may occasionally be necessary for family to return home to establish the facts.

In the case of overdose or poisoning, it is essential to obtain some baseline investigations including:

- Full blood count, renal and liver function, electrolytes, coagulation studies and blood sugar
- A blood gas will provide rapid overview of acid base balance and essential electrolytes
- Toxicology screen – blood and urine
- Saved serum for further toxicology
- ECG.

Specific management is needed for many of the drugs implicated in her overdose and there are multiple sources to find specific information.

- National Poisons Information Service (NPIS) UK number: 03448920111
- Toxbase.org – online resource and primary toxicology database of the NPIS
- Toxicology team at local hospital or nearby tertiary centre.
- Local PICU/retrieval service
- Children's Hospital of Philadelphia (www.chop.edu).

Consulting Toxbase will give you valuable information about the toxicity of the medications she has ingested at the doses that she has ingested them.

Amlodipine is very toxic in large doses and in this case would be of most significant concern. However, she had taken a multiple agent overdose of several antihypertensive agents and the potential cumulative effect could not be ignored.

Amlodipine is a dihydropyridine class calcium channel blocker, used in the treatment of hypertension and angina and for angina prophylaxis. It is **highly toxic** in large overdoses, due mainly to antagonism of calcium channels in smooth muscles causing peripheral vasodilation and **severe hypotension**. High doses can cause blockade of calcium channels in the heart, leading to **bradyarrhythmias** including junctional escape rhythms, atrio-ventricular conduction block and **asystole**. Blockade of calcium channels in the pancreas causes **hyperglycaemia**.

In children ingesting more than 10mg, 11% developed clinically important features of overdose. Peak plasma concentrations are reached 6–12 hours after ingestion with a therapeutic elimination half-life of 35–50 hours.

Doxazocin The expected toxicity is hypotension. Peak plasma concentration may be delayed up to 9 hours (sustained release preparation) after ingestion and the elimination half-life is 16–30 hours.

Perindopril is an angiotensin converting enzyme (ACE) inhibitor with toxicity manifesting clinically as drug-induced hypotension. Other features include bradycardia, hyperkalaemia, hyponatraemia, acute kidney injury, metabolic acidosis, headache, dizziness, gastro-intestinal disturbance, coma and abnormal liver function tests (LFTs). Peak plasma concentrations are at 1–4 hours with a half-life of 17 hours.

2. What would be your initial management and stabilisation priorities?

This child was still verbally responsive at the time of presentation; however, the risk of deterioration and airway compromise was significant. There could be an argument for elective intubation prior to transfer; however, this is not without risk given her cardiovascular instability, which is likely to get worse on induction of anaesthesia.

The following should be your immediate concerns and must be considered as part of initial stabilisation before transfer.

- Refractory hypotension
- Low Glasgow Coma Score (GCS) (drowsiness)
- Electrolyte abnormalities and arrhythmias
- Liver dysfunction – due to paracetamol ingestion
- Acidosis – due to methylated spirits intake – and potential need for haemofiltration.

Ensure early discussions are had with the local Poisons Information team as well as the local paediatric retrieval team.

- **Maintain a clear airway and ensure adequate ventilation**:
  - Monitor GCS and ensure airway remains protected.
  - Gastric emptying may be delayed by the overdose and put her at increased risk of vomiting/ aspiration.
  - The multi-drug overdose may put her at risk of seizures.

- **Gastric decontamination** with activated charcoal, for drug adsorption, may have a role in the first hour after ingestion, provided the airway remains protected. Efficacy declines rapidly with time except in the case of sustained release preparations or large ingestions.
- **Monitor vital signs and check cardiac rhythm repeatedly**:
  - Check cardiac rhythm, QRS duration and QT interval. Repeat 12-lead ECGs are recommended, especially in symptomatic patients or in those who have ingested sustained release preparations.

- **Check blood sugar** and ensure adequate **hydration** to maintain a good urine output.
- **Establish baseline electrolytes and biochemistry** with regular blood gas monitoring.

Patients are at high risk of sudden deterioration if they have any one of the following features:

- Hypotension and bradycardia
- New hyperglycaemia
- Rising blood lactate concentration.

The following treatment is recommended in the presence of bradycardia; hypotension, depressed cardiac function and vasodilatation.

- **Bradycardia** Give atropine intravenously, dosed at 20mcg/kg for a child. Repeat doses may be necessary. Dobutamine or isoprenaline may be considered if bradycardia is associated with hypotension. Temporary pacemaker insertion may be required, alternatively external pacing may be used.
- **Hypotension:**
  - **Calcium treatment** Give 10% calcium chloride 0.2mL/kg up to 10mL over 5 minutes. To achieve the intended effect, high doses may be required. Repeat the dose of calcium every 10–20 minutes to a maximum of four doses or consider an infusion at 0.2mL/kg/hour (maximum 10mL/hour). Monitor the calcium level aiming for high normal concentration. Ionised calcium concentration (gas result) may be a more accurate measure.
  - **High dose insulin** In severe cases, an insulin and dextrose infusion has been shown to improve myocardial contractility and improve systemic perfusion. It is particularly useful in the presence of acidosis. Often very high doses are needed, up to 10 units/kg/hour to improve cardiac output and clinical state.
  - **Glucagon** Glucagon is a treatment option for severe hypotension, heart failure or cardiogenic shock. A bolus of 50–150mcg/kg IV should be administered over 1–2 minutes, followed by an infusion of 50mcg/kg/hour, titrated to clinical response. Adverse effects of IV administration include vomiting, hyperglycaemia, hypokalaemia and hypocalcaemia. If this therapy is used, consider prophylactic treatment with an antiemetic.
  - **Inotropes** An adrenoceptor agonist should be instituted if hypotension fails to respond to the above measures. Adrenaline has both alpha- and beta- adrenergic effects and may improve both cardiac dysfunction and decreased systemic vascular resistance. If hypotension is mainly due to decreased systemic vascular resistance, drugs with mainly alpha-adrenergic activity, such as noradrenaline, are more beneficial. If hypotension is secondary to the negative chronotropic and inotropic effects of the calcium channel blockers with little evidence of systemic vasodilation, beta adrenergic agonists such as dobutamine, isoprenaline or low dose dopamine (2–10 mcg/kg/min) may be of benefit.
  - **Lipid emulsion therapy (intralipid)** In cardiac arrest or life-threatening cardiotoxicity where other therapies have been ineffective, consider the use of IV lipid emulsion therapy, but the evidence of benefit is weak. It is thought lipid may reduce free concentrations of active drug and therefore improve myocardial function, although other mechanisms are also postulated.
  - **Mechanical cardiac support – veno-arterial (VA ECMO)** may be a bridge to recovery in patients with life-threatening haemodynamic instability where other measures have failed and when cardiovascular arrest or shock persists despite volume administration, inotropes and vasoconstrictors, and (if appropriate and available) intra-aortic balloon counterpulsation. There are no randomised controlled trials of ECMO in poisoned patients with refractory shock. ECMO is discussed further in Chapter 26.

3. What would be the key priorities for facilitating a safe transfer of this patient?

Safety of the child and anticipation of deterioration is key. With multidrug overdose, the potential for continued and progressive deterioration is magnified.

A systematic plan to mitigate this deterioration must be in place.

A & B: Should the child be intubated before transfer? The response would be yes in the presence of

- A decreased GCS
- Risk of aspiration, or respiratory failure
- Seizures
- Non-compliance with medical intervention due to mental state, aggression or agitation.

C: Adequate access for multiple infusions and monitoring must be sited:

- Multiple large bore peripheral access or central access if requiring inotropes.
- Arterial line for continuous blood pressure monitoring during transfer.

The receiving PICU should be forewarned of the information from Toxbase and the potential need for:

- **Cardiac/ECMO centre:** The receiving PICU should have onsite paediatric cardiology and ECMO capabilities. In the situation where the child cannot be stabilised locally despite all medical therapy, consideration should be given to mobile ECMO.
- **Liver centre:** If the overdose she has taken included toxic doses of paracetamol with evidence of acute liver failure.

4. Should this child have a psychiatric assessment prior to transfer?

This child certainly needed psychiatric input and review during this admission; however, at the time of referral the medical emergency took priority unless the child was refusing treatment.

Gillick competence is a term used in medical law in the UK to decide whether a child (16 years or younger) is able to consent to his or her own medical treatment without the need for parental permission or knowledge.

Children over the age of 16 are presumed to be Gillick competent. Children under the age of 16 can be deemed Gillick competent – if they can show sufficient maturity to make the decision, then the child can provide legal consent for medical treatment.

Given the nature of this case, and the effect of the drugs, this child would not be in the position to be deemed Gillick competent, and treatment should be initiated in the best interests of the child.

There would be wider psychosocial implications if the child survived, and it is important to consider how you would support the child and her parents both in the acute setting and in the future.

Further Reading

Children's Hospital of Philadelphia:
www.chop.edu.

National Poisons Information Service (NPIS)
UK number: 0344 892 0111. www.npis.org.

www.toxbase.org – online resource primary toxicology database of the NPIS.

Chapter

45

Death Is a Possible Outcome

Dawn Knight and Shelley Riphagen

A 17-month-old little girl was referred to the regional retrieval service for urgent transfer. She was normally fit and well and had presented 3 hours previously to A&E at her local district general hospital with a 1-day history of diarrhoea and vomiting with intermittent fever (although she had been apyrexial for the past 8 hours). During her wait in A&E she had deteriorated and been moved to the resuscitation bay.

Based on her clinical examination and initial venous gas results, the A&E team managed her as septic shock with her abdomen considered a possible source, due to significant distension.

Only the venous blood gas results shown in Table 45.1, were available at the time of referral.

The child was accepted for transfer and PICU admission and the retrieval team set off after giving further advice to the local team to continue fluid resuscitation, proceed to intubate and ventilate as soon as possible with peripheral dopamine on standby and to obtain central venous access for inotropes and ongoing resuscitation after intubation.

At the time of referral, she was apyrexial and self-ventilating in 15 L face mask oxygen with saturations of 98%. She had a persistent tachycardia of 180 bpm and BP of 119/83. Her hands, feet and ears were all cold and described as 'purple'. Although her abdomen was distended, it was soft with no urine in the bladder on catheterisation. The local team had one IV access through which she had been given antibiotics and 30 ml/kg volume boluses by the time of the call. On presentation she had been hypoglycaemic, but this had resolved after one glucose bolus.

When the retrieval team arrived 70 minutes later, she was intubated with a 4.0-mm endotracheal tube and ventilated on high pressures 30/10 in 100% oxygen with saturations of 94%. CXR showed diffuse bilateral opacification. She had been given a total of 90 ml/kg volume resuscitation and started on dopamine 15 mcg/kg/min and adrenaline 0.2 mcg/kg/min. Her heart rate was still 180 bpm with no recordable blood pressure on cuff measurements. Her abdomen was tense and distended. She was sedated with morphine and midazolam with sluggishly reactive pupils.

The local team had tried to secure central venous access in both groins, but she had significant bleeding at the sites and the attempts were unsuccessful. The retrieval team lead joined the attempts to gain vascular access. All four senior clinicians were unsuccessful except for establishing one intra-osseous line.

Working together over the next 70 minutes the referring team and retrieval team sought to resuscitate and stabilise her. She was given packed red cells, cryoprecipitate, fresh frozen plasma and dextrose for low blood sugar through the intra-osseous needle. She also received aciclovir and vitamin K.

Table 45.1. Venous blood gas

pH	7.09	Lactate	9.4 mmol/L
pCO_2	4.3 kPa	Glucose	4.1 mmol/L
pO_2	5.1 kPa	Na	131 mmol/L
HCO_3	9.7 mmol/L	K	4.0 mmol/L
Base excess	−19 mEq/L		

During this time her condition continued to worsen with increasing difficulty in ventilation until a point of tenuous stability was achieved with ETCO2 9.0, HR 180, BP 106/44(60) and 3-mm equal sluggishly reactive pupils on adrenaline and dopamine. A repeat blood gas showed a pH of 6.85, pCO_2 of 7.3 and lactate of 24 mmol/L.

Questions

1. Should this child be moved in this condition or not?
2. If she were to have a cardiac arrest at the referring hospital, who should take the lead?
3. In the event of death of a child with the retrieval team present, what are the useful learning points in optimising and managing the situation?

1. Should this child be moved in this condition or not?

This is a complex decision which ultimately is made by the retrieval team present supported by a retrieval consultant, but working closely with the referring team, including both referring paediatric and anaesthetic consultants.

There are two possible options:

One option is to undertake the transfer at this point, knowing that the child may have a cardiac arrest in the ambulance. During the transfer there are often only two competent clinical team members to undertake CPR. A parent is also usually present during transfer and in this setting there would be no spare team member to support the parent. Considerations to address include:

- **Prepared and 'hands-free' as practicable:** Discussion about the likely course of events needs to be had between the retrieval team and ambulance technician and parents: what the parents and technician would be expected to do, and what role and actions would each of the two clinical team members undertake. The retrieval team needs to be as prepared and 'hands-free' as practicable in the back of the ambulance, including prepared rounds of age-specific arrest drugs and resuscitation fluids drawn up and ready to run; noradrenaline attached and pre-programmed, crystalloid in a pressure bag to infuse rapidly; and defibrillation pads on and connected.

- **Having a Do-Not-Attempt-CPR (DNA-CPR) order in place or not:** This child's parents must be made fully aware of the situation before leaving. They need to be informed a cardiac arrest is a real possibility. A DNA-CPR order needs to be discussed with them and, if agreed to, completed before leaving. The referring team's consultant, should sign a DNA-CPR order if agreed. If the child arrests in the back of the ambulance without a DNA-CPR order in place and the retrieval team does not include a doctor (e.g.

is led by a retrieval nurse practitioner), the retrieval team will be obliged to continue CPR in a moving ambulance to the PICU or nearest A&E, unless authorised telephonically by the retrieval consultant to discontinue. Should the child die in transit, her death would have to be certified by a doctor who attended her during this episode of illness. This could be at the referring hospital, a doctor involved in the retrieval or the retrieval consultant on the call if taken to the PICU. Her death would also have to be referred to the Coroner for two reasons; the cause of death is unknown, sudden or unexplained and death within 24 hours of admission to hospital.

- **The parents' demeanour as determined by the retrieval team:** It may be more appropriate to have parents follow the ambulance in a police escort. Should the ambulance have to stop to give treatment, the retrieval team will keep them informed with the assistance of the police escort. Many parents would still prefer to accompany their child, even in the knowledge the child may have a cardiac arrest. The parents must be fully informed of the possibilities.

The other option is to remain at the district general hospital for a limited period to see if the child has genuinely stabilised and in that time undertake additional actions to further optimise stabilisation. Such actions could include: more attempts at central access; further inotropic support (e.g. noradrenaline to address her wide pulse pressure), further fluid resuscitation, and following up and acting on abnormal blood test results. A problem with this strategy is that it delays getting the child to a PICU where treatments (such as haemofiltration or extra-corporeal life support) can be initiated to address ongoing shock and multi-organ failure. At some point, however, the decision has to be made that the child is either (a) to be moved with or without a DNA-CPR order in place and parents fully aware of the risks of cardiac arrest; or (b) life-sustaining treatments are no longer in her best interests and should be withheld, withdrawn or limited and palliative care commenced locally.

Fortunately, in the United Kingdom (b) above is permitted using the framework produced by the Royal College of Paediatrics and Child Health.

The guiding principle is to determine the child's best interests with great consideration of the interests of the child, the family and their rights. This is a complex decision and should be made using the decision-making guidance set out in this framework. The consultant at the referring hospital should lead the process and ultimately make the decision, in partnership with the child's parents, the rest of the referring hospital team and retrieval team. Her parents will need to be fully informed of the best information available, in a manner and at a pace they can comprehend with great weight given to their views. Ideally, all participants involved in the process should feel comfortable with the decision made.

If the decision is made to follow the palliative care route, the retrieval team will seek to support the referring hospital team as much as possible with this process, including after death.

2. If she were to have a cardiac arrest at the referring hospital, who should take the lead?

The answer to this is clear: the person with the most situational awareness and ability to direct the team. The more difficult part of the solution is understanding who that person is when not everyone is familiar with individuals in other teams. The leader may or may not be the most clinically competent professional present. S/he should not assume a hands-on role, but stand in an optimal position to assess the situation and gather information about the child's condition, often at the bed end. Frequently the referring hospital consultant or retrieval lead will assume the role.

The leader needs to:

- Ensure compliance with the cardiac arrest algorithms
- Ensure the quality of CPR is good with adequate ventilation and good quality cardiac compressions
- Optimise the use of the team by allocating roles appropriately
- Be a central information gathering and relay point for the team of clinical information
- Lead the evaluation and likely cause-specific treatment of the arrest (4 Hs and 4Ts)
- Ensure accurate recording of events by a designated scribe
- Ensure appropriate care and communication with the parents.

Throughout the arrest the leader will be seeking input and checking out thought processes with the rest of the team.

Ultimately, spontaneous circulation will return or, liaising with other clinicians present, the leader will decide to stop the resuscitation, usually after at least 20 minutes of commencing good quality CPR and once all reversible causes have been adequately addressed.

3. In the event of death of a child with the retrieval team present, what are the useful learning points in optimising and managing the situation?

After any critical incident, resuscitation or death, a **Hot Debrief** primarily provides a semi-formal opportunity to ascertain the facts and check-out the emotional impact on, and support of, all concerned. Learning points may become apparent, but this should **not** be the primary aim.

Ideally all involved, however peripherally, should be invited to attend. It should take place shortly after the event (at least in the same shift), so involved individuals are available and events are fresh in their minds. It should be held in a quiet area, away from where the event took place. The leader (hopefully with some debriefing training) should make it clear that participation from all is highly valued.

The aims are to clarify the facts and support each other.

Each in turn should be invited to add to the factual picture, and then to share what they were thinking at any point in the event and, if they feel able, to share their feelings (during the event and now). Key for the hot debrief is that participants have had some space to clarify the facts, air their emotions and know they are not alone in coming to terms with the emotional impact of the event.

To finish, **discussion should be had of 'what next'.** At the very least contact details should be collated of all present for future support and information of changes following the event. If time and emotions permit, it may be possible to consider learning points thinking of (a) what went well, (b) what did not go well and (c) what can be done differently in future.

If not, **learning points** can be sought once each key participant has had the time and space to give a written statement of his/her perception of the event. Most hospitals will have a Clinical Governance team who will co-ordinate statement collection and subsequent meetings to consider learning points from the event.

Outcome: This little girl was a normally fit and well child. She died of her rapidly progressive toxic shock within 7 hours of arriving in A&E, just before the retrieval team planned to leave. A hot debrief was held with many staff feeling traumatised at the loss of a child who had been admitted talking 7 hours previously. Post debrief staff follow up and counselling was provided locally

Further Reading

Academy of Medical Royal Colleges (2008) *Code of practice for the diagnosis and confirmation of death.* www.aomrc.org.uk/reports-guidance/ukdec-reports-and-guidance/code-practice-diagnosis-confirmation-death/.

Advanced Life Support Group (ALSG) 6th Edition *Advance Paediatric Life Support. A practical approach to emergencies.* Wiley: Chichester, 2016.

BMA, Resuscitation Council (UK) and Royal College of Nursing. 3rd ed. *Decisions relating to cardiopulmonary resuscitation.* www.bma.org.uk/advice-and-support/ethics/end-of-life/decisions-relating-to-cpr-cardiopulmonary-resuscitation.

Larcher V, Craig F, Bhogal K, et al. Making decisions to limit treatment in life-limiting and life-threatening conditions in children: a framework for practice. *Arch Dis Child* 2015;100(Suppl 2):s1–23.

Linney M, Hain RDW, Wilkinson D, et al. Achieving consensus advice for paediatricians and other health professionals: on prevention, recognition and management of conflict in paediatric practice. *Arch Dis Child* 2019;104(5):413–6.

Medical Defence Union. 14 August 2018 *Signing death certificates and cremation forms.* www.themdu.com/guidance-and-advice/guides/signing-death-certificates-and-cremation-forms.

Paediatric FOAMed 'Hot debrief' www.paediatricfoam.com/2017/01/the-hot-debrief/.

46

A Cold, Unconscious 12-Year-Old Girl

Louisa Brock and Marilyn McDougall

A 12-year-old girl was referred to your service after being found collapsed and unresponsive in the bathroom at home by her parents at 07:00 on the morning of referral, and brought in by ambulance to A&E.

She was previously fit and well but on direct questioning her parents had noticed weight loss and compulsive drinking in the previous few months. Her mother had ascribed it to the stress of changing schools. She also had a recent history of earache associated with offensive discharge from the right ear which had been treated with antibiotics and eardrops from her GP.

The ambulance personnel reported that when they arrived about 10 minutes after the 999 call, the patient was breathing spontaneously with good respiratory effort, but she had poor peripheral pulses and an unrecordable blood pressure. Her blood glucose was noted to be 25 mmol/L and she was cold to touch with a temperature of 31°C. She remained unresponsive during transfer to her local A&E, where, on arrival, her Glasgow Coma Score (GCS) was recorded as 10/15 (E4 V2 M4). Her initial blood gas results were:

pH <6.8, pCO_2 1.9 kPa, Bicarbonate unrecordable, lactate 2.0, base excess −26.

In light of the history, the high glucose, acidosis and elevated blood ketones (6 mmol/L), the A&E team were able to diagnose the first presentation of diabetic ketoacidosis (DKA). Due to her reduced GCS and history of ear infection a CT scan was undertaken to exclude complications of otitis media, such as a cerebral abscess. An anaesthetist accompanied the child to scan and she remained self-ventilating throughout.

The scan demonstrated no evidence of cerebral oedema and no other intracerebral abnormality apart from opacification of the right mastoid air cells.

The referring registrar was seeking retrieval and further management advice while they awaited retrieval.

Questions

1. How do you evaluate and manage shock in severe DKA?
2. How would you manage the depressed level of consciousness in this patient?
3. How would you manage the acidosis in this case?
4. How would human factors affect this particular retrieval situation?

1. How do you evaluate and manage shock in severe DKA?

Recognition and management of shock in DKA is exceptionally challenging. Understanding and consideration of the pathophysiology is essential to guide appropriate management.

There are a number of key factors which contribute to the signs of poor peripheral perfusion in DKA:

- the profound metabolic acidosis (pH <6.8) caused by high ketone levels
- the marked hypocapnia (pCO_2 frequently <2 kPa)
- dehydration which has developed over several weeks.

For these reasons, children with DKA may appear mottled, cold and have prolonged capillary refill time due to peripheral vasoconstriction. In the majority of cases, despite these changes, the intravascular volume and blood pressure have been preserved and majority of children with DKA are not shocked, with no lactic acidosis. Children with DKA may even be hypertensive on presentation due to the profound peripheral vasoconstriction and consequent appearance of poor perfusion.

In this particular case, the child had an unrecordable blood pressure and persistent tachycardia despite the documented hypothermia. It was therefore appropriate to conclude that child was shocked and required restoration of the intravascular volume and perfusion pressure to restore blood flow to vital organs. This creates a conundrum in the setting of DKA because of the concern regarding large volume resuscitation and the incidence of cerebral oedema in DKA.

The retrieval team should specifically say to the referring team that this degree of hypotension in DKA is unusual and reflects shock, which requires urgent resuscitation. This is despite the appearance of low lactate, which may be expected to rise with warming and restoration of peripheral perfusion. It is always important when communicating with a team via telephone not to make any assumptions. Identifying both **shock** and **DKA** as emergencies requiring treatment is important.

The initial resuscitation with both 20 ml/kg of saline and 5 ml/kg of hypertonic saline was appropriate. However, as the patient remained hypotensive and tachycardic further resuscitation including more cautious fluid boluses (absolute maximum 40 ml/kg) and early initiation of inotropes is essential. In addition to concerns regarding cerebral perfusion, renal perfusion is also fundamental. Ketones are most effectively cleared by renal excretion, therefore maintaining urine output is an important part of the therapy of DKA.

The retrieval service would recommend starting low dose peripheral adrenaline (<0.05–0.1 mcg/kg/min) or dopamine (5–10 mcg/kg/min) to restore organ perfusion. It would be even more effective to deliver the inotropes centrally, because of the presence of peripheral vasoconstriction, but the lack of central venous access should not delay starting inotropes. The retrieval team would suggest placing a central line (femoral) or intra-osseous access as soon as possible.

In this particular case it is likely that the cause of the hypotension and shock is infection in addition to the DKA. It is important to provide broad spectrum antibiotics, such as ceftriaxone and metronidazole, to cover both gram-positive, gram-negative and anaerobic infections. Inclusion of a third generation cephalosporin would provide CNS cover for potential meningitis as a complication of the primary ear infection.

2. How would you manage the depressed level of consciousness in this patient?

Many children presenting in DKA may have a reduced level of consciousness due to:

- **Hypocapnia /vasogenic cerebral ischaemia** (low pCO_2) which causes cerebral vasoconstriction and focal or generalised ischaemia

- **Intracellular hypoglycaemia** whereby neurons are dependent on glucose as their primary source of energy; however, in the absence of insulin, glucose is unable to enter the cells. This is in part compensated by ketones which are the only alternative energy source that can be utilized by neurons but are less effective than glucose as a neuronal energy source.
- **Osmotic oedema** due to the prolonged high serum osmolarity (caused by high levels of glucose in the serum). Neurons develop idiogenic osmoles to compensate and prevent extreme intracellular fluid losses and maintain brain cellular volume.

Cerebral oedema is a rare complication (less than 1% of all cases) but remains the leading cause of death in paediatric DKA, with a mortality rate of up to 25%. Cerebral oedema in DKA is multifactorial, with the highest risk for development of cerebral oedema in the first 8–12 hours following presentation and initiation of treatment. Specific risk factors for the development of cerebral oedema have been identified in large retrospective studies and include:

- Age below 2 years at onset
- pCO_2 <2 Kpa
- pH <7.1 at presentation
- >40 ml/kg in first 4 hours of therapy
- Rapid fall in serum glucose
- $NaCO_3$ therapy or raised urea
- Hyperventilation post intubation.

Signs of DKA-related cerebral involvement may include: headache, vomiting, fluctuating level of consciousness, irritability, agitation or incontinence. Neurological signs and symptoms, such as abnormal posturing, irregular respiratory pattern and unequal or abnormally responsive pupils should prompt urgent assessment and management.

If cerebral oedema is suspected in DKA, it should be treated with osmotherapy. Hypertonic saline (2.7%) at 3–5 ml/kg is highly effective with a measurable response of rapidly improving neurology. A response should be expected within 10–15 minutes and the dose can be repeated if necessary. The biochemical effect of hypertonic saline can also be tracked using serum sodium levels, and it is interesting anecdotally that the serum sodium from a hypertonic saline bolus alone does not rise more than 1–3 mmol/L per dose.

In this case, the patient continued to have a depressed level of consciousness (GCS 10) despite fluid resuscitation, inotropes and hypertonic saline treatment. At this stage, it would be necessary to intubate the patient. Intubation in this case would not only protect the patient's airway but also maintain optimal oxygenation and normalise the pCO_2 to improve cerebral perfusion, albeit at the cost of a fall in pH as the compensatory hypocarbia should not be maintained.

Careful preparation and planning is essential to optimise the safety in this situation. The whole team should discuss the plan for intubation prior to induction of anaesthesia with clear role allocation. A safety checklist should also be completed to ensure that all the correct equipment and drugs including those to manage a cardiac arrest are available at the start of the anaesthetic induction process.

Two important considerations should be highlighted and discussed prior to induction in this case:

1. **Avoid hypotension:** all induction agents are likely to aggravate the hypotension by reducing the patient's natural stress response. To avoid this, ensure that there has been a

good response to inotropes prior to administration of any induction agents. The inotrope therapy should be titrated upwards until the systolic blood pressure is >95–120 mmHg which is the normal range for this 12-year-old child.

2. **Normalise pCO$_2$ level:** Once the patient is sedated and muscle relaxed, the CO$_2$ should be maintained in the normal range 3.5– 5 kPa to optimise the cerebral blood flow, expecting that initially the pH will be worse.

After the child has been intubated and ventilated, it is essential to monitor her pupillary reactions regularly. As she had a very low pH and pCO$_2$ at the time of presentation she was in a high-risk category for development of cerebral oedema even though the initial CT scan was unremarkable. In the setting of a profoundly dehydrated child, with dehydrated brain, the diagnosis of cerebral oedema by CT scan in DKA is fraught with difficulty. Other cerebral complications of profound dehydration and DKA, including sagittal and other venous sinus thrombosis and cerebral infarction, should be specifically excluded.

The next few hours of resuscitation should include careful titration of therapy to avoid precipitous falls in the serum osmolarity, checking the pupils hourly and maintaining the blood pressure.

A useful calculation to ensure that the serum osmolarity is maintained is the 'corrected sodium calculation'. In order to ensure that the sudden fall in serum glucose as insulin is provided doesn't cause all the fluid to shift into brain cells, it is necessary to counter-balance the fall in glucose with a moderate rise in the serum sodium in the ratio of approximately 2:1, i.e. a fall in glucose of 10 mmol/L should be concurrent with a rise in serum sodium of 5 mmol/L.

Corrected sodium calculation = Plasma sodium + (0.4 × (Glucose − 5.5 mmol/L)

The corrected sodium would be expected to rise by about 5 mmol in 4–8 hours. If the corrected sodium does not rise at this rate the fluid rate should be reduced, and it may be necessary to provide hypertonic saline boluses to ensure this rise if fluid balance alone is unable to achieve the desired goals. National guidance is available for managing the rate of fluid administration through NICE (National Clinical Institute of Excellence) and BSPED (British Society of Paediatric Endocrinology and Diabetes).

If the corrected sodium rises too quickly (>5 mmol every 4 hours) it would indicate that the patient may need a faster rate of rehydration.

3. How would you manage the acidosis in this case?

Following initial stabilisation, the principles of DKA management are to correct the ketoacidosis with careful titration of insulin and glucose therapy. It is very tempting to try to fix the acidosis as quickly as possible. It is important to remember that both the dehydration and ketoacidosis in these children have developed over an extended period and a more gradual approach to recovery is entirely appropriate.

The predominant cause of acidosis in this case is ketones. Insulin inhibits ketone production from fat cells. There is however, evidence to suggest that early initiation of insulin in DKA is associated with an increased risk of cerebral oedema, which is why the insulin should only be started 1 hour after the initiation of IV fluid therapy, particularly in the high-risk cases. IV fluid alone, especially resuscitation boluses can result in a precipitous drop in glucose (by dilution) even without insulin.

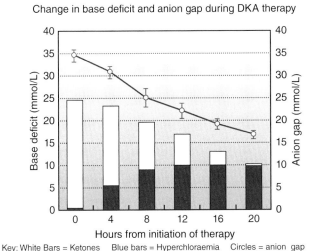

Change in base deficit and anion gap during DKA therapy

Figure 46.1 Change in base deficit and anion gap during DKA therapy.

Key: White Bars = Ketones   Blue bars = Hyperchloraemia   Circles = anion gap

The insulin infusion should be started at a dose of 0.05–0.1 units/kg/hour and continued until blood ketone levels are below 1 mmol/L. If blood ketone measurement is unavailable, the anion gap can be used as a weak surrogate targeting a level of 18 mEq/L.

The patient should be catheterised to ensure that she continues to pass urine at the rate of at least 1 ml/kg/hour to clear the ketones.

Base excess is not a reliable indicator of acidosis, since children presenting with DKA develop hyperchloraemia during the recovery phase. This alone causes a degree of acidosis.

Figure 46.1 demonstrates the correlation between the drop in ketones and anion gap and highlights the lag in the base deficit due to a rise in the serum chloride. This hyperchloraemic acidosis has not been shown to cause harm in children and usually resolves spontaneously over the following 48–72 hours.

4. How would human factors affect this particular retrieval situation?

Emergency resuscitation of children often brings together groups of individuals who don't usually work together, such as emergency department staff, paediatricians, paediatric nurses and anaesthetic teams. In this case, the parents are likely to be very anxious, and possibly upset that the GP had not identified the problem earlier. This combination of multiple teams, a patient who remains critically unwell despite treatment and anxious family may result in a distracting environment which could impact decision making and increase the risk of error.

It would be important for a leader to be identified to manage the situation and patient effectively. Role allocation would help to ensure that all tasks are completed in a timely manner. In particular, an individual should be assigned to explain to the parents what the next steps of treatment will involve. Also by having a team leader, they can ensure regular reviews are conducted, this being especially important in a case such as this when regular small adjustments may need to be made.

In this case, conflicting priorities of rapid fluid resuscitation of children with shock and the risk of developing cerebral oedema in children with DKA who receive fluid boluses >40 ml/kg could make the decision making and management particularly difficult. Early involvement of the retrieval service who are experienced in the management of these complex cases can help to prioritise the tasks. It is important in complex situations, such as this one, to carefully reassess the patient after each intervention. In this particular case, monitoring the blood pressure, pupillary responses, blood glucose and corrected sodium could be used to guide each step of the therapy.

Finally the use of checklists and guidelines is specifically designed to reduce the risk of errors in complex situations. In this case, communicating the plan with the whole team and using a safety checklist prior to induction of anaesthesia would be essential. Monitoring the DKA therapy using a published guideline would also be particularly helpful in this complex high-risk child and can give all those caring for the child a reference point.

Outcome

This child took three days to recover normal consciousness. She had *Streptococcus pneumoniae* cultured from blood and an ear swab, and she received a week of antibiotics. Lumbar puncture performed on day 4, when her neurology had returned to normal, showed no cells. Her acidosis took over 48 hours to resolve although ketones were completely normal by 18 hours. The presentation of septic shock in DKA is unusual and made this a complex and interesting case.

Further Reading

BSPED (British Society for Paediatric Endocrinology and Diabetes) Integrated Care Pathway for the management of children and young people with Diabetic ketoacidosis. www.bsped.org.uk/media/1742/dka-icp-2020-v1_1.pdf.

Clinical Guidance. Paediatric critical care: Diabetic ketoacidosis www.evelinalondon .nhs.uk/resources/our-services/hospital/ south-thames-retrieval-service/diabetic-ketoacidosis-jan-2018.pdf.

Glaser, N. Treatment and complications of diabetic ketoacidosis in children and adolescents. Up To Date. www.uptodate .com/contents/diabetic-ketoacidosis-in-children-treatment-and-complications.

Mahoney CP, Vlcek W, DelAguila M . Risk factors for developing brain herniation during diabetic ketoacidosis. *Pediatr Neurol* 1999;21(4):721–7.

Another Collapsed Neonate

Hannah Hayden and Maja Pavcnik

You have been referred a 3-day old, 4.1 kg baby who was born by normal vaginal delivery after an uncomplicated antenatal course. Her parents had attended the A&E the day before with concerns regarding poor feeding but were discharged home, as first-time parents, with advice. They re-presented the following day with increasing concern regarding lethargy and not feeding. On admission to A&E the baby was grunting but had no other signs of respiratory distress. He was mottled and cool peripherally, with normal heart sounds and palpable femoral pulses. He was floppy and very difficult to rouse, only crying feebly to painful stimuli. On arrival in A&E he had capillary glucose and gas performed. The glucose was just in normal range at 2.8 mmol/L but lactate was elevated at 4.3 mmol/L. Initial management in A&E comprised of starting the baby on high flow nasal cannula oxygen, IV access was sited and he was given three 10 ml/kg boluses of normal saline as volume resuscitation. The local team remained concerned and had escalated management to an anaesthetic review but felt he would need transfer to somewhere with a higher level of care, hence the referral.

His observations at the time of referral are noted in Table 47.1 and initial laboratory blood results and venous gas in Table 47.2.

Questions

1. What would be your advice to the referring team?
2. What additional investigations and management would you suggest?
3. What are your considerations around transfer and communication with the receiving unit?

1. What would be your advice to the referring team?

As a retrieval team triaging referral calls that range from advice regarding electrolyte correction to management of the sickest children, it is most important to try and distill the essence of the clinical problem being referred.

Triaging by phone is more difficult than seeing the child yourself and requires developing the ability to see a child through someone else's eyes.

When any child is referred to you, in any setting, the first fact to establish is whether this is an acute emergency that is being described. If the answer to that question is yes, then what is the emergency?

At first glance at the clinical parameters reported by the referring registrar, none are strikingly abnormal or concerning; however, the baby is profoundly encephalopathic, responding only to pain and needs emergency management in this regard.

Table 47.1.

Heart rate	162 bpm
Respiratory rate	53 breaths per minute
Blood pressure	87/51 mmHg
Saturations in air	98%
AVPU	P

Table 47.2.

Na	148 mmol/L	pH	7.21
K	5.2 mmol/L	pCO$_2$	4.6 kPa
Urea	1.6 mmol/L	pO$_2$	5.9 kPa
Creatinine	47 U/L	Base excess	−6.7 mEq/L
ALT	61	Lactate	4.3 mmol/L
CRP	2 mg/L		
Haemoglobin	198 g/L		
White cell count	12.8 × 10^3/mm^3		
Plts	650		

In any encephalopathic child, the presence of raised intracranial pressure (RICP) as an immediate life-threatening problem needs to be actively excluded by critically examining heart rate, blood pressure, respiratory pattern and pupils, and the fontanelle in infants. These questions need to be asked of the local team, and if any concern remains, it is better to assume and treat RICP with a bolus of hypertonic saline and assess the response (improved level of consciousness) than to not treat.

This baby is identified as a collapsed neonate with encephalopathy as the overriding clinical emergency.

There are many differential diagnoses of a collapsed neonate with encephalopathy; however, the usual causes of a collapsed neonate with shock are not identical to those presenting with encephalopathy, although the presence of encephalopathy with shock may muddy the differentiation.

In neonatal collapse with encephalopathy:

- CNS infection remains the most common cause and requires urgent treatment with appropriate antibiotics and antivirals. Lumbar puncture should not be undertaken until the baby has been resuscitated and intracranial hypertension excluded. Blood and urine cultures and herpes PCR should be sent.
- Cardiac disease is unlikely to be causal in this group unless the child is profoundly shocked.
- Metabolic conditions causing 'intoxication' must be actively excluded with an urgent blood ammonia level sent locally, and request for it to be run immediately through the

lab and reported within the hour. Blood glucose, ketones and acyl carnitine level should also be sent.
- Intracranial bleeding secondary to trauma has to be excluded by urgent neuroimaging, either by screening ultrasound if there is a low index of suspicion, or more definitive CT head.

Cultures, viral PCR, echocardiogram (if available locally), ammonia, ketones, acyl carnitines and repeat blood gas all need to be included in investigations performed urgently.

While taking the referral call, the registrar reported that the baby appeared to be seizing. The initial ammonia level had just been phoned down as 640 µmol/L.

2. What additional investigations and management would you suggest?

This is most likely a metabolic condition with hyperammonaemia causing encephalopathy.

The main aims of treatment should be airway protection; cardiovascular stability; seizure management, prevention or treatment of cerebral oedema, clearing of toxic metabolites – in this case ammonia; stopping catabolism and if possible, promotion of anabolism.

As the child appears to be seizing, the usual advanced paediatric life support measures should commence including use of lorazepam to terminate the seizure. Intubation and ventilation should be undertaken to ensure airway protection, help seizure control, facilitate neuroprotection due to risk of cerebral oedema and for subsequent retrieval.

The clinical presentation and high ammonia make a metabolic cause most likely so emergency metabolic medications – sodium benzoate, sodium phenylbutyrate, arginine and carnitine should be commenced as soon as possible in order to start reducing the ammonia.

The regional metabolic team should be contacted for guidance, but this should not delay commencing treatment.
- The child should be made nil by mouth as protein ingestion can worsen ammonia production.
- IV fluids should be commenced 0.9% sodium chloride and 10% dextrose initially to avoid catabolism but keeping a close eye on the blood sugar noting that once specialist advice is sought, the glucose infusion rate may need to change. The metabolic team may request glucose infusion of 6–10mg/kg/min.
- Broad spectrum antibiotics should also be commenced as sepsis can run concurrent with or be a cause of a metabolic decompensation.

Some children with known metabolic conditions may have an emergency decompensation plan that they carry with them or that their local hospital has easy access to. In these circumstances, follow these guidelines and get help from the local metabolic team early.

Many guidelines for stabilisation and early management of individual metabolic conditions are available including those from the South Thames Retrieval Service website.

3. What are your considerations around transfer and communication with the receiving unit?

The child was grunting at presentation, was unconscious and having seizures and required intubation and ventilation for airway protection and to ensure adequate ventilation for neuroprotection.

This would also facilitate a safer transfer.

The child has evidence of cardiorespiratory decompensation and some metabolic conditions can cause a cardiomyopathy and myocardial depression. In these cases, induction of anaesthesia for intubation carries additional risk, and caution should be exercised with provision and plans made with entire team involvement prior to intubation. The use of an inotropic agent in the peri-intubation period may be appropriate. In older children with metabolic conditions manifesting with myopathy, depolarizing neuromuscular blockers should be avoided due to the risk of hyperkalaemia. In children with significant haemodynamic instability or suspected cardiomyopathy, the cardiology team should be forewarned at the receiving centre and given an estimated time of arrival of the child.

Adequate glucose delivery is key to promoting anabolism and thus preventing further production of ammonia thus patients should be transferred with IV fluids containing dextrose, such as 0.9% sodium chloride with 10% dextrose. Sodium benzoate, sodium phenyl butyrate and arginine will also need to continue throughout transfer thus it is imperative to ensure the child has adequate IV access which may be central or peripheral.

If the ammonia is over 350umol/L for 4 hours (consult local guidelines for figures relevant to your local centre) or rising rapidly, continuous veno-venous haeomofiltration (CVVH) should be commenced as soon as possible to avoid further cerebral insult. Transfer to an appropriate centre to commence this should not be delayed and the accepting PICU should be forewarned and ready to establish vascular access and start CVVH as soon as possible. Placing a CVVH catheter in smaller babies and achieving adequate flows, once CVVH is commenced, can be challenging. Peritoneal dialysis can be considered, although this is not as effective at clearing toxic metabolites.

This child will be best managed in a unit with a specialist metabolic team. The metabolic team should be made aware, if possible prior to admission, once a metabolic condition is suspected, and if possible given an expected time of admission.

Often the history, examination findings, glucose and presence or absence of ketones can suggest a specific diagnosis. Some hospitals can offer rapid testing in order to pinpoint the specific disease and thus management. They may suggest further disease specific treatment based on presumed or confirmed diagnosis of a specific metabolic condition.

Further Reading

British Inherited Metabolic Disease Group. Emergency guidelines. www.bimdg.org.uk/guidelines/guidelines-child.asp.

British Inherited Metabolic Disease Group. Intravenous drug calculators for hyperammonaemia. www.bimdg.org.uk/tempdoc/02062021_203201_Drug_Calculator_Index_743383_12042017.pdf.

British Inherited Metabolic Disease Group. Undiagnosed hyperammonaemia diagnosis and immediate management. www.bimdg.org.uk/store/guidelines/Hyperammonaemiaand_manage_2016_415469_09092016.pdf.

The Challenges of Chemotherapy

Heather Burnett and Maja Pavcnik

A 5-year-old boy with acute myeloid leukaemia presented to A&E at his local hospital with a 1-week history of diarrhoea and a 1-day history of fever. Members of his family had also been unwell.

He was attending his district general hospital for weekly surveillance under guidance of the Primary Treatment Centre. The last dose of consolidation chemotherapy had been 6 days earlier via the single lumen Hickman catheter he had placed during induction chemotherapy 3 months ago.

By the time of referral to the retrieval team, additional peripheral access had been gained, and blood and culture investigations sent. He had been given 50 ml/kg of 0.9% sodium chloride as fluid resuscitation and had been commenced on broad spectrum antibiotics as per the oncology shared care protocols.

The local team had already contacted his tertiary oncology centre, who had advised that he be transferred to the tertiary oncology HDU by the regional retrieval team and hence this referral.

During the initial phone-call the local team gave the clinical information seen in Table 48.1 and results of special investigations (including venous gas) as seen in Table 48.2.

Questions

1. Based on the information presented, what is your assessment of the situation and advice to the referring team?
2. What would be your management plan for transfer?
3. What information would you give to the parents?

1. Based on the information presented, what is your assessment of the situation and advice to the referring team?

The child presented shocked – he was tachycardic, hypotensive and had a raised lactate. The local team had already given a significant amount of fluid resuscitation to which they reported only a transient response. This suggests that the child has fluid responsive shock but is not fully resuscitated by fluid alone. He needed urgent escalation of shock management.

The child was febrile. In children with cancer, fever is often the first indication of what can progress to life-threatening infection. The white cell count (WCC) is only 1.4 with a total absence of neutrophils. This lack of defence against both bacterial and fungal infection

Table 48.1. Clinical observations

Heart rate	142 bpm
Respiratory rate	31 breaths per minute
Saturations	97% (in air)
Blood pressure	62/30 mmHg
Temperature	38°C
AVPU	A

Table 48.2. Investigations including venous gas

Haemoglobin	55 g/L	pH	7.46
White cell count (Neut)	1.4×10^9/L 0.0	pO$_2$	3.6 kPa
Platelets	15×10^9/L	pCO$_2$	3.2 kPa
Na	131 mmol/L	HCO$_3$	19.7 mmol/L
K	2.3 mmol/L	Base excess	−6.1 mEq/L
Cr	24 μmol/L	Lactate	4.7 mmol/L
Urea	3.1 mmol/L	Glucose	6.2 mmol/L
ALT	46 U/L		
ALP	222 U/L		
CRP	108 mg/L		

leaves the child at significant risk. The combination of shock, fever and neutropenia is highly suggestive of neutropenic sepsis and this is a medical oncological emergency.

Neutropenic sepsis is the most frequently encountered complication of childhood cancer and is a significant source of morbidity and mortality. Prompt and effective management is therefore imperative. Neutropenic sepsis should be suspected in anyone receiving anti-cancer treatment who presents with a temperature of 38°C or higher and has either a neutrophil count of less than 0.5×10^9/L or other clinical signs of sepsis.

In addition to neutropenia, anaemia and thrombocytopenia are also present leaving the child at risk of bleeding. Pancytopenia can be a result of myelosuppression by cytotoxic agents, as a result of the malignant disease process invading the bone marrow or as a result of overwhelming sepsis with multi-organ failure.

Although this child with neutropenic sepsis presented critically unwell with neutropenic septic shock, there are many others that are relatively well with neutropenic sepsis and can be managed with outpatient antibiotics.

A very important aspect of care of these children is identifying the source rapidly (blood cultures from both lumens of indwelling line plus peripheral) and achieving source control as soon as possible (antibiotic treatment through the indwelling line). In a child with an indwelling line, line sepsis must be actively excluded and treated, and response to treatment critically reviewed on a frequent basis with appropriate blood tests tracking inflammation and infection (CRP, procalcitonin and ESR).

Early administration of antibiotics is the mainstay of treatment of neutropenic sepsis. Appropriate antibiotics should be administered to children within 60 minutes of presentation. Empiric antibiotics for this group of children must cover both gram-positive and gram-negative infection. Piptazobactam is broad spectrum and adequate for the relatively well children with febrile neutropenia; however, in the extremely unwell child, the addition of gentamicin will ensure excellent gram-negative cover.

In this case, an anaesthetic review and consideration of intubation and ventilation is an important early step. Although the child was self-ventilating in air and maintaining good oxygen saturations, the child was shocked with ongoing need for cardiovascular support. If the response to inotropic support through the indwelling line did not achieve good haemodynamics, the child should be progressed to intubation and ventilation to help facilitate cardiovascular support.

Active resuscitation should continue until the blood pressure and heart rate are normal for age, once other confounders have been accounted for (e.g. temperature). Further fluid boluses should be given as long as there remains a positive response and inotropic/vasopressor support commenced. A bolus of hypertonic saline could be considered as good low volume resuscitation which will also partly address the hyponatraemia. Ongoing volume resuscitation with Hartmann's solution rather than normal saline may also be considered in view of the low potassium and to avoid exacerbating hyperchloraemia. Hypokalaemia is significant and needs to be addressed specifically with potassium replacement. Most children with neutropenic sepsis present with warm shock (peripherally warm with wide pulse pressure and good cardiac output). Noradrenaline is therefore, most commonly, the drug of choice if central access is available, as in this case.

Clinical judgement must be used to assess use of the Hickman line. If the line is infected, bolus administration using the line may cause septic showers and destabilise the child further, but this may not occur if the infected line is used for low volume inotrope infusions.

Anaemia and thrombocytopenia should be corrected (which will also aid resuscitation) ideally prior to intubation, both to aid the maintenance of cardiovascular stability and to minimise the risk of bleeding caused by the procedure. Nasal intubation should be avoided. The oncology team may have special requests regarding the use of blood products, and the decision to transfuse should be across teams.

2. What would be your management plan for transfer?

Transfer destination should be to a PICU with on-site oncology support and appropriate isolation facilities for the degree of immunocompromise.

On arrival at the referring hospital the child had not been intubated, although the anaesthetic team were present. His saturations were 90% in air and crackles were audible on auscultation. He had received 70 ml/kg of crystalloid resuscitation, had 20 ml/kg of packed red blood cells and 12 ml/kg of platelets. A dopamine infusion was running at 10 mcg/kg/min. The referring team reported an ongoing transient response to fluid boluses, but he remained tachycardic (heart rate 137). His blood pressure had normalised (93/44).

In view of the volume of fluid given, the low saturations in air (and therefore new oxygen requirement), the presence of crackles and the ongoing need for cardiovascular support, this child should be ventilated. Application of non-invasive ventilatory support may be attempted.

Careful consideration should be given as to whom should intubate. The potential for further instability on induction of anaesthesia, necessitates the most experienced operator. Consideration should also be given to how and what anaesthesia to administer. Children with septic shock have a low tolerance for vasodilating or negatively inotropic induction agents. Ketamine, given in small aliquots, is the most likely anaesthetic agent to maintain cardiovascular stability, combined with rocuronium for muscle relaxation. Noradrenaline infusion can be commenced at low dose, in addition to the dopamine or low dose adrenaline infusion to continue until the child is safely anaesthetised. Additionally, it is prudent to prepare for cardiac arrest on induction. Arrest drugs should be drawn up and roles allocated.

It is also essential to update the receiving hospital on the child's condition so that they can ensure the right team, equipment and medications are ready for when the child arrives.

3. What information would you give to the parents?

It is important to establish the parents' understanding of their child's illness and prognosis and of what the acute problem is. They will be used to their child feeling unwell, and so may be shocked by how quickly this has escalated and by how different it is to previous presentations. It is also important to establish whether the possibility of admission to intensive care has been discussed with them by their oncologist.

In this case the child was extremely unwell. It is imperative to prepare parents for deterioration en route to the receiving hospital. Remember that acceleration and deceleration of movement of the ambulance can have profound effects on a cardiovascularly unstable child and it may be necessary to request a steady journey rather than fast journey from the ambulance crew. All team members should be pre-drilled for a cardiac arrest scenario in the ambulance.

The outcome from septic shock in ventilated children with an underlying malignancy but who have not had a bone marrow transplant is only marginally worse than for other children; however, all septic shock in children carries a significant risk of mortality so the parents should not be promised a guaranteed good outcome at this point.

Further Reading

Davies K, Wilson, S. Febrile neutropenia in paediatric oncology. *Paediatr Child Health* 2020;30(3): 93–7.

Fletcher M, Hodgkiss H, Zhang S, et al. Prompt administration of antibiotics is associated with improved outcomes in febrile neutropenia in children with cancer. *Pediatr Blood Cancer*, 2013;60(8): 1299–1306.

National Institute of Health and Care Excellence (2012). Neutropenic sepsis: prevention and management in people with cancer. www.nice.org.uk/guidance/cg151.

Diarrhoea and Vomiting

Georgina Humble and Shelley Riphagen

Chapter

49

A 14-year-old girl presented to her local A&E with vomiting and blood-stained loose stools. Up until a week before presentation, she had been a completely well child with no previous significant illnesses and no known allergies.

The family had recently returned from a holiday in rural France. In the week following their return she had begun to feel generally unwell, and for the past 6 days had developed loose stools containing blood and mucus. Three days before presentation she had also experienced some non-bilious vomiting, which had largely subsided, but, as she admitted, she had not felt like eating or drinking much in the past week and was feeling very unwell and without 'energy'. Her last bloody stool was the previous afternoon, but since then she had not passed any urine or stool. She did not report any fever.

At presentation her observations were recorded as follows: temperature 36.5°C, HR 127 bpm, blood pressure 86/60 mmHg, RR 22 breaths per minute, sats 100% in air. The A&E registrar felt she had normal cardiorespiratory examination and her abdomen, though slightly distended was soft and non-tender. He felt there was nothing significant to find on full clinical examination. Because of the history of diarrhoea and vomiting and poor intake, some baseline blood tests were taken from surprisingly good sized veins, dispelling his concerns she may be dehydrated. She was asked to wait for the results, as well as given a stool sample bottle.

The following blood results seen in Table 49.1 including a venous blood gas were phoned down to A&E 2 hours later.

The A&E registrar referred the child to the regional renal team, who asked the registrar to refer the child to the regional retrieval service to assist with transfer in view of the very deranged biochemistry. The renal team had accepted the child for admission.

Questions

1. Do you think this child's clinical condition warrants use of the critical care retrieval service?
2. What emergency management would you suggest to the local team?
3. Based on the most likely diagnosis, would you recommend starting antibiotics for this child?

1. Do you think this child's clinical condition warrants use of the critical care retrieval service?

With all referrals to the critical care transfer service, no matter what the referrer is asking, it is important to ask yourself the question whether there is an established or

Table 49.1.

Na	131 mmol/L	Haemoglobin	89 g/L
K	6.7 mmol/L	White cell count	$10 \times 10^3/mm^3$
Ca	2.26 mmol/L	Platelets	$85 \times 10^3/mm^3$
PO^4	2.8 mmol/L	pH	7.24
Urea	56 mmol/L	pCO_2	5.1 kPa
Creatinine	1097 μmol/L	pO_2	3.7 kPa
Albumin	35 g/L	HCO_3	16 mmol/L
ALT	122 U/L	Base excess	−10 mEq/L
Lactate dehydrogenase	3550 U/L	Lactate	2.8 mmol/L
CRP	4 mg/L	Glucose	4.5 mmol/L

likely- to- develop emergency. High dependency referrals and transfers are often more difficult to triage and sometimes to transfer.

With children, this is particularly important when there are significant derangements in physiological parameters, blood results, X-ray or ECG findings but the child, at first glance, does not appear that unwell, and is felt to be fit for ward admission.

The most difficult evaluation in sick children is not the child who is obviously critically unwell, and where the decision making is clear, but rather the child who fits into the above category and is not triggering a significant level of concern locally.

There are limited emergency presentations in children and your approach to evaluation should be undertaken in a systematic manner.

- Airway emergencies like upper or lower airway obstruction
- Respiratory emergencies causing impending or established respiratory failure
- Cardiovascular emergencies with established or developing shock
- Neurologic emergencies which can include encephalopathy with or without raised intracranial pressure, status epilepticus or dystonicus, or profound weakness
- Electrolyte and metabolic emergencies involving major electrolyte disturbances or likely inborn errors of metabolism
- Fluid balance abnormalities including emergency renal presentations
- Glucose emergencies related to high or low levels and other endocrine emergencies
- Haemato-oncological emergencies
- Injuries related to trauma emergencies, or other non traumatic surgical emergencies

In this child, there are a few concerning features.

Cardiovascular Status

This is a stressed and unwell teenager who is significantly tachycardic for age with a borderline blood pressure. Teenagers are notoriously difficult to evaluate accurately as they will often 'soldier on' despite being severely unwell. In this setting it is important to ask the question whether this child has any other signs of shock.

In the setting of a history of 6 days of diarrhoea and vomiting, does this child have hypovolaemic shock? A normal teenager is unlikely to progress to this level of illness without being incredibly thirsty and wanting to drink.

In the setting of established renal failure, significant cardiovascular compromise can be caused by uremic pericardial effusion or myocardial dysfunction.

Potential Metabolic Emergency

The potassium is elevated and the cardiovascular effect this is having on rhythm has not been documented. An urgent ECG should be performed and critically evaluated. The child is possibly anuric or severely oliguric. The hyperkalaemia will have to be managed with this in mind.

This child has enough concerning features to warrant critical care retrieval and admission to a HDU/PICU setting with full cardiovascular monitoring until the potassium can be brought under control and the aetiology of the cardiovascular compromise established.

2. What emergency management would you suggest to the local team?

The local team should:

- Record an ECG and then continue with continuous ECG monitoring while hyperkalaemia is actively managed.
- With the high phosphate, additional cardioprotective calcium would not be recommended.
- Salbutamol can be nebulised or given IV at 4 mcg/kg over 5 minutes; however, the response rate is only 50%, so should not be used as monotherapy.
- An insulin dextrose infusion must be delivered through the same cannula, to a maximum of 0.2 U/kg/hr insulin and targeting a glucose of ≥ 6 mmol/L with IV 10% dextrose infusion and regular blood glucose monitoring.
- If it's possible to obtain an echocardiogram, while awaiting the retrieval team, this would be helpful to determine the aetiology of the cardiovascular compromise and rule in or out pericardial effusion or myocardial dysfunction.

3. Based on the most likely diagnosis, would you recommend starting antibiotics for this child?

The child has established renal failure. The history does not suggest the child has had any long-standing health problems, and this most likely represents an acute presentation.

- The commonest cause of acute kidney injury (AKI) in children is haemolytic uraemic syndrome (HUS), affecting 1 in 100,000 children. In the setting of recent exposure to 'rural' setting, with subsequent bloody diarrhoea, and with accompanying thrombocytopenia, diarrhoea positive (D+) HUS is a possibility. The age of the child is unusual, however, as this is a disease more commonly of young children under 5 years old.
- Thrombotic thrombocytopenic purpura usually presents with neurological symptoms and fever with a lesser degree of AKI. Although it is rare in children, it presents most often in adolescence. Testing for ADAMTS 13 will exclude this diagnosis.

- Sepsis with disseminated intravascular coagulation is unlikely as the child would be profoundly shocked with multi-organ failure and an elevated CRP.

Thus the most likely diagnosis is HUS which requires a triad of haemolysis, renal failure and thrombocytopenia. A blood smear would demonstrate haemolysis and fragmented red cells, but in the absence of this, the increased lactate dehydrogenase is suggestive.

In HUS the need for intensive care is based around:

1. Complications of renal failure including pulmonary oedema, hypertensive cardiac failure and uraemic pericardial effusion.
2. Electrolyte emergencies related to renal failure and requiring active management while awaiting renal replacement therapy
3. Neurological symptoms and complications related to HUS, which occur in up to 50% cases and increase morbidity and mortality significantly.

D+ HUS is responsible for 90% of cases and the peak incidence is in the under-5s. It is caused by shiga-toxin producing bacteria.

    E. coli 0157:H7 accounts for 80% of D+HUS in the UK. although less than 10% of children with *E. coli* infections will progress to HUS. *E. coli* is transmitted through undercooked meat, particularly beef and pork; vegetables contaminated with bacteria shed in animal waste and by faecal–oral transmission.

    The pathophysiology is based on toxin-mediated endothelial cell damage, resulting in thrombotic microangiopathy and intraluminal thrombosis of small vessels with subsequent tissue ischaemia and necrosis and the typical clinical presentation affecting mainly kidneys and brain.

Two important points in the management of D+ HUS relate to:

i. Management of anaemia and thrombocytopenia

    The aim is to avoid transfusion until at a renal centre with dialysis available because of the risk of the transfusion-related exacerbation of hyperkalaemia, fluid overload and possibility of acute haemolysis.

    If severe (Hb<50) and symptomatic anaemia, consider transfusion only under direction of the renal team.

    Platelet transfusion should be avoided, unless there is active bleeding, as transfusion may exacerbate the formation of intravascular micro thrombi.

    Plasma should also be avoided if possible, due to naturally occurring IgM antibodies in plasma and the risk of triggering an acute haemolytic crisis.

ii. Antibiotics are contra-indicated in D+HUS as they have been implicated in worsening disease severity, especially neurological involvement. This is not the case in D−HUS (often related to pneumococcal infection) where children can be severely unwell due to bacterial infection with shock and should receive appropriate antimicrobial therapy in this setting.

Specialist interventions includes the use of eculizumab

- This is now first line treatment in atypical HUS.
- Currently it is being trialled in a multicentre study (ECUSTEC Trial) looking at its effectiveness in D+HUS.

Outcome

This girl underwent a successful transfer. Her potassium was down to 5.8 mm/L by the time she was admitted to PICU. An echocardiogram had not been possible locally but was performed on admission to PICU. Echo confirmed a large pericardial effusion pre-tamponade, with a degree of right atrial collapse and she underwent placement of a pericardial drain and vascath after 600 ml of pericardial effusion was drained. Haemofiltration was started that evening and she was discharged to the renal ward the following morning with a potassium of 4.7 mmol/L and feeling significantly better. She continued to be dialysed but made steady progress towards recovery. Her stool culture yielded *E. coli.*

A significant learning point for the local team was that her clinical picture did not reveal how close she was to a severe cardiovascular and metabolic crisis, and without careful supported review and collaboration with the renal and retrieval team, her outcome might have been very different.

Further Reading

ECUSTEC Trial: national multicentre study.

Fakhouri F, Zuber J, Frémeaux-Bacchi V, Loirat C. Haemolytic uraemic syndrome [published correction appears in *Lancet.* 2017 Aug 12;390 (10095):648]. *Lancet.* 2017;390(10095):681–696, doi:10.1016/S0140-6736 (17)30062-4.

Loirat C, Saland J, Bitzan M. Management of hemolytic uremic syndrome. *Presse Med.* 2012;41(3 Pt 2):e115–e135, doi:10.1016/j.lpm .2011.11.013.

A Life-Threatening Sickle Cell Crisis

Juan Ramon Valle Ortiz and Shelley Riphagen

A 10-year-old, 45 kg boy with a background of sickle cell disease had presented to his local A&E with a 5-day history of abdominal pain, and a more recent 2-day history of back and shoulder pain. The morning of the presentation, he had started vomiting and was noted to be jaundiced by his accompanying parent. His mum reported he normally had a haemoglobin of 80–90 g/L and he had had no in-patient hospital stays previously.

A&E was very busy and he was seen and admitted by the paediatric consultant. On arrival in A&E he was self-ventilating with moderate work of breathing, saturating 89% in air but 95% in 15 L/min via face mask. His respiratory rate was 48 breaths per minute with a heart rate of 140 bpm, and blood pressure of 136/69 mmHg. He looked warm and well perfused but noticeably very pale. His abdomen was soft on examination with 5-cm palpable hepatomegaly and 2-cm splenomegaly. He was alert but tired and once settled on the A&E bed was noted to be drowsy.

His initial management included facemask oxygen, establishing IV access and taking some initial blood tests including a cross-match, as shown in Table 50.1. A CXR was also performed in view of the respiratory symptoms and was reviewed as normal. The blood tests took over 2 hours to be processed, while the child waited in A&E on oxygen.

The blood results were reported by telephone to the A&E registrar by the laboratory who also reported they were having difficulty cross matching the sample, and requested a repeat cross-match sample.

Having reviewed the results, the A&E registrar discussed the child with the consultant who was dealing with another ventilated child in A&E. The two senior clinicians decided to give 20 ml/kg of normal saline to the boy and cover with antibiotics. The consultant advised referral was made to the regional retrieval service to transfer the child to the tertiary hospital HDU. The child remained drowsy but rousable.

At the time of referral, 3 hours after the child had first arrived in A&E, the two main questions posed by the A&E registrar to the regional retrieval team were:

1. Request for transfer to a tertiary centre HDU as the blood results were all very abnormal and more than could be managed locally.
2. In a child with sickle cell disease, would it be permissible to use O-negative blood in view of the fact that the cross match was taking such a long time and the child was anaemic.

The retrieval team immediately accepted the child for transfer and advised that the local team wait for cross matched blood.

Table 50.1. Admission blood results

Biochemistry		Haematology		Venous blood gas	
Na	130 mmol/L	Haemoglobin	48 g/L	pH	7.21
K	6.5 mmol/L	White cell count	11.6	pCO$_2$	4.02 kPa
Cl	83 mmol/L	Platelets	131	pO$_2$	7.9 kPa
Creatinine	283 U/L			HCO$_3$	12.8 mmol/L
Bilirubin	408 μmol/L			Base excess	−14.4 mEq/L
ALT	3428 U/L			Lactate	13.9 mmol/L
				Glucose	3.6 mmol/L

Questions

1. How would you evaluate this child's clinical picture?
2. What emergency management would you suggest to the local team?
3. In view of the outcome of this child, what could be done differently, considering the departmental, interdepartmental, hospital-wide and retrieval service perspectives?

1. How would you evaluate this child's clinical picture?

This child was awake and talking on admission despite being breathless and desaturated which probably led the team to consider that his situation was not alarming. However, he was critically ill with a number of identifiable emergencies. It is striking that the blood results were much worse than the clinical appearance of the child. On reflection, the patient had shock with multi-organ failure and should have been treated as a time-critical emergency case.

He had **respiratory failure** with tachypnoea, work of breathing and significant desaturation requiring a large amount of oxygen therapy.

He was **shocked** with tachycardia (despite normal blood pressure, and reportedly being warm and well perfused), high lactate (13.9 mmol), altered level of consciousness (reported as drowsiness, which is unusual in an 10 year old) and biochemical evidence of renal and hepatic dysfunction.

He was also developing a **metabolic emergency** with hyperkalaemia in the setting of renal failure and probable active haemolysis.

Any of these emergencies individually have the potential to deteriorate quickly but together in one child would make this an incredibly difficult stabilisation and resuscitation scenario.

The most likely explanation for this constellation of signs and symptoms is septic shock in the setting of sickle cell disease. In a critically ill child with sickle cell disease, significant **infection** with encapsulated organisms (including salmonella) should be considered and appropriate cultures taken. Antibiotics must be started at the earliest opportunity.

2. What emergency management would you suggest to the local team?

From a **respiratory** point of view, this child has responded well to oxygen. The cause of the respiratory embarrassment does not appear to be lung pathology and may well be secondary to anaemic cardiac failure and shock.

In terms of managing this child's **shock**, this scenario is incredibly challenging. This child is clearly very anaemic and volume resuscitation with further crystalloid will only serve to further haemodilute the child. The blood bank were having trouble cross matching the child because of antibodies, and with active haemolysis clearly evident by falling haemoglobin and rising bilirubin, it would not be without significant additional risk of catastrophic haemolytic transfusion reaction to use non cross-matched blood. The high potassium is already a problem, without the risk of sudden severe haemolysis.

While awaiting cross-matched blood, it may be better to use a small volume (3–5 ml/kg) of hypertonic saline and commence low dose inotropic support, despite the blood pressure, to support the cardiac function. The child needs to be intubated to support shock management and reduce oxygen consumption, but anaesthesia will be poorly tolerated without concurrent inotropic support.

The **hyperkalaemia** is significantly problematic in a child in renal failure and shock, and probable active haemolysis, and the initial management will need to focus on relocating potassium to the intracellular space while more definitive treatment such as continuous venovenous haemofiltration or equivalent can be instituted. This child should be fully monitored on continuous ECG with a defibrillator checked and stationed nearby. Managing the hyperkalemia is the first priority to enable blood transfusion. Transfused packed red cells can have potassium levels of 20 mmol/L or more by the end of the pack life, and transfusion of red cells over 8 days post donation, in the setting of hyperkalaemia should be undertaken with extreme caution.

Interventions to reduce potassium levels in this child would include nebulised salbutamol (with a 50% response rate) and a continuous infusion of glucose and insulin. Calcium should be given as a cardiac membrane stabiliser and magnesium levels should be optimised above 1 mmol/L. It would not be of benefit in this child to try and diurese the potassium out as the child is in renal failure and shocked and likely unresponsive to diuretic at this time.

Arrival of Retrieval Team

The retrieval team arrived 35 minutes after accepting the call to find A&E still very busy. The child was in a cubicle with ECG and saturation monitoring. On examination the child was unrousable, pupils were fixed and dilated. His heart rate was 156 and his blood pressure was unrecordable. The retrieval team asked the attending nurse to summon help immediately and aggressive resuscitation measures began, including immediate intubation and ventilation; arrest doses of adrenaline and a bolus of hypertonic saline were prepared. A repeat blood gas done at that time was largely unchanged except for potassium of 7 mmol/L, lactate of 14.1 mmol/L and haemotcrit of 105 with haemoglobin on the gas of 34 g/L. Bilirubin on the gas had increased to 504. During resuscitation there were intermittent episodes of pulseless ventricular tachycardia. All resuscitation efforts were unsuccessful and the child was declared dead 48 minutes after initiating CPR.

3. In view of the outcome of this child, what could be done differently, considering the departmental, interdepartmental, hospital-wide and retrieval service perspectives?

This child presented in a profoundly unwell state but this was not recognised and therefore he did not get the help he needed immediately.

Children with sickle cell disease are a high-risk group of children who deserve the same degree of caution and surveillance that children receiving chemotherapy are treated. They are more often unwell, frequently in pain when unwell, and both they and their parents are more used to them feeling unwell. Slowly worsening problems can creep up on children and families without the individual or parents being aware of any significant change. These children need to be regarded with a high degree of clinical concern when they present urgently for help, and it is always safer to overestimate the severity of illness.

At the time that this child presented to A&E, all paediatric support had been called to help with three acutely unwell children. This child was the only child who did not need intubation to maintain a safe airway. Once the other two children had been intubated, they both required both paediatric and anaesthetic attention until the retrieval service arrived. This is a rare situation, even in large A&E departments, and would certainly warrant additional support. In an individual paediatric department under these circumstances where can help be summoned from?

Although this child required assistance from his parents to walk in, he was talking and co-operative. He did not have the clinical appearance of a desperately ill child that his blood results would later reveal, and thus was triaged as a lower acuity than the other children. His blood gas, however, was extremely concerning.

- When the clinical picture or blood results are highly discrepant, it is important to review the child in detail again.
- When A&E does become very busy and there are multiple demands on senior clinicians, it is imperative to actively seek additional help within the hospital or from colleagues at home.

What contributed to the severity of this child's illness being unrecognised by the referring team?

- The child walked in and was talking.
- Besides the tachycardia and respiratory distress, which settled on oxygen, the rest of the clinical examination was not obviously concerning without careful scrutiny and questioning.
- The gas results may not have been reviewed immediately because attention was being deflected to other sick children.
- The competing interests of other sick children, made it much more challenging to keep this child under constant review.

What contributed to the severity of this child's illness being unrecognised by the retrieval team?

- When the referral call was made, the questions were a request to move to HDU and about O-negative blood. The referral team did not specifically ask for resuscitation advice.
- The retrieval team did not look beyond the questions asked and failed to identify the emergency need for resuscitation to the local team.

Outcome

Post mortem examination showed this child had salmonella and enterobacter septic shock with evidence of multiorgan ischaemia, and he might not have survived even under the best resuscitation circumstances. However, every hour of unresuscitated shock is associated with two-fold increase in the risk mortality in children with sepsis. Therefore, early recognition and appropriate therapy are fundamental. Recognising the emergency and the time-critical nature of resuscitation in this type of case may help to mobilise the right additional support when there are many competing emergency cases.

Further Reading

1. Han YY, Carcillo JA, Dragotta MA, et al. Early reversal of pediatric-neonatal septic shock by community physicians is associated with improved outcome. *Pediatrics* 2003;112(4):793–9, doi: 10.1542/peds.112.4.793.

A Baby with Acute Liver Failure

Marilyn McDougall

A 7-day-old term baby girl presented to her local A&E with a brief history of poor feeding associated with breathing pauses (apnoeas). She was hypothermic (skin temperature 34.9° C) and had a mixed metabolic and respiratory acidosis pH 7.21, pCO$_2$ 8.8 Kpa on a venous gas with a lactate level of 4.5 mmol/L. Heart rate and blood pressure were within normal limits and there were no signs of respiratory distress. Although saturations were difficult to measure due to temperature, the baby appeared pink in between apnoeic pauses.

She was assumed to have an infection and was admitted to the local paediatric ward. She was warmed by environmental measures and treated with benzyl penicillin and gentamicin for a possible bacterial infection. In addition, continuous positive pressure (CPAP) non-invasive respiratory support was started in view of the apnoea.

These interventions resulted in a transient improvement in her condition. Twenty-four hours later her condition deteriorated with further apnoeas and increasing lethargy and drowsiness to the point that she was only opening her eyes to vigorous stimulation, having previously been alert. Her fontanelle had started to bulge, but there were no abnormalities detected on a cranial ultrasound scan. Prolonged bleeding from venepuncture sites was noted. Her heart rate has increased significantly to 180 bpm, but blood pressure was well preserved 86/38mmHg and stable since admission.

In view of the clinical deterioration, a referral was made to the regional retrieval team for advice regarding further management. At the time of referral, her clinical observations were as shown in Table 51.1. Blood tests from earlier in the day were also reported, as shown in Table 51.2.

Questions

1. What was the identified clinical emergency in this baby?
2. Which other investigations should be undertaken urgently?
3. What are the specific considerations for induction of anaesthesia in acute liver failure, and how will you best manage this patient for transfer?
4. What would you explain to the parents of the patient prior to transfer?

1. What was the identified clinical emergency in this baby?

This baby was encephalopathic with bleeding. She was only rousable with vigorous stimulation and there were clinical signs of raised intracranial pressure with a bulging fontanelle and relatively high blood pressure for such a sick neonate. The combination of encephalopathy with bleeding with biochemical evidence of elevated liver enzymes (ALT) and

Table 51.1.

Heart rate	130 bpm
Respiratory rate	30 breaths per minute
Sats	99% in air
Blood pressure	71/44 mmHg
Temperature	35.8°C
AVPU	P

Table 51.2.

Biochemistry		Haematology	
Na	133 mmol/L	Haemoglobin	123 g/L
K	5.3 mmol/L	White cell count	$3.7 \times 10^3/mm^3$
Creatinine	37 U/L	Platelets	$18 \times 10^3/mm^3$
ALT	52 1 U/L	INR	5.3
CRP	5 mg/L	Albumin	25 g/L

deranged liver function (coagulopathy, lactic acidosis and hypoalbuminaemia), would suggest the baby has acute liver failure until proven otherwise. Although the blood pressure is preserved, the increasing tachycardia is unexplained especially in the setting of hypothermia and the presence of shock, in addition to the above must be considered. Occasionally tachycardia is an outstanding feature of babies with acute severe raised intracranial pressure.

Clinical signs associated with the deranged coagulation may include bleeding from an umbilical stump, easy bruising and excessive bleeding from venepuncture sites. An INR >4 is associated with an increased mortality in children.

Vitamin K should be administered to all patients with liver failure. Clotting factors should only be replaced if invasive procedures are planned or there is evidence of active bleeding. A cross-matched sample of blood should be available to treat large haemorrhage.

The falling level of consciousness may indicate hepatic encephalopathy, one of the life-threatening presentations of acute liver failure, especially when associated with cerebral oedema causing raised intracranial pressure.

Hepatic encephalopathy can be classified into four grades (Table 51.3) Distinguishing grades can be more challenging in infants. This patient would be categorised between grade 3 and 4. Patients with Grade 3 and 4 encephalopathy often go on to require liver transplantation. If this diagnosis is considered, the patient should be transferred to an appropriate liver specialist centre for assessment as soon as possible.

In this setting with a week-old infant, vertically transmitted infection and metabolic conditions feature high on the list of differential diagnoses, with other non-specific features of sepsis present including low serum sodium levels (Na 133), low white cell count (WCC 3.7) and thrombocytopenia (platelets 18).

Table 51.3.

Encephalopathy grade	Clinical signs
Grade 1	Confusion & mood changes
Grade 2	Drowsy, inappropriate
Grade 3	Sleepy but arousable
Grade 4a	Coma but responsive to painful stimuli
Grade 4b	Deep coma not arousable with any stimuli

2. Which other investigations should be undertaken urgently?

Blood glucose levels must be measured urgently. In this patient, the level was 5.3mmol/L and therefore not a concern. Hypoglycaemia is a recognised complication of acute liver failure due to the loss of gluconeogenesis in the liver. Hypoglycaemia further increases the risk of brain injury associated with liver failure. Adequate supply of glucose in the form of IV dextrose 6–8 mg/kg/min must be provided throughout the transfer and blood glucose level must be checked at regular intervals.

Serum ammonia level should be checked as a matter of absolute urgency in all cases of suspected acute liver failure. Liver failure results not only in loss of synthetic function of the liver but also in the capacity to filter waste products. Raised ammonia levels contribute to encephalopathy and brain injury and need to be identified as early as possible. Ongoing protein administration and protein catabolism should be prevented by providing IV dextrose only for energy supply until the elevated ammonia can be treated. Details of therapy for hyperammonaemia are covered in Chapter 47.

As a specific cause for liver failure had not been identified in this patient, a broader septic screen for potential viral infections (e.g. herpes and other congenital infections) and metabolic causes of liver failure (e.g. galactosemia or urea cycle defects) should be undertaken to direct ongoing treatment once the baby is stabilised. Up to 40% of cases of liver failure in infants are due to metabolic conditions. An additional 15% of cases of infantile liver failure are due to viral infections, including herpes in the neonatal group. Aciclovir should be added to the treatment of all cases of acute liver failure in neonates even in the absence of a clear history of herpes contact. In fact, all shocked or encephalopathic neonates presenting critically ill, without a clear cause of collapse should be covered with aciclovir until herpes infection can be positively excluded. This is a potentially treatable infective cause of neonatal collapse and liver failure, but treatment must be instigated early to avoid a fatal outcome.

3. What are the specific considerations for induction of anaesthesia in children with acute liver failure, and how will you best manage this patient for transfer?

The baby has an unexplained tachycardia, altered level of consciousness and apnoea with bulging fontanelle. The possible scenario of shock with raised intracranial pressure should be considered. This scenario is compounded by signs of active bleeding. This baby would require intubation and ventilation for safe transfer. Shock and raised intracranial pressure should both be managed prior to anaesthesia. Hypertonic saline in this setting would treat both clinical emergencies. Owing to the ongoing risk of bleeding, an oral endotracheal tube would be a safer option than nasal.

Optimising the patient's clinical and particularly cardiovascular status prior to induction of anaesthesia is essential. Adequate vascular access must be established to allow administration of fluid boluses and inotropes to support anaesthesia.

Patients with liver failure are more sensitive to the sedative and cardio-depressant effects of anaesthetic agents, as they are unable to metabolise drugs at the same rate as well children. Lower doses should be used. Ketamine can be used as it maintains cardiovascular stability but is metabolized in the liver, thus should not be used as an infusion or with repeated doses. Fentanyl is a suitable opioid to use in this context as it does not have an active metabolite and is renally excreted. Volatile agents should be used with extreme caution as hypotension can already be challenging to manage in this group due to vasodilatation (already apparent with the wide pulse pressure 86-38).

The onset of action of muscle relaxant drugs may be delayed due to the increased volume of distribution and altered protein binding. Atracurium can be safely used as it does not rely on hepatic excretion. Rocuronium and vecuronium are both steroid based and may therefore have delayed elimination in the setting of liver failure.

4. What would you explain to the parents of the patient prior to transfer?

It is important to be honest with the parents and explain that their baby may not survive even if they are safely admitted to a PICU. The patient is in a high risk category and will be best managed in an intensive care with specialist facilities. If the patient does survive, they are likely to require prolonged intensive care and more extensive tests to determine the cause of the liver failure.

Due to the critical nature of the patient's illness it would be appropriate to offer both parents the opportunity to travel with the baby. It would not be appropriate to discuss consideration of liver transplant at this stage.

Outcome

This baby was diagnosed with acute fulminant neonatal herpes infection and despite heroic measures in intensive care proceeded to brain death with unmanageable cerebral oedema and bleeding from all puncture sites. Neither the baby nor mother had any external evidence of herpetic infection, but the mother had immunologic evidence of acute herpetic infection and the baby was PCR positive for herpes.

Further Reading

Davies JH, McDougall M. *Children in Intensive Care a Survival Guide,* 3rd ed. Elsevier, 2019.

Cochran JB, Losek JD. Acute liver failure in children. *Pediatr EmergCare* 2007;23 (10):129–35.

Vaja R, McNichol L, Sisley I, Anaesthesia for patients with liver disease, *Cont Ed Anaesthes Crit Care Pain* 2010;10(1):15–19.

Chapter

52

Air Transport of a Critically Ill Baby

Joanna Davies and Shelley Riphagen

A 13-day old baby presented to her local hospital with respiratory distress and a history of poor feeding for a few days. The baby had no history of maternal risk factors for infection and had normal antenatal scans. At the time of referral, she was self- ventilating in air with sternal and subcostal recession. She had a 2/6 systolic murmur and a firm liver, enlarged to her umbilicus. Pre- and post-ductal saturations were 92% on admission with upper limb/lower limb blood pressure as shown in Table 52.1. CXR identified cardiomegaly and opacification of the right lung fields. Her abdomen was distended but soft. She had microscopic blood present on urine bedside testing. She was sleepy but responsive with a flat fontanelle. The referring hospital had sent relevant blood tests as noted in Table 52.2 and commenced IV cefotaxime.

In view of the cardiomegaly, respiratory distress and hepatomegaly, the referral hospital requested transfer of this baby with a presumed diagnosis of congenital cardiac disease. Their location was several hours' flight from the paediatric tertiary services provider.

Questions

1. What advice would you give about the management of this baby while awaiting transfer? What other medication should be advised? What further investigations are required urgently?
2. What are your priorities for management by air transfer?
3. What do you need to do prior to leaving hospital to board the flight?
4. After an hour of trying you are unable to site central access – what potential options do you have?

1. What advice would you give about the management of this baby while awaiting transfer? What other medication should be advised? What further investigations are required urgently?

Important prior to any advice being given is to try and identify the urgent presenting clinical problem, which in this case appears to be progressive cardiac failure with respiratory distress. The baby has a cardiac murmur, cardiomegaly and hepatomegaly with signs of pulmonary oedema. Untreated cardiac failure may progress to cardiogenic shock.

Although this baby is well saturated self-ventilating in air, she has significant tachypnoea and work of breathing with both subcostal and sternal recession. It is evident that the baby will require some type of respiratory support as left unsupported, she will likely

Table 52.1. Initial observations

Respiratory rate	120 breaths per minute
Heart rate	136 bpm
Blood pressure	Right arm 103/76 mmHg; Left arm 100/69 mmHg
	Right leg 100/66 mmHg; Left leg 83/55 mmHg
Sats	92% (right hand and left foot)
Capillary refill time	4sec

Table 52.2.

Blood tests		Venous blood gas	
Na	136 mmol/L	pH	7.32
K	5.1 mmol/L	pCO$_2$	6.8 kPa
Urea	2.5 mmol/L	pO$_2$	5.4 kPa
Creatinine	35 U/L	HCO$_3$	25.7 mmol/L
CRP	0.5 mg/L	Base excess	0.3 mEq/L
		Lactose	2.6 mmol/L
		Glucose	5.8 mmol/L

progress to respiratory exhaustion and arrest. Young children have reduced respiratory reserve as a result of a number of developmental factors including alveolar number and lung surface area, along with a higher baseline metabolic rate with increased oxygen consumption and carbon dioxide production from tissue metabolism. Under conditions of extreme respiratory compromise, apnoea (respiratory arrest) is not an uncommon response in babies under 2 months of age, where the fetal life-preserving 'diving reflex' is still active. Factors affecting the decision to support ventilation invasively are centred around knowledge that this level of work of breathing is not sustainable, and the baby needs to be transported a considerable distance to a tertiary centre, by air in this instance. Were she not in need of undergoing transfer, non-invasive respiratory support could be attempted as a temporary measure; however, the amount of support delivered by nasal CPAP or high flow oxygen is unlikely to reverse this level of respiratory work, and the baby would still be at risk of respiratory arrest.

The most senior anaesthetic doctor in the hospital (preferably with paediatric experience), and a senior neonatal or paediatric doctor should be called to attend this baby. There are a number of factors to consider prior to anaesthesia for intubation:

- This baby is critically ill and at the limit of physiological reserve. It is imperative that this is not only recognised by the referring team but stated out loud so that the whole team is focused, alert and prepared prior to intervention.
- The choice of drugs for intubation needs to be carefully considered and openly discussed, led by the senior clinical team.

- It is likely that this baby has an undiagnosed cardiac condition (although other diagnoses have not been ruled out). This will affect optimal resuscitation strategy with respect to fluid boluses, inotropic support and the need to be prepared for cardiac arrest during induction of anaesthesia.
- Inotropic drug infusions should be prepared, connected and correctly programmed to run or already running prior to intubation (usually diluted so it can be given via a peripheral cannula as no central access is available).
- Adrenaline, atropine, calcium doses and small aliquot volume resuscitation boluses should be prepared in case of cardiac arrest during induction and intubation.
- As a cardiomyopathy is a possibility, defibrillation pads should be correctly sited on the baby, connected to the defibrillator with the energy dose agreed and a competent operator appointed.

Drugs for Intubation

The recommended drugs for intubation for critically ill babies and children are ketamine 1–2 mg/kg, fentanyl 0–2 mcg/kg and rocuronium 1 mg/kg. In critically ill and shocked children, smaller doses of ketamine and fentanyl can be used, anticipating that children in this condition need lower doses to achieve an appropriate level of anaesthesia, before muscle relaxation. It is also anticipated that time to achieve anaesthesia would be prolonged in this setting and bag valve mask ventilation, to ensure good oxygenation, should be managed by a competent airway operator during induction. Propofol is **not** recommended in cardio-vascular unstable patients, as this may precipitate cardiac arrest due to hypotension. The stomach should be actively decompressed via nasogastric tube during mask ventilation.

a. What other medication should be advised?

It is likely that this baby has a cardiac diagnosis, but the referring hospital did not have access to personnel to perform a neonatal echocardiogram. All neonates who present with cardiac symptoms, where structural congenital heart disease cannot be excluded, should be commenced on prostaglandin E2 (Prostin/dinoprostone) in case of a possible duct dependent lesion.

The ductus arteriosus usually closes in the first few days of life but may remain patent well beyond the first 2 weeks of life in children with congenital structural heart disease. Duct-dependent congenital heart lesions are dependent on the duct remaining patent to supply pulmonary or systemic blood flow or to allow mixing between the pulmonary and systemic circulations. In the event that the duct starts closing in neonates with these lesions, they will present with significant compromise. Remember that this drug is delivered in nanograms/kg/min. Recommended starting dose of Prostin in nanograms/kg/min:

-	If clinically well -	5 ng/kg/min
-	If unstable or absent femoral pulses	20 ng/kg/min
-	If no response or under consultant guidance	50–100 ng/kg/min

Prostin-related apnoea is common in the first hour of administration, with increased doses and in extremely ill neonates. At high dose, the vasodilatory properties of the drug that results in ductal muscle relaxation also compromises blood pressure, which may need to be supported with inotropes. (Details are given in the STRS Neonatal Collapse Guideline 2017.)

b. What further investigations are required urgently?

Although it seems most likely that the baby has a cardiac diagnosis, it is important to exclude other causes of cardiomegaly and hepatomegaly. In neonatal collapse, the most likely diagnoses include sepsis, cardiac causes, respiratory disease, metabolic abnormalities or trauma. When giving advice to a referring centre or on a paediatric transport in such a scenario, the aim is to:

- Provide supportive care to whichever organ is dysfunctional
- Diagnose and treat all life-threatening problems
- Exclude and treat likely possible differential diagnoses including taking blood and other cultures and establishing baseline parameters suggestive of infection (white cell and platelet count, CRP and procalcitonin) prior to starting antibiotics and anti-virals; undertaking a basic metabolic screen with blood glucose, ketone and ammonia testing, while ensuring the baby is kept nil by mouth with glucose maintained in the high normal range with glucose infusion; performing CXR and other imaging as indicated, to exclude trauma as a cause of collapse.

It is unlikely that the tertiary centre will be able to accurately specify the cause of the cardiac failure until further investigations are carried out.

2. What are your priorities for management by air transfer?

It will be 4 to 6 hours before the retrieval team reach this baby. In the event of significant delay in retrieval, clear and detailed advice needs to be given.

1. Identify three urgent actions in order of priority; e.g. in this situation:
   - Start Prostin
   - Proceed to intubation with the most senior anaesthetist
   - Send relevant blood tests to exclude other diagnoses, e.g. metabolic prior to commencing antibiotics, antivirals and glucose infusion.
2. Arrange air ambulance and team to collect baby as soon as possible. This will take several hours.
3. If crossing borders, the neonate is unlikely to have a passport but will need some form of travel documentation/urgent birth certificate/urgent passport to be arranged to allow travel with mum. Ensure the mother is fit to fly. The travel documentation must be cleared by the air ambulance company and national immigration services.
4. Start preparations for flight transfer – personnel, medical equipment (see below for further detail).
5. Follow up calls to referring centre to check on progress of baby and give further advice as required.

   For flight checklists and logistics consult Chapter 3 Air Retrieval.
   Additional considerations include:

- Fixed wing flight retrievals are used when journey times are longer. This must be considered when preparing documentation for contemporaneous record keeping with regard to observations and medical and nursing notes during transfer.
- There is usually a requirement for transport team passport or travel documents and air tickets if a commercial carrier is used.

- Also a letter is required from the service medical lead, with relevant contact details, regarding controlled drugs if these are taken. These will need to be cleared through airport security, and it is worthwhile having a discussion with this team prior to flying to ensure there are no surprises.
- Calculate oxygen requirements:
  - Total journey time in minutes × ventilator or flow metre usage (litres/minute) and then double the total, to allow for delays/flight re-routing.
  - Do not forget the travel time to and from the airport with the patient, the flight waiting time as well as the in-flight time.
  - Discuss the oxygen requirement with the carrier to ensure that the cylinder capacity is adequate, as well as smaller cylinders for transport to and from the airport. Data regarding medical gas cylinder capacity is available from www.bochealthcare.co.uk.
  - Not all cylinder heads are the same and the cylinder ventilator interface must be checked. Also ensure you have a spanner key to change a pin index cylinder if those are the only ones available.
  - Remember too that the ambulance pick-up at the destination may also need compatibility check with your ventilator.

Status of Baby on Arrival of Retrieval Team

The baby was intubated and ventilated with an appropriate-sized tube, situated high on CXR. Right-sided consolidation and progressive cardiomegaly were noted on CXR. Heart rate and blood pressure were in acceptable range, however, despite normothermia, the baby remained cold to touch and very poorly perfused with weak central pulses and gallop rhythm. The baby was comfortably sedated and muscle relaxed.

The baby only had two peripheral cannulae in situ. Internal jugular access had been attempted unsuccessfully by the local team. Nasogastric tube was well positioned on CXR and on free drainage.

Prostin 20 nanograms/kg/min, morphine 20 mcg/kg/hour and maintenance fluids 0.9% saline and 10% dextrose 12 ml/hour were all in progress. The baby had also received 10 ml/kg bolus of fluid, IV cefotaxime and intermittent doses of rocuronium.

3. What do you need to do prior to leaving hospital to board the flight?

Use a structured ABCDE approach again, then reassess:

A: Ensure the endotracheal tube position is optimised and firmly secured.

B: Perform airway suctioning with physiotherapy manoeuvres, if possible, to improve air entry to right side.

C: Check Prostin dose (as this is the commonest drug error in emergency paediatrics due to the triple dilution required). Ensure vascular access is patent and secure. Obtain further IV access if possible due to long flight and difficulty establishing access at altitude. Re-attempt central access using ultrasound guidance. Prepare inotrope infusions, and have connected and programmed to run if required. Prepare emergency drugs for flight. Site arterial line if time permits.

D: Check adequate sedation and make provision for ongoing sedation and muscle relaxation. Check blood sugar prior to flight and ensure glucose saline maintenance running to maintain blood sugar in 5–8 mmol/L range in sick neonate.

E: Prepare baby for flight. Temperature control is more challenging at altitude because of the associated environmental temperature fall. Use warming transport blanket, hat, mittens, booties. Ensure baby has ear defenders for flight transfer.

F: Catheterise baby.

Most important is to update the parents on baby's condition, find out if they are travelling with their baby and to explain the risks of transporting a very sick and fragile baby. There is a possibility she may deteriorate or even die during transfer.

4. After an hour of trying you are unable to site central access – what potential options do you have?

You have now been with the baby at the hospital for an hour. You have repositioned and secured the endotracheal tube, suctioned large quantities of thick secretions and carbon dioxide clearance has improved, allowing reduction of ventilator settings.

You and the senior anaesthetist have only managed to site one further peripheral line. Despite using ultrasound, attempts for central access by senior personnel have been unsuccessful. The flight crew inform you that you need to be in the aircraft with patient ready to take off within 1 hour, otherwise they will be grounded until the following day, having exceeded flying hour allowances.

Do you:

- a. Keep trying for central venous access as you are concerned that this baby will deteriorate during the flight and need inotropes?
- b. Keep trying for arterial access as it is essential to have accurate blood pressure monitoring?
- c. Prepare dilute inotropic infusions and transfer with three peripheral lines?
- d. Plan to stay overnight and establish both central and arterial access before boarding a flight to the tertiary centre?

Difficult decisions should be discussed with the PICU consultant/transport consultant on call. None of the options is ideal. It is most important to get the baby to a tertiary centre where a diagnosis can be made with appropriate specialist input. However, the baby needs to reach the tertiary centre alive and in good condition for this to happen.

The baby's condition has deteriorated significantly in the 12 hours since admission. The decision is taken to fly with three peripheral cannulas and an intra-osseous needle set to hand. Arterial access is not a life-saving measure so extra time trying to secure this is not warranted. Non-invasive blood pressure monitoring will be used.

Important discussion with pilots must occur prior to take off to update them of any anticipated complications/specific requests regarding altitude/potential need to divert.

Inform the tertiary centre of baby's condition, current support required, and expected time of arrival at destination, prior to take-off to ensure an ambulance will be waiting airside to collect baby and team on arrival.

The Flight to the Tertiary Centre

Due to anticipated instability on take-off and at altitude, and on discussion with the consultant, peripheral concentration of an inotrope, e.g. dopamine is commenced at low dose of 5 mcg/kg/minute prior to take-off.

This was increased to 10 mcg/kg/minute during the flight due to hypotension. Oxygen was also increased for the duration of the flight due to desaturation despite increased airway pressures.

The baby was safely transferred to the tertiary centre where she was diagnosed with obstructive hypertrophic cardiomyopathy.

Further Reading

South Thames Retrieval Service 2017 Neonatal Collapse Guideline. STRS Evelina London Children's Hospital.

Medical gas cylinder capacities:- www.bochealthcare.co.uk

Crew Resource Management

Sam Fosker

Winter has come!

   You have just started your shift and been handed five referrals of children that need transferring. The human resources available to you at your transfer hub are as follows.

Teams

   Retrieval lead: Potential three retrieval teams (including yourself) with fully stocked kit. Retrieval leads within each team are one consultant, two retrieval fellows.

   Retrieval nurses: two retrieval-trained nurses to support the retrieval leads.

   Ambulance technicians: two blue light trained technicians. Service manager is also blue light trained.

   Vehicles: three working and road-tested ambulances, 1 air ambulance rotary service.

   Weather: Generally sunny day with some patchy cloud.

Child 1

   Locality: 24 miles away at local hospital with no Special Care Baby Unit. Helipad on site.

   Referral: Female premature 30-week neonate who has returned at day 8 of life. The baby is shocked and has poor femoral pulses. Prostin has been started at 10 nanograms/kg/min with some initial response; however, the local team has increased the infusion to 20 nanograms/kg/min on advice from cardiology. Bloods have been taken, antibiotics have been given and glucose started to maintain glucose level 4–8 mmol/L. There is no concern from ECG or CXR. The baby needed to be intubated for ongoing management of shock and possible prostin related apnoea. The local neonatal team should be called to assist anaesthesia.

   Working diagnosis: Shock due to coarctation of the aorta possibly precipitated by ductal closure.

Child 2

   Locality: 90 miles at local hospital. Nearest PICU full. Nearest helipad 5 miles away at the local airfield.

   Referral: 4-year-old child who has had cough and coryzal symptoms for 4 days. He had been given antibiotics by the GP but not improved and today was brought into the A&E as he was worsening and becoming more lethargic. Due to the fact that the saturations remained below 90% in 15 L/min facemask oxygen, with ongoing significant work of breathing, the local team made the decision to proceed to intubation and ventilation.

CXR showed extensive right-sided consolidation. The child has been given appropriate antibiotics and 60 ml/kg fluid resuscitation in A&E. Blood test results are awaited. The child remains shocked with current observations HR 150, BP 62/35, capillary refill 6 seconds.

Working diagnosis: Septic shock due to pneumonia.

Child 3

Locality: 48 miles away at local hospital. Nearest helipad 10 miles away.

Referral: 8-year-old with brittle asthma who had a sudden severe attack at school. He deteriorated further when he arrived in A&E and despite optimal medical therapy, CO_2 levels continued to rise with no improvement in clinical status and the child was intubated by the anaesthetic team. The local team are having some difficulty ventilating the child as the high-pressure alarm keeps sounding on the ventilator, and ending the breath prematurely.

Working diagnosis: Life-threatening asthma.

Child 4

Locality: Currently at your local PICU. Helipad on site.

Referral: 15-month-old. Brought to PICU due to needing intubating and ventilating for severe bronchiolitis. Now improved and extubated for 48 hours. Needs repatriating back to same hospital as Child 2. Transfer was due for yesterday but delayed due to no team being available. Single mum is with other child at home and will meet you at the local hospital.

Child 5

Locality: PICU 40 miles away. Helipad on site.

Referral: Neonate treated for meconium aspiration but has worsening ventilation and latest CXR this morning shows ARDS-type picture. Current calculated oxygen index is 36 despite optimal therapy. Would like consideration and urgent transfer for ECMO.

Questions

1. What are your potential options for obtaining additional resources?
2. What are your initial thoughts on the locality and urgency of each child?
3. How would you organise your current resources to deal with the referrals, assuming no new more urgent referrals come in?

1. What are your potential options for getting other resources?

When approaching these problems, it's important to establish and understand what your current resources are and also how you may be able to source others. Most retrieval teams will cover a specific geographic area and so will have neighbouring teams which may be able to cross cover across borders. In times of resource scarcity, it is not uncommon for teams to help each other out with transfers outside of their normal area.

There may also be other resources closer to home. For retrieval teams that are co-located with a PICU, it may be possible to create an extra retrieval team for the time of the retrieval only, from those on shift, if transport and equipment allows. Other retrieval teams, such as neonatal or adult retrieval teams, may be able to assist with children within the age and size of their team confidence and competence. Most teams will have an escalation plan or major incident plan to utilise when resources become overwhelmed.

Local teams are usually required to transfer children with time critical conditions, so although this is not the default position for other children, it is well within the local team's capability to undertake transfer. To utilise this resource means depleting the team locally and will place additional pressure on local resources. In the case of a critically ill child, where the local team cannot leave the child's bedside, and retrieval is likely to be delayed >120 minutes, and no other paediatric team is available, the option of local team retrieval of the child to a pre-arranged PICU bed, should be discussed.

2. What are your initial thoughts on the locality and urgency of each child?

When faced with this number of urgent retrievals, it is important to triage the cases based on:

1. Clinical acuity of the child
2. Predicted natural progression of the disease or condition
3. Ability of the local team to stabilise the child
4. Local resources, confidence and competence of the local team in dealing with the specific condition of the child

The cases should be stacked in order of priority, with the decision at the outset to continue to review the triage order and to modify based on additional clinical information. It is sometimes easier to see this decision making in tabular form as shown in Table 53.1. These decisions are based on clinical judgement which may vary between operators, but should be transparent and justifiable, no matter the decision.

Child 1

The prostin will likely act as a holding measure and may even improve the situation. There will be local paediatric (neonatal) resources to assist with stabilisation. If available and due to anticipated delay in transfer, the neonatal transport team can be approached to transfer this baby.

Child 2

This child is severely unwell and resuscitated. The natural history is one of deterioration before improvement. The local team needs directed advice. This is a challenging situation and the local team will need on-site support urgently. This child is transfer priority.

Child 3

Life-threatening asthma can be extremely challenging to ventilate even in PICU. The local team will need careful guidance about ventilation prior to arrival of the retrieval team. High

Table 53.1.

	Severity of illness/ clinical acuity	Natural progression	Local team location	Local team resources	Distance and likely delay	Triage decision
Child 1 COA with shock	4	4	3	4	24 miles	Approach neonatal team for transfer. Give advice
Child 2 Pneumonia with septic shock	1	1	1	1	90 miles	Air retrieval team 1. Advice re resuscitation while en route
Child 3 Life threatening asthma	2	2	2	2	48 miles	Team 2. Give advice re management and ventilation
Child 4 Recovered bronchiolitis	5	5	5	4	Local miles	Air takeback to location 2 Team 1
Child 5 Meconium aspiration /ARDS for ?ECMO	3	3	4	3	40 miles	Neighbouring PICU team or first team back. Give advice

pressure ventilation puts this child at risk of pneumothorax and this should be considered in retrieval equipment. This child is the second priority.

Child 4

This child is stable and in a place of safety, but as the awaited repatriation is the destination of the first retrieval, this can be achieved at the same time, as retrieving child 2.

Child 5

This child is severely ill, but in a place of safety. The local team have exhausted all their resources. Review of management may allow additional treatment suggestions. There are three or four options for transfer, as the retrieval is going to be delayed. A neighbouring paediatric retrieval team can be asked to help; the local team can transfer or the local team can wait until the first team arrives back from Child 2 or 3. Alternatively the service retrieval consultant can attend the NICU and use the local team, with a frontline ambulance, to transfer the child.

3. How would you organise your current resources to deal with the referrals, assuming no new more urgent referrals come in?

If child 2 and child 3 can be stabilised after retrieval team advice, then it may be possible to re-prioritise child 5 into first position. However with the current information:

Child 4 is repatriated by air to Child 2's hospital with team 1.

Child 3 is transferred by team 2

Team 1 or team 2 (whichever returns first) will transfer Child 5, if not already moved.

Next team back will transfer Child 1 if not moved by neonatal transport team.

These decisions are all clinical and logistic decisions based on critical evaluation of the child's condition, the likely course and progress of disease and the local team resources, and should be open to challenge and re-ordering based on new or additional information.

Chest Drain Insertion

Marilyn McDougall

Fortunately, the need to insert a chest drain during paediatric retrievals is rare ($<$1% of retrievals). However, when necessary, a chest drain may need to be inserted quickly and safely, to prevent further deterioration. Pleural collections can compromise both the respiratory and cardiac systems. Most children with a chest drain will subsequently require transfer to a tertiary PICU or respiratory centre for ongoing management of their chest drain.

Chest drain insertion can be associated with harm. There was an alert in 2008 regarding 12 deaths and 15 serious harm events related to chest drain insertion in children and adults. Many of the complications were related to incorrect site of insertion, inadequate staff experience and supervision, and failure to follow manufacturer guidelines. Ideally a local checklist should be used if available to ensure that all the necessary equipment and safe monitoring are available. It is important to discuss the planned steps of chest drain insertion with the team supporting the medical lead who will perform the procedure. At least one person should be assigned to monitor the patient carefully during the drain insertion to detect any clinical change or concern. An assistant should be designated to support the person performing the drain insertion.

Most children will require general anaesthesia or deep sedation to facilitate chest drain insertion. In shocked patients good IV access with ongoing fluid resuscitation and inotropes are essential to facilitate safe induction prior to drain insertion.

This does not apply to tension pneumothorax which should be urgently decompressed with a needle before any analgesia or sedation administered.

In a medical emergency consent for the procedure may not be necessary; however, it would be appropriate to explain the planned procedure to parents or carers in advance.

Sterile precautions are essential at all stages of chest drain insertion to avoid local infection.

Indications for Chest Drain Insertion on Retrieval

Clinical signs and symptoms are more important than the radiological features when deciding about drain insertion. Ultrasound guidance improves success and reduces complications of chest drain insertion.

1. Pneumothorax

   - Tension pneumothorax (following needle decompression)
   - Symptomatic: hypoxia or respiratory distress
   - Any size in a patient who requires air transfer
   - Patient on positive pressure ventilation.

2. Haemothorax: blunt or penetrating chest injury

3. Pleural effusion or empyema leading to difficulty providing adequate ventilation

- Empyema usually need drainage for infection management.

Tension Pneumothorax Is a Medical Emergency

Clinical signs include:

- Hypoxia, hypotension and tachycardia
- Ipsilateral (on the side of the pneumothorax): hyper-resonance, reduced breath sounds, hyperexpansion with reduced chest movement
- Tracheal deviation in a unilateral pneumothorax and distended neck veins.

In ventilated patients: reduced tidal volume, elevated central venous pressure and surgical emphysema may develop.

Treatment includes urgent needle decompression:

- Insert 14–18 gauge cannula in the second intercostal space, mid-clavicular line.
- Immediate egress of air confirms the position.
- Chest drain should be inserted immediately after needle aspiration. The needle should remain in place until the chest drain is bubbling continuously.
- If second decompression is needed you can go in the same place (cannulas can become kinked easily and pneumothorax may re-accumulate).

Paediatric scenarios that can lead to tension pneumothorax include:

- Trauma patients
- Obstructive lung diseases including asthma and bronchiolitis
- Patients receiving non-invasive or invasive ventilation
- Blocked, clamped or misplaced chest drains.

Equipment Required for Chest Drain Insertion

Sterile gown and gloves
Skin cleaning solution
Sterile drapes
Syringe, needle and local anaesthetic
Scalpel and blade
Sutures (silk 2/0 or 3/0) and needle holder
Curved Kelly clamp (for blunt dissection)
Appropriate bore chest drain (10–32F) with guidewire (Table 54.1).

Table 54.1.

Age (weight)	Chest tube size (French gauge)
Neonate (2–5 kg)	10–16
6 months (6–8 kg)	14–18
1–2 years (10–20 kg)	14–20
5 years (16–18 kg)	14–24
8 years (30 kg)	16–32

- Lateral borer of pectoralis major (anteriorly)
- anterior border of latissimus dorsi (posteriorly),
- line superior to 5th rib and at the level of the nipple.
- Apex of triangle below axilla

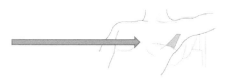

Figure 54.1 Site for chest drain insertion: SAFE triangle.
Source: London School of Paediatrics part task guide

Tubing to connect to underwater drain
Underwater drain or Heimlich valve and collection bag
Adhesive dressing
Ultrasound machine and sterile cover for probe

Site for Chest Drain Insertion: SAFE Triangle

This area is considered the 'safe triangle' as it is the least muscular surface of the chest wall and if appropriately adhered to will avoid injury to organs such as the heart, liver and spleen (Figure 54.1).

Seldinger Drain Insertion

1. The patient should be lying on their back. Position patient with arm extended or folded behind head on the side of the drain insertion.
2. Check equipment assembled, patient fully monitored and team aware of procedure and timing.
3. Confirm presence of fluid or air with ultrasound, mark the appropriate drain insertion site.
4. Scrub and put on sterile gloves, gown and mask.
5. Clean skin with antiseptic solution or swabs and apply sterile drapes. Remember that the neurovascular bundle runs under the rib therefore the needle and drain should be inserted along the upper border of the lower (4th or 5th rib) (Figure 54.2).
6. Infiltrate site with local anaesthetic, aspirating as you advance and then infiltrate the pleural space. Remember to check the maximum local anaesthetic dose that can be safely administered (e.g. 3 mg/kg for lidocaine).
7. Attach 5 ml syringe to introducer needle, gradually advance the needle at the same site that the local anaesthetic was applied. Advance until air or fluid is aspirated, a 'pop' or loss of resistance is noted when crossing the pleura.
8. Detach the syringe from the needle (aspirated fluid should be retained for investigations, such as microbiology) and insert the Seldinger wire through the needle into the pleural space. There should be no resistance until the wire has passed several centimetres. Stop when resistance is encountered. Early resistance would reflect malposition of the needle, usually into the intercostal muscle layer.
9. Once the wire is in the correct place, carefully withdraw the needle ensuring that the wire is not dislodged.

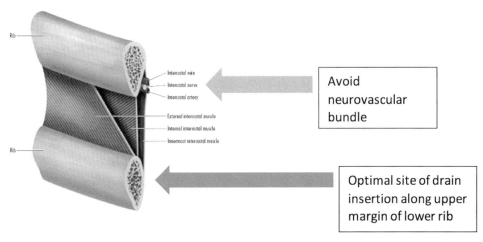

Rib

Intercostal vein
Intercostal nerve
Intercostal artery

External intercostal muscle
Internal intercostal muscle
Innermost intercostal muscle

Rib

Avoid neurovascular bundle

Optimal site of drain insertion along upper margin of lower rib

Figure 54.2 Single handed technique for forced expiration of non-dependent lung in babies and small children.

10. Use the scalpel to make a small horizontal incision along the upper border of the lower rib through the skin and subcutaneous tissue to the level of the skeletal muscle.
11. Advance a dilator over the wire and using a firm gentle pressure, dilate to the level of the pleural space. Serial dilators may be necessary to make an appropriate size hole for a particular chest drain.
12. Once the site has been dilated appropriately, remove the dilator and pass the chest drain over the wire. Remove the guidewire. Pleural fluid should begin to drain. Clamp the drain and suture into position. The drain should be well secured using a stay suture on the chest wall which is then tied around the chest drain.
13. Attach the drain to the underwater drain or Heimlich valve and release the clamp. Check that the drain is swinging or bubbling. Apply dressing to the drain insertion site and tape the drain to the abdomen securely at a site distant from insertion.
14. When draining a large effusion the drain should be clamped for 1 hour after 10 ml/kg of fluid is initially removed. A bubbling drain should never be clamped.
15. CXR is necessary to confirm appropriate drain position prior to transfer.
16. Any acute change in the patient's condition after drain insertion should include consideration of drain occlusion and pneumothorax.

Blunt Dissection Method

Steps 1–7 as per Seldinger technique.

8. Use the scalpel to make a small horizontal incision along the upper border of the lower rib (usually 5th rib) through the skin and subcutaneous tissue to the level of the skeletal muscle. A 0.5–1 cm incision is adequate for a small child, larger 1–2 cm incision required for an older child.
9. Closed curved clamp or straight mosquito forceps (or equivalent dissecting clamp) inserted into the incision and blunt dissection is performed by gently advancing and opening the clamp dissecting layers of fascia and muscle until the pleura is breached. Do not close the blunt dissection forceps in the tissue tunnel. A pop or sudden loss of resistance is felt when the pleura is punctured. A rush or air or fluid usually ensues at this point.

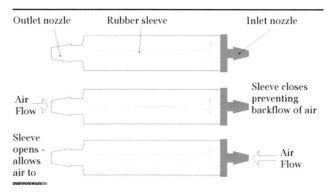

Figure 54.3 Heimlich (flutter) valve mechanism.

10. The forceps should be spread widely at this point to ensure adequate opening for chest drain insertion. In an older child it may be possible to place a finger in the space to strip any adhesions between lung and pleura. The chest tube is then advanced into the pleural space. If the child is too small to allow a finger to the placed into the space the chest drain can be inserted through the tips of the open curved forceps.

The same steps (12–16) are used to secure and check the position of this drain as for the Seldinger method.

Heimlich Valve

A Heimlich valve is a flutter valve which can be used for transport situations when an underwater system is not practical. The Heimlich valve creates a one-way valve that allows air or fluid to escape from the pleural space but prevents re-entry during inspiration.

In a pneumothorax cessation of the fluttering either indicates resolution of the pneumothorax or obstruction of the drain. A small bag (such as a bile bag) can be applied to the outlet nozzle if there is fluid draining from the chest during transfer until a more definitive underwater system can be applied (Figure 54.3).

Complications of Chest Drain Insertion

Careful cleaning of the site and dissecting close to the upper border of the lower rib can reduce the incidence of complications.

1. During blunt dissection:
   - Bleeding due to injury to intercostal artery
   - Injury to neurovascular bundle causing pain or numbness.

2. During drain placement:
   - Penetration of lung parenchyma, mediastinal contents, diaphragm.
   - Most organ injury can be avoided by using blunt dissection without insertion of a trocar
   - Abdominal penetration, increased risk if hemi diaphragm paralysis.

3. Complications due to location of drain:
   - Cardiogenic shock due to right atrial compression

- Horner syndrome due to pressure by the drain tip on the inferior cervical ganglion
- Surgical emphysema: may be concerning for patient or their family, but it usually resolves spontaneously without any long-term consequences. May be caused by blocked, kinked or malpositioned drain with the last holes close outside the pleural space. It can sometimes be due to the imbalance between a relatively large pneumothorax and small bore chest drain.

4. Ongoing complications after insertion:

- Infection
- Bronchopleural fistula
- Pain at insertion site can lead to splinting of the chest and pneumothorax
- Drain disconnection or obstruction.

Further Reading

Henretig FM, King C. *Textbook of paediatric emergency procedures*. Williams and Wilkins 1997.

Lamont T. Insertion of chest drains: Summary of the safety report from National Patient Safety Agency. *BMJ* 2009;339:b4923.

MacDuff A, Arnold A, Harvey J, et al. Management of spontaneous pneumothorax: British Thoracic Society pleural drain guideline 2010. *Thorax* 2010;65(Suppl 2) ii:18–31.

Maskell N, British Thoracic Society Pleural Disease Guideline Group. British Thoracic Society Pleural Disease Guidelines 2010 Update. *Thorax* 2010;65 667–9.

Chapter

55

Paediatric Airway Clearance for Acute Management on Retrieval

Rosalie Summers

The techniques outlined below should only be used by practitioners clinically trained in their use by a competent physiotherapist. Preparation by contacting local physiotherapy service is advisable. If a local physiotherapist is available they should be contacted for assistance. The procedures outlined below should only be employed when the patient's respiratory status demands it to optimise clinical condition for transfer.

This guidance for airway clearance using saline lavage is only for use with intubated and ventilated patients or those with a tracheostomy who are in acute respiratory failure e.g. hypoxia +/- hypercapnia. Other patients should await the availability of a qualified physiotherapist.

Typical patient conditions where these techniques are useful include:

- Bronchiolitis, where there is secondary pneumonia, dense consolidation or mucus plugging with atelectasis and collapse
- Acute asthma exacerbation
- Pneumonia
- Respiratory deterioration in patients with background medical history that makes their airway clearance poor (i.e. neuromuscular weakness).

It is important to remember that in a retrieval situation, these contraindications may be disregarded due to necessity for life-saving interventions.

Indications
- Central airway obstruction
- Focal consolidation or collapse of a lung or lobe of a lung.

Safety Contraindications
- Pulmonary haemorrhage
- Rib fractures
- Undrained pneumothorax
- Foreign body aspiration
- Frank bleeding from the airway
- Raised intracranial pressure.

Safety Precautions
- Lung bullae
- Pneumothorax

- Impaired cardiac function, e.g. cardiomyopathy, myocarditis or post cardiac surgery
- High oxygen requirements
- High positive end-expiratory pressure (PEEP)
- Osteopenia.

Prior to any treatment, review post-intubation CXR to check endotracheal tube position, exclude any air leaks and identify the target areas for treatment. Ensure the stomach contents have been aspirated and the patient is cardiovascularly capable of tolerating a level of treatment.

There are two main situations that occur where airway clearance techniques can be very beneficial and effective.

Central Airway Secretion Obstruction

The aim of the technique in this situation is to clear central secretions, increase tidal volume and hence improve oxygenation and ventilation. Two experienced practitioners are required. Normal isotonic (0.9%) saline is instilled via the endotracheal tube or tracheostomy, 1 ml/kg up to a maximum of 10 ml. Manual hyperinflation (MHI), e.g. a slow and steady breath aiming for a 50% larger than normal tidal volume, should be performed by one practitioner to a maximum pressure of 30–40 cm/H_2O with an inspiratory hold as tolerated by the patient for a total of 5–6 breaths to aid the dispersal of saline.

Immediately following this procedure, airway clearance should be commenced using the following technique. Bagging should be carried out at a 2:1 ratio of normal tidal volume breaths followed by one MHI breath again to a maximum pressure of 30–40 cm/H_2O, i.e. two small breaths followed by a large breath. An inspiratory hold should be provided as tolerated by the patient, followed by quick release of the bag.

At the start of the expiration of the larger breath, the second practitioner provides additional expiratory flow by manually compressing the rib cage with a moderate force in an inward and upward direction, spread evenly across the surface of the hands. This technique is used for all age groups (See Figure 55.1 for details of technique). Only moderate force is required. Timing of forced expiration is the key to success. This force should not be applied until the MHI inspiratory breath is completed to avoid excessive airway pressure. The practitioner who is performing the MHI should give vocal cues as to when inspiration is completed; this will assist in co-ordinating the timing of forced

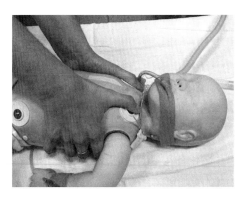

Figure 55.1 Position of hands for forced expiration in central airway clearance. Note full hand contact with the chest wall.

expiration and make the treatment far more effective. The three-breath cycle should be performed typically 5–6 times. The key is fast expiratory flow to aid secretion movement to a point in the airway where suction can effectively remove them. Suctioning should be performed to the local the guideline standard. On completion, MHI for approximately 5–10 breaths is very useful in minimising the effects of de-recruitment.

The patient's cardiovascular and respiratory status must be monitored throughout. Treatment should be suspended if the patient suffers from treatment-related adverse effects, e.g. significant decrease in blood pressure.

This technique can be repeated if required. If, however, there is combined central airway secretions and more focal problems, the more appropriate follow up treatment would be as described in section 2 below.

Significant Lung or Lobar Collapse

This technique is a variation on the lavage technique previously described. This is a simplified version of a physiotherapy technique; therefore if qualified physiotherapy assistance is available, it should be utilised. Two experienced practitioners are required for this technique. Normal respiratory assessment is used to determine the lung causing the respiratory compromise.

The aim is to clear secretion plugging and restore function to this lung. Gravity is used to assist in instillation of the lavage. This is done by positioning the patient in side lying so that the target area of lung is dependent. Normal isotonic (0.9%) saline is instilled via the endotracheal tube or tracheostomy, 1 ml/kg up to a maximum of 5 ml. Following instillation, a series of 5–6 increased MHI breaths are given, e.g. a slow and steady breath aiming for a 50% larger than normal tidal volume, to a maximum pressure of 30–40 cm/H_2O with an inspiratory hold as tolerated by the patient in order to increase dispersal of the saline.

Following instillation, the patient must be repositioned in order to put the affected side in a drainage position, i.e. affected lung non-dependent.

Chest clearance is commenced by bagging at normal tidal volume for two breaths followed by one MHI breath to a maximum pressure of 30–40 cm/H_2O, i.e. two small breaths followed by a large breath. An inspiratory hold should be given with the MHI as tolerated by the patient, followed by a quick release of the bag. On expiration of the MHI breath, the second practitioner provides manual compression of the lung to aid the speed of expiration. Only a moderate force is required as timing of forced expiration is the key to

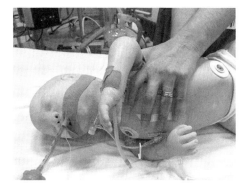

Figure 55.2 Single-handed technique for forced expiration of non-dependent lung in babies and small children.

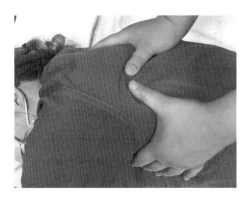

Figure 55.3 Double-hand positions for forced expiration of non-dependent lung in adolescents and large children.

success. The force should not be applied until the MHI inspiratory breath is completed, with PEEP at 0 cm H_2O, to avoid excessive airway pressure. Verbal cues by the practitioner providing the MHI will make the treatment safer and more effective. Figure 57.2 shows single-handed technique for babies and small children and Figure 57.3 shows the recommended hand position for adolescents and larger children for forced expiration.

The three-breath cycle should be performed typically 5–6 times. Suctioning should be performed to the local guideline standard. On completion, MHI for approximately 5–10 breaths is very useful in minimising the effects of de-recruitment.

This technique can be repeated if required; generally, a maximum of two treatments is sufficient. In extreme cases three treatments can be safely performed but patient fatigue will follow.

If patients are muscle relaxed, mild or moderate manual abdominal support can also assist in increasing expiratory flow.

The patient's cardiovascular and respiratory status must be monitored throughout. Physiotherapy causes large changes in intrathoracic pressures, which may not be tolerated very well by children with significant cardiac impairment or severe air trapping disease. Treatment should proceed cautiously and should be suspended if the patient suffers from treatment-related adverse effects, e.g. significant decrease in blood pressure. In some cases where treatment is essential to optimise ventilation, but poorly tolerated from a cardiovascular point of view, additional volume boluses and pressors may be required to support the child until airway clearance and lung optimisation is complete.

Further Reading

Galvis AG, Reyes G, Nelson WB. Bedside management of lung collapse in children on mechanical ventilation. *Pediatr Pulmonol* 1994; 17:326–30.

Gregson RK, Shannon H, Stocks J, et al. The unique contribution of manual chest compression-vibrations to airflow during physiotherapy in sedated, fully ventilated children. *Paed Crit Care Med* 2012;13(2): e97–102.

Nyman A, Puppala K, Colthurst S, et al. Safety and efficacy of intratracheal DNase with physiotherapy in severe status asthmaticus. *Crit Care* 2011; 15:(Suppl 1):P185.

Chapter 56

Use of Ultrasound for Paediatric Retrieval

Ariane Annicq

Point-of-care ultrasound (POCUS) is real time bedside use of ultrasound by the clinician to answer a focused diagnostic question, achieve a specific procedural goal or track clinical progression. It has been widely established in adult emergency medicine and intensive care. Increasingly it is also becoming an integral part of paediatric emergency medicine and most recently paediatric intensive care.

POCUS can be seen as an extension or enhancement of the clinical exam and stethoscope. Scanning of the lungs, heart and abdomen are the three main areas where POCUS is useful in acute and critical care medicine and therefore also in retrieval medicine. This brief expose will use some real examples of how it can be used in the hands of a skilled operator.

Lung ultrasound is a handy tool to detect pneumothorax, pleural effusions, pneumonic consolidation or collapse. It has been shown to be superior to CXR as a diagnostic tool. Additionally, it is instantaneous, at the bedside and free of radiation.

When the retrieval team find themselves with a child who has a pleuropneumonia and is difficult to ventilate, they need to consider drainage of the effusion to stabilise the patient prior to transfer. Ultrasound can be used to make a detailed assessment of the size of the effusion, location and whether it is septated or not. The best drainage site can be identified, while remaining within safe anatomical landmarks. Ultrasound-guided drainage further reduces the risks of the procedure and minimises complications.

Retrievals are often delayed by waiting in a district general hospital for a CXR after intubation to confirm tube position or repositioning of tube. Although there is still limited usage of this in the paediatric population, position on ultrasound appears to correlate with CXR in 73–100% of the cases. This could significantly improve stabilisation times, one of the key performance indicators in retrieval medicine.

Sudden desaturation in the back of an ambulance is of the highest concern for retrieval teams. After running through a systematic DOPES (Displacement, Obstruction, Pneumothorax, Equipment, Stomach) assessment, POCUS can be of added value to help rule out pneumothorax or tube displacement.

Cardiac ultrasound: Respiratory disease accounts for the highest proportion of retrievals (41% in 2019 for STRS) with the majority of these being infants with bronchiolitis. Data shows that up to 10% of the apparently 'simple bronchiolitis' cases admitted to PICU are actually undiagnosed pertussis, cardiovascular disease, airway disease or neuromuscular diseases. A rapid review of the heart, using POCUS, prior to retrieval can easily identify reduced function (suggesting myocarditis or cardiomyopathy) or significant anatomical intra-cardiac defects like septal defects. This can guide management, avoid arrest on intubation, direct inotropes and ventilation strategy, help decide retrieval destination and/ or avoid secondary transfers between PICU's for specialist services.

It is important to highlight that POCUS needs to be used as a goal-directed tool. Clinicians can become expert at using ultrasound to examine a particular organ or disease of interest relevant to their area of expertise. However, an imaging specialist will typically perform a more comprehensive examination. Clinicians should use ultrasound only to rule out or rule in a specific diagnosis, with the acknowledgement that they are not expert ultrasonographers.

Procedures: Ultrasound guidance for procedures may improve success and decrease complications. Clinicians are widely using ultrasound for IV access (central or peripheral), arterial lines and drainage of pleural collections (fluid or air).

Use of ultrasound for central line insertion has been rated by the Agency for Healthcare Research and Quality as one of the highest patient safety practices designed to decrease medical errors, and it is now accepted as standard of care for central venous line insertion. Numerous articles have proven that ultrasound has been associated with a reduction in the relative risk of complications, failed attempts and failed first attempt. The success is dependent on the skill, training and learning curve of the operator as well as the anatomical site.

Retrieval teams often arrive at the bedside of a critically ill child where IV access has proven difficult because of their shocked condition. The child will usually have had multiple attempts at peripheral IV access before resorting to intra-osseous access. In order to safely retrieve a child, the policy is to have two working vascular access sites. Ultrasound is a helpful aid in achieving this, in the hands of a skilled operator. An ultrasound probe with the smallest footprint and highest frequency is needed to establish IV access in neonates and infants as the vessels are often less than 3–4 mm in diameter and very superficial. Often these specialised probes are not available in the referring hospital. It is best if the retrieval team arrives with their own ultrasound. Familiarity with the machine and setup will also help to increase success rate and reduce complications.

In conclusion, ultrasound in retrieval medicine is still an emerging field but has great potential.

Safe transport of the critically ill child requires accurate assessment and stabilisation prior to transport and tracking of progression during transport. Ultrasound can improve the care delivered by assisting early diagnosis at the bedside, guiding clinical management, potentially reducing complications from invasive procedures and shortening stabilisation times.

Previously the impact of ultrasound in retrieval has been limited mainly due to technical factors. New compact, robust and portable ultrasound machines have been developed and well tested in the field, mainly by military teams. Ultrasound can be advocated in the retrieval setting if used by ultrasound competent retrieval physicians with appropriate governance in place.

Further Reading

Brass P, Hellmich M, Kolodziej L et al. Ultrasound guidance versus aatomical landmarks for subclavian or femoral vein catheterization. 1:CD011447, *Cochrane Database Syst Rev*, 2015.

Caballero AF, Villarreal K. Ultrasound for central vascular access. A safety concept that is renewed day by day: review. *Colombian J Anesthesiol* 2018; 46:32–8.

Jaeel P, Sheth M, Nguyen J. Ultrasonography for endotracheal tube position in infants and children. *Eur J Pediatr* 2017;176: 293–300.

Moore CL, Copel JA. Point-of-care ultrasonography. *N Engl J Med*;2011;364 (8):749–57.

Singh, Y., Tissot, C., Fraga, M.V. et al. International evidence-based guidelines on Point of Care Ultrasound (POCUS) for critically ill neonates and children issued by the POCUS Working Group of the European Society of Paediatric and Neonatal Intensive Care (ECPNIC).*Crit Care* 2020;24:65.

Shojania KG, Duncan BW, McDonald KM, et al, eds. Rockville, MD: Agency for Healthcare Research and Quality; July 2001. AHRQ Publication No. 01-E058.

Xirouchaki, N., Magkanas, E., Vaporidi, K. et al. Lung ultrasound in critically ill patients: comparison with bedside chest radiography. *Intensive Care Med* 2011; 37:1488–93.

Vasoactive Drugs on Retrieval

Benedict Griffiths

The commonest reason for retrieval to a PICU in the UK is respiratory failure; however, a smaller percentage of children present with isolated or concurrent cardiovascular collapse. These children are often described as 'Shocked' that is to say there is inadequate oxygen delivery and utilisation by cells of the body. There are multiple causes of shock in paediatric patients with different treatment approaches; however, the ultimate goal is to restore oxygen delivery to the organs in need.

Improving the balance between oxygen delivery and utilisation is one of the cornerstones of critical care medicine and is the basis for the interventions in stabilising a critically ill patient. Note in this equation, PaO_2 is measured in kPa.

Oxygen delivery = cardiac output X arterial oxygen content
Or in more detail
Oxygen delivery = cardiac output $\{(1.31 \times Hb \times SaO_2 \times 0.01) + (0.0225 \times PaO_2)\}$

Equations in medicine can be long and daunting; however, the oxygen delivery equation succinctly describes what most will recognise in their clinical practice. For oxygen to be effectively delivered, there needs to be enough haemoglobin in the blood, the haemoglobin needs to be well saturated with oxygen (arterial saturations) and that saturated haemoglobin has to be pumped around the circuit (cardiac output) effectively. There is one other consideration not alluded to in the equation and that is that the oxygen pumped around the circuit must be at a high enough pressure in the blood vessels to reach the end organs (blood pressure).

The relationship between blood pressure (BP), systemic vascular resistance (SVR) and cardiac output (CO) is described in just one more equation:

BP $= SVR \times CO$

This highlights that blood pressure is not just dependent on CO. Blood pressure is determined by the CO and the resistance in the vascular system. So even in a low CO state blood pressure can be preserved with increased SVR, and equally you can have a high CO with low blood pressure. Therefore assessment of CO requires more than simply measuring blood pressure and forms the basis of everything we do when we reach the 'C' of our ABC assessment. We feel for a pulse; we look for pallor; we check capillary refill and we measure blood pressure trying to populate these equations in our mind to determine the best therapeutic intervention.

If we are concerned that CO is inadequate we need to consider therapies to augment it. Ok then, just one more equation:

Table 57.1. Vasoactive drugs

Receptor	Action	Location
Alpha 1	Vasoconstriction – increased vascular tone and increased blood pressure	Vascular smooth muscles, sphincters of gastrointestinal tract, renal and coronary circulation
Beta 1	Increased myocardial contraction, increase in heart rate, atrioventricular conduction	Heart and kidney
Beta 2	Vasodilation, bronchodilation	Blood vessels, bronchial smooth muscle, uterus, myocardium but much less than beta 1
Dopaminergic receptors (D1 to D5)	D1 and D4 increased contraction of the myocardium D1 activation cause vasodilatation – renal and	
Vasopressin receptors V1 to V2	Vasoconstriction	V1 Smooth muscle, myocardium V2 in renal collecting duct

$$CO = HR \times SV$$

So, we can either increase heart rate (HR) or the stroke volume (SV). The stroke volume is the volume of blood ejected with each cardiac contraction and is influenced by how 'full' (or preloaded) the heart is, how hard the heart contracts (contractility) and how much resistance there is to pump against (afterload).

Vasoactive Drugs

Inotropes are a group of medications which aim to increase the force of contraction of the heart. They also have other effects on the cardiovascular system including vasoconstriction, cardiac relaxation and vasodilatation. Vasoactive drugs is a better term to describe this group of drugs. Vasoactive drugs can be potent manipulators of a patient's physiology and require a sound knowledge of their basic pharmacological properties. These properties are dependent largely on the receptors with which they bind in the cardiovascular system. These are summarised in Table 57.1.

Vasoactive Drugs

Dopamine

Dopamine acts on both **dopaminergic** and **adrenoreceptors**. At low doses it predominantly causes some vasodilation in the renal system with only a mild increase in CO, but at higher doses it increases the contraction of the heart due to activation of B-adrenoreceptors and causes some vasoconstriction of the vascular beds associated with alpha-1-adrenoceptor activation. On retrieval it is used at a dose between 5 mcg/kg/min and 10 mcg/kg/min with the aim to predominantly improve CO. Dopamine does have chronotrophic effects and can increase the HR. HR is a key component of CO and one of the body's key responses to stress. It is important to note, however, that at extreme tachycardia, cardiac function is impaired and therefore heart rate response must be monitored.

Adrenaline

Adrenaline is a potent agonist at all adrenoceptors but beta effects are most prominent at the lower levels and at higher dose, it has more alpha effect causing vasoconstriction. Adrenaline has significant metabolic effects as a stress hormone and can cause a raised lactate and glucose.

Noradrenaline

The main effect of noradrenaline is on the alpha-1 adrenoreceptors, causing vasoconstriction. This increases the systolic and diastolic blood pressure and subsequently increases blood flow through the coronaries which are protected from the alpha-1 effects. Improved coronary blood flow may improve contractility. Noradrenaline has minimal chronotrophic effect and does not increase heart rate significantly.

Milrinone

Milrinone inhibits the enzyme phosphodiesterase, thereby increasing levels of the energy precursor cAMP. This improves cardiac relaxation thus improving diastolic function without increasing heart rate, and increases cardiac contractility by both better diastolic function and better cardiac filling. It also acts as a vasodilator, thereby reducing afterload, with improved contractility. It is commonly used in the care of patients undergoing congenital cardiac surgery but is occasionally used on retrieval. It has a long half-life and takes time to reach therapeutic levels in the patient when infused. Loading of the drug can cause hypotension with low diastolic blood pressure and reduced coronary perfusion. In critically ill children, this should only be undertaken by those familiar with the drug.

Vasopressin

Vasopressin is a posterior pituitary peptide hormone with actions on the kidney and the systemic vascular bed. Stimulation of V1a receptors leads to contraction of vascular smooth muscle increasing systemic vascular resistance and blood pressure. There is also an effect at the renal collecting duct level leading to increased water reabsorption via V2 receptors.

Practical Application of Vasoactive Drug Knowledge

The evidence base for the use of vasoactive drugs in paediatric shock is extremely limited and relies on clinical assessment, application of basic pharmacology and practical considerations with knowledge of side effects.

Sepsis still carries significant mortality and morbidity in paediatrics and is often associated with septic shock. Sepsis is an inappropriate immune response to an infective pathogen which causes widespread cardiovascular dysfunction. Classical teaching describes children with poor peripheral perfusion, cold extremities with tachycardia and hypotension. As this state persists, signs of end or organ failure present including anuria with renal failure, ischaemic hepatitis, confusion and stupor with brain hypoxia. Lactate is produced as the body deals with this body wide metabolic stress. Acidosis is evident on blood gas analysis.

Fluid resuscitation is the first step in the management of septic shock in children. The aim is to increase the circulating volume and increase the cardiac preload with secondary increase of the contractile force by increasing stroke volume. This alone can be effective treatment; however, as detailed in the Frank-Starling law, a point is reached where further cardiac preload is detrimental and further fluid will not improve the clinical condition. At this point in the management, a vasoactive drug is indicated.

Sepsis manifests in many ways in children and there have been attempts to classify the shocked phenotype – the terms 'warm' and 'cold' shock have been used in the literature. The terms have been disputed but are helpful in thinking about the clinical course of sepsis. In early sepsis as the immune response builds, the patient becomes vasodilated – looking warm and flushed as the blood vessels dilate. In order to maintain a perfusion pressure the CO increases by increase in HR as the heart pumps vigorously. The decreased vascular tone will be evident in a blood pressure which may be maintained in the normal range but with an increased pulse pressure as the elastic recoil that generates the diastolic pressure is lost. At this stage, to improve oxygen delivery, and maintain blood and perfusion pressure a vasopressor such as noradrenaline would be appropriate.

As the inflammatory storm progresses the cardiac function starts to deteriorate with a septic myocarditis related to various circulating myocardial depressant factors'. Cardiac output falls. The patient becomes hypotensive and tries to preserve perfusion pressure with vasoconstriction. Poor peripheral perfusion develops with resulting cold, mottled extremities. This presentation is described as cold shock and vasoactive drugs, such as dopamine or adrenaline, are started to try and improve stroke volume by increasing the strength of the heart's contraction.

Very often the clinical entities are not as clearly defined but with careful assessment, an attempt to prioritise inotropes can be made. Very often the picture is mixed and a combination of vasoactive drugs is required. Doses can, of course, be titrated up, but it must be remembered that at higher doses the affinity of inotropes for certain receptors changes and unwanted side effects may become more apparent. A child started on dopamine may become increasingly tachycardic with a worsening of the clinical condition and a drop in blood pressure. Reassessment may lead to the introduction of a second agent, such as noradrenaline. Noradrenaline increases vascular tone and therefore perfusion pressure but you must be aware that there is an increased afterload of the heart. The left ventricle has to contract against increased resistance and at the extreme too much afterload could induce cardiovascular compromise.

As much as clinicians love to label and group patients together, real life is seldom that simple or clear; thus the importance of reassessment cannot be overstated.

Practical Considerations

There is a long-held belief that vasoactive drugs given by peripheral infusion had a high risk of extravasation and serious tissue damage. It has long been practiced that all vasoactive drugs (except milrinone) be given by a central venous catheter. However in children, placement of central venous catheter is not always practically possible without sedation/anaesthesia which carries inherent risks, magnified in the presence of shock. In paediatrics in the UK, to deliver inotropes in situations where a central line was not possible diluted infusions were used via a peripheral line. Dopamine was previously the first choice to give in this manner; however, more recently adrenaline has been delivered in this way. Early evidence in the literature suggests no increase in the number of extravasation injuries.

Most vasoactive agents (except milrinone) have very short half-lives and therefore any interruption in delivery can cause severe cardiovascular instability. Where possible a central line provides the most secure form of access. Knowing which line is required and when is part of the skill of retrieval practitioner. Pick the most appropriate line for the situation, remembering that with critically ill children, where peripheral vascular access is extremely challenging, and central venous access usually requires some form of anaesthesia, the use of intra-osseous lines has a significant role in initial resuscitation and stabilisation.

Index

ABCDE protocol
  cardiogenic shock
    management, 113–14
  critically ill baby, 285–6
  intracranial pressure
    assessment, 155–6
  referral procedures, 102–3
  spelling in CHD patients
    and, 91–2
  time-critical neurosurgical
    transfer, 166–8
abdominal malignancies,
  abdominal sepsis,
  differential diagnosis,
  179–81
abdominal/pelvic surgery, small
  bowel obstruction risk
  and, 187
abdominal sepsis
  bilious vomiting and, 178–84
  septic and hypovolaemic
    shock, 181–3
abdominal ultrasound (US),
  intracranial pressure
  assessment, 155–6
abdominal x-rays
  fall injuries, 237–42
  tachycardia and irritability
    and, 99–104
abuse/neglect, fall injuries, 163–4
acidosis
  management in diabetic
    ketoacidosis, 256–7
  Tetralogy of Fallot
    management, 92
acute abdomen
  abuse assessment, 237–42
  bilious vomiting and,
    178–84
  differential diagnosis,
    178–81
  extra-abdominal
    considerations, 179–81
  haemodynamic support and
    electrolyte management,
    181–3
  possible causes of, 238–40
  sickle cell crisis, 272–6
acute liver failure, 277–80

acute lymphoblastic leukaemia
  (ALL), presenting clinical
  emergencies with, 135–8
acute myeloid leukaemia,
  chemotherapy
  management of, 263–6
acute myocarditis/
  cardiomyopathy, acute
  abdomen and, 179–81
acute respiratory distress
  syndrome (ARDS)
  criteria for paediatric ARDS,
    141–3
  diagnosis and management,
    128–32
  evidence-based management,
    129–32
  retrieval *vs.* resuscitation
    decision, 132–3
adenosine, tachycardia
  management, 119
adrenaline
  in cardiogenic shock
    patients, 114
  congenital heart disease
    patients, 86–7
  guidelines for using, 308
adrenaline nebulisers, stridor
  management, 65–9
agitation, Tetralogy of Fallot
  management and
  avoidance of, 92
air transfers. *See* flight retrieval
  and transfer
airway management
  in acute management on
    retrieval, 299–302
  cardiogenic shock, 113
  fall injuries, 160–1
  hypovolaemic shock,
    173–4
  indications and
    contraindications,
    299–302
  multidrug overdose, 245–6
  during transfers, 218, 221–4
Alisio, Michelle, 122–6
ambulance kit bag, storage and
  restocking of, 13–14

ambulance transfers
  crew resource management
    guidelines, 288–92
  palliative care transfers,
    232–3
  protocols for, 7
aminophylline infusion, asthma
  management, 72–3
amiodarone treatment,
  tachycardia, 120
amlodipine, 244–5
amoxicillin, anaphylactic
  reaction, 127–33
anaemia, tumour lysis
  syndrome patients, 139
anaesthesia
  acute liver failure, 279–80
  asthma management and
    risk of, 71
  in cardiogenic shock
    patients, 113
  in critically ill infants, 281–3
  guidelines for, 19–28
  inhaled foreign body,
    44–5
  oxygenation and, 20
  in pneumonia/empyema
    shock patients, 56–7
  upper airway obstruction
    and, 32–3
analgesia
  abdominal sepsis, 182, 188–9
  Tetralogy of Fallot
    management, 92
Annicq, Ariane, 191–6, 303–4
antibiotics
  for abdominal sepsis, 181
  bronchiolitis and
    co-infection, 37
  neutropenic sepsis, 263–5
  renal disease management,
    269–70
anti-diuretic hormone release,
  bronchiolitis and, 37
antihypertensive agents,
  multidrug overdose from,
  243–7
antimicrobial therapy, septic
  shock, 125, 229

anti-NDMA encephalitis,
212–13
aortic covered stent, foreign
body ingestion and, 176–7
aorto-oesophageal fistula,
foreign body ingestion
and, 176
APLS algorithm
cardiac arrest procedures,
148–53
haemorrhage as PEG
insertion complication,
204–5
apnoeic episodes
acute liver failure, 277
retrieval and transfer
processes, 35–40, 218–19
arrhythmia, transfer procedures
with, 97–8, 115
asthma management, 70–3
complications, 71
differential diagnosis, 70–1
rescue measures during
retrieval, 72–3
atrial flutter, tachycardia
diagnosis, 118
atropine, pulmonary
hypertension and
avoidance of, 77–8
autoimmune encephalitis,
212–13
AV re-entry tachycardia
(AVRT), 116–18

back bruising, abuse
assessment, 237–42
bag mask ventilation
pertussis patients, 62–3
upper airway obstruction, 33
bat wing markings, chest
x-rays, 96
Berlin criteria, adult ARDS,
128–32
beta-2 agonist infusion, asthma
management, 72–3
beta blockers, Tetralogy of
Fallot management,
91–2
Bickell, Fiona, 207–9
bilious vomiting
differential diagnosis, 178–81
extended abdomen and,
178–84
bleeding
fall injuries, 162–3
vomiting with, 171–7

blood pressure
assessment of, 17–18
intubation in pneumonia/
empyema patients, 56–7
neurosurgical emergency
targets, 168–9
blood products
complications from, 174
resuscitation in gastro-
intestinal bleeding and,
172–4
sickle cell crisis and, 274
blood sugar levels
cardiac arrest assessment,
148
cyanotic baby, 84
multidrug overdose, 245–6
blood tests and blood gas
results
abdominal sepsis and, 185
acute liver failure, 277
anaphylactic reaction,
127–33
anesthestisation and, 19
apnoeic episodes and, 35–40
bilious vomiting, 178
bronchiolitis patients, 59
cardiomegaly and
opacification, 281–7
chemotherapy management
and, 263–4
in collapsed neonate, 259–62
COVID-19 assessment, 227
COVID-19 results, 227
diarrhoea and vomiting and,
267
facial swelling, 48
fall injuries, 159, 237–42
functional decline
assessment, 94
lethargic patients, 109–11
pneumonia/empyema, 53
pulmonary hypertension, 74
respiratory failure, 221–6
shock and cyanosis
assessment, 84–8
sickle cell crisis, 272
spelling episodes and, 89–93
tachycardia, 116
upper airway obstruction, 29
blue baby assessment and
transfer, 79–83
blunt dissection, chest drain
insertion, 296–7
boot-shaped cardiac shadow,
89–93

bougie, 21–2
bradycardia
antenatal diagnosis and
treatment, 108
intubation guidelines, 105–6
multidrug overdose, 245–6
pharmacological treatment,
107
transcutaneous pacing, 107
brain death. See hypoxic
ischaemic brain injury
breathing management
in cardiogenic shock
patients, 113
hypovolaemic shock, 173–4
neonatal air transfers, 218
Brock, Louisa, 253–8
bronchiolitis
co-infection with, 37
diagnosis and management,
35–40, 59–62
outcomes, 40
white cell count and, 59–64
bronchodilators, asthma
management and,
70–1
bronchopulmonary dysplasia
(BPD), 74
Burkitt's lymphoma, acute
abdomen and, 179–81
Burnett, Heather, 263–6
burn injuries
inhalation injuries,
191–6
paediatric burns centres,
193–6

cABDE assessment, fall
injuries, 162–3
Cadman, Emily, 185–90
cannot intubate, cannot
ventilate (CICV) scenario,
33
carbon dioxide trace, CPR
monitoring, 149–50
carbon monoxide poisoning,
inhalation injury, 192–3
cardiac arrest
Four Hs and Ts aetiology
moniker with, 150–2
management of, 148–53
prognosis, 152–3
septic shock and, 202–6,
227–9
swallowed foreign body, 171
team approach to, 250–1

cardiac conditions. *See also*
    acute myocarditis/
    cardiomyopathy;
    congenital heart defects
    (CHD)
    acute abdomen and, 179–81
    mediastinal mass and,
        48–50
cardiac death, organ donation
    following, 201
cardiac rhythm assessment,
    multidrug overdose,
    245–6
cardiac ultrasound, 303–4
cardiogenic shock
    differential diagnosis, 111–13
    emergency intervention with,
        95–6
    preventive measures for,
        281–3
cardiomegaly, clinical
    assessment, 281
cardiopulmonary resuscitation
    (CPR). *See also* Do Not
    Attempt
    Cardiopulmonary
    Resuscitation (DNAR)
    cardiac arrest procedures,
        148–53
    indications for stopping,
        152–3
cardiorespiratory monitoring
    intubation, 22
    mediastinal mass, 48–50
cardiovascular support
    abdominal sepsis, 182
    acute liver failure, 279–80
    neutropenic sepsis,
        263–5
Carter, Michael, 48–52, 127–33
ceftriaxone, 125
Ceftriaxone, 229
central airway secretion
    obstruction, manual
    hyperinflation, 300–1
central venous access,
    abdominal sepsis and,
    188–9
cerebral edema, diabetic
    ketoacidosis, 254–5
cerebral ischaemia, diabetic
    ketoacidosis, 254–5
checklists
    of ambulance equipment,
        13–14
    of processes tasks, 4–5

chemical burn, foreign body
    aspiration, 43
chemotherapy, management
    protocols for, 263–6
chest drain insertion
    blunt dissection, 296–7
    complications, 297–8
    equipment, 294–5
    Heimlich valve, 297
    indications for, 293–4
    in pneumonia/empyema
        shock patients, 57
    protocol for, 293–8
    SAFE triangle, 295
    Seldinger drain insertion,
        295–6
    tension pneumothorax, 294
chest x-rays (CXR)
    apnoeic episodes and,
        38–40
    bat wing markings in, 96
    bronchiolitis patients, 59
    congenital heart defects,
        79–81
    foreign body aspiration, 41–2
    functional decline
        assessment, 94
    intubation/ventilation
        assessment, 224
    pneumonia/empyema, 53
    respiratory failure, 221–6
    respiratory failure and
        deterioration, 141–2
    shock and cyanosis
        assessment, 84–8
    tachycardia and irritability
        and, 99–104
chickenpox
    concomitant severe bacterial
        infection with, 126
    diagnosis and management,
        122–6
    non-steroidal anti-
        inflammatory drugs and,
        124
Children's Acute Transport
    Service (CATS),
    establishment of, 1
children's hospice, 233–4
chronic infective foreign body,
    44
circulation management
    in cardiogenic shock
        patients, 114
    in hypovolaemic shock,
        173–4

neonatal air transfers,
    218–19
coagulation derangement, acute
    liver failure and, 277–8
Co-amoxiclav, 37
    bronchiolitis patients, 59
collapsed neonate
    differential diagnosis of,
        217–18
    management during transfer
        of, 216–20
    metabolic disorders and,
        259–62
    signs and symptoms of,
        217–18
    Total Anomalous Pulmonary
        Venous Drainage, 84–8
COMET management
    acronym, upper airway
    obstruction, 66–8kk
community paediatric palliative
    care team, 233–4
compartment syndrome,
    abdominal injury, 240–1
compensated shock, differential
    diagnosis, 111–13
congenital heart block
    antenatal diagnosis and
        treatment, 108
    fetal bradycardia and, 105–8
    pharmacological treatment,
        107
    transcutaneous pacing, 107
    transfer of neonates with,
        106–7
congenital heart defects (CHD)
    acute abdomen and, 179–81
    air transfers of neonates with,
        218–19, 281–7
    in collapsed neonate, 217–18
    epidemiology, 82–3
    extracorporeal membrane
        oxygenation and, 143–5
    management principles,
        81–2
    pulmonary hypertension
        and, 75
    shock and cyanosis in, 84–8
    testing for, 79–81
    transfer procedures for
        infants with, 82–3
continuous/bilevel positive
    airway pressure (CPAP/
    BiPAP), transfer airway
    management, 223–4
continuous capnography, 22

continuous positive airway pressure (CPAP)
apnoeic episodes, 35–40
bronchiolitis patients, 59–62
inhaled foreign body and avoidance of, 44–5
Tetralogy of Fallot management, 91–2
upper airway obstruction and weaning of, 29–33
continuous veno-venous haemofiltration (CVVH), metabolic condition in collapsed neonate, 261–2
contralateral lung collapse, intubation and risk of, 20–1
controlled drugs, kit bag storage and monitoring, 15–16
Cormak and Lehane grade 4, upper airway obstruction, 33
COVID-19 (SARV-CoV2)
clinical condition/syndromes in children, 229–30
fever in children and, 227–30
cranial ultrasound (CrUSS), for ECMO patient transfers, 143–5
cricoid pressure, limited value of, 20
croup, incidence and aetiology, 65–6
CRP levels, apnoeic episodes and, 36–7
CT angiogram, foreign body ingestion and, 176–7
CT scan
fall injuries, 159
intracranial pressure assessment, 155–6, 166–8
CVS administration, abdominal sepsis and, 181–2
cyanide poisoning, inhalation injury, 192–3
cyanosis
assessment and management, 79–83
congenital heart disease testing, 79–81
pulmonary causes of, 79
shock and, 84–8
spelling episodes and, 89–93

data quality and audit, Paediatric Critical Care Retrieval and, 5–6
Davies, Joanna, 65–9, 79–83, 281–7
decompensated shock, differential diagnosis, 111–13
delayed transfers
critically ill infants, 284–5
team performance and, 17–18
tumour lysis syndrome patients, 139–40
dexamethasone, stridor management, 65–9
diabetic ketoacidosis (DKA), diagnosis and management of, 253–8
diarrhoea, renal disease and, 267–71
Difficult Airway Society (DAS) guidelines, team briefings, 25–7
Dinoprostone, for critically ill babies, 283–4
direct current (DC) cardioversion, 120
diving reflex, critically ill infant, 281–3
donation following circulatory death (DCD) procedures, 231–2
Do Not Attempt Cardiopulmonary Resuscitation (DNAR), 248–52
palliative care transfers, 233
dopamine
ARDS patients, 132–3
in cardiogenic shock patients, 114
congenital heart disease patients, 86–7
guidelines for using, 307–8
septic shock, 227–9
DOPES protocol
point of care ultrasound, 303–4
ventilation emergencies, 38–40
doxazocin, 244–5
drowning
organ donation and, 197–201
prognosticators for outcome, 199–201

drug ingestion
encephalitis and, 213
multidrug overdose, 243–7
Dunn, Elizabeth Daisy, 53–8
Dyer, Jo, 59–64, 135–40
dynamic hyperinflation, ARDS and, 129–32

echocardiogram
cardiogenic shock, 111–13
for ECMO patient transfers, 143–5
functional decline assessment, 97–8
renal disease assessment, 269
tachycardia diagnosis, 116–18
eculizumab, haemolytic uraemic syndrome, 269–70
electrolyte abnormalities
abdominal sepsis, 182–3
Tetralogy of Fallot management, 92
emergency care plan, palliative care transfers, 233
emergency drugs, intubation, 23
encephalitis
autoimmune disorders, 212–13
encephalopathy diagnosis and management, 209
investigation and management protocols, 213–14
meningitis and, 212
metabolic causes, 213
seizures and, 210–15
space occupying lesions, 213
toxin ingestion/poisoning, 213
encephalopathy
acute liver failure and, 277–8
in collapsed neonate, 259–61
diagnosis and management, 207–9
seizure management with, 154–8
sudden onset differential diagnosis, 212–13
tachycardia with, 102–3
endobronchial intubation, contralateral lung collapse and, 20–1

end-of-life care. *See* hospice care
endotracheal intubation, inhalation injury, 192
end-tidal CO2 monitoring, pulmonary hypertension intubation, 77–8
ENT surgeons
cannot intubate, cannot ventilate (CICV) scenario, 33
upper airway security and, 32–3
equipment
airway management during transfers, 221–4
ambulance storage and monitoring of, 13–14
checklists, 13–14
chest drain insertion, 294–5
complications management and, 12
flight transfers, 9–11, 284–5
intubation, 19–20
for palliative care patients, 234
ETT (endotracheal tube). *See also* intubation
management of, 17–18
size and position assessment, 38–40
Evelina PICU, STRS integration with, 1–2
extracorporeal membrane oxygenation (ECMO). *See also* veno-venous extracorporeal membranous oxygenation (VV-ECMO)
asthma management, 73
cardiac arrest and, 152–3
cardiac diagnoses requiring, 143–5
indications and exclusion criteria for, 143–5
pertussis patients, 63

facemask ventilation, intubation, 20
facial bruising, abuse assessment, 237–42
facial swelling
assessment and management guidelines, 48–52
mediastinal mass, 48

failure of medical therapy standard, intubation indications and, 66–8
fall injuries
abuse assessment, 237–42
management of, 159–64
non-accidental injury, examination for, 241–2
FAST scan, abdominal injuries, 238–40
fentanyl
acute liver failure, 279–80
intubation, 23
fever in children
COVID-19 and, 227–30
diagnosis and management, 122–3
Fine-Goudlen, Miriam, 89–93, 231–6
fixed wing transfers, 7–8
tumour lysis syndrome patients, 139–40
flexible bronchoscopy, foreign body aspiration, 45
flight bag size and contents, air retrievals, 9–11, 284–5
flight equipment, air retrievals, 9–11, 284–5
flight retrieval and transfer. *See also* delayed transfers
collapsed neonate, 218–19
complications in, 286
considerations in, 8
crew resource management guidelines, 288–92
critically ill baby, 281–7
flight equipment, 9–11, 284–5
incidence of, 7
in-flight patient complications, 12
landing sites, 8–9
logistics overview, 7–12
parent accompaniment, 9
patient safety, 11–12
pre departure checks, 11–12
rotary (helicopter) transfer, 7–8
team communication and management during, 219
team composition, 9
tumour lysis syndrome patients, 139–40

fluid resuscitation
abdominal injury, 240–1
in abdominal sepsis, 181–2
in cardiogenic shock patients, 114
in chemotherapy patients, 263–5
septic shock and, 308–9
fluid status, Tetralogy of Fallot management, 92
foreign body aspiration, 41–6
airway obstruction, 41–3
chemical burn, 43
chronic infective foreign body, 44
clinical observation and chest x-ray, 41–2
inhaled foreign body, 44–5
intubation guidelines, 44–5
non-pharmacological soothing of patient, 45
novel techniques and issues, 45
safeguarding issues with, 45–6
swallowed foreign body, 45
foreign body ingestion. *See* swallowed foreign body
Fosker, Sam, 35–40, 159–70, 221–6, 288–92
Four Hs and Ts moniker, cardiac arrest aetiology, 150–2
fractures, assessment and management, 159–64
fridge drugs, transfer storage and monitoring, 15–16
functional decline, assessment of, 94–8

gastric decontamination, multidrug overdose, 245–6
gastric loss, abdominal sepsis and, 181–2
gastro-intestinal bleeding
aetiology and management of, 172–4
Sengstaken-Blakemore intubation, 175
GCS score, fall injuries, 162–3
general practitioner (GP), palliative care and involvement of, 233–4
Gillick competence, 247

Glasgow coma score, encephalopathy diagnosis and management, 207–9
glucagon, multidrug overdose, 148
glycaemic control, neonatal air transfers and, 219
Goldilocks Phenomenon, 38–40
Gomez, Xavier Freire, 178–84
Goulden, Miriam Fine, 116–20
Group A streptococcus, 229
group A streptococcus (GAS)
 antimicrobial therapy, 125
 chicken pox and, 126
 diagnosis and management, 122–3
 non-steroidal anti-inflammatory drugs and, 124

haemolysis, sickle cell crisis and, 274
haemolytic uraemic syndrome (HUS), 269–70
haemorrhage
 classification, 172–4
 fall injuries, 162–3
 as PEG insertion complication, 202–6
Hall, Alexander, 41–6
Hands, Christopher, 70–3
Hardwick, Sarah, 116–20
Hayden, Hannah, 259–62
Heimlich valve, chest drain insertion, 297
helicopter transfers. See flight retrieval and transfer
hepatic encephalopathy, 277–8
hepatomegaly, clinical assessment, 281
herpetic infection, acute liver failure, 279–80
Herring, Sasha, 210–15
Hickman line, neutropenic sepsis and, 263–5
high dose insulin, multidrug overdose, 245–6
High Flow Nasal Canula (HFNC)
 bronchiolitis patients, 59
 equipment, 223–4
 respiratory failure, 221–6

high frequency ventilation (HFOV), respiratory failure, maximum support protocols, 141–6
Hodgkin lymphoma, mediastinal mass with, 48
hospice care
 children's hospice, 233–4
 transfer procedures for, 231–6
hot debrief
 cessation of CPR decisions, 152–3
 death during transfer, 251–2
Humble, Georgina, 267–71
hyperammonaeamia
 acute liver failure, 279
 in collapsed neonate, 261
hyperkalaemia
 abdominal sepsis, 182–3
 bilious vomiting, 178
 in cardiac arrest, 150–1
 haemorrhage complications, 174
 renal disease assessment, 269
 sickle cell crisis and, 274
hyperleucocytosis
 pertussis and, 59–62
 pre-retrieval therapy, 135–8
hyperthermia, neonatal air transfers and, 219
hyperventilation, pulmonary hypertension intubation, 78
hypocalcaemia, haemorrhage complications, 174
hypocapnia, diabetic ketoacidosis, 254–5
hypoglycaemia
 acute liver failure, 279
 diabetic ketoacidosis, 254–5
hypokalaemia, in cardiac arrest, 150–1
hyponatraemia
 apnoeic episodes and, 37
 shock and, 56–7
hypotension
 diabetic ketoacidosis, 255–6
 multidrug overdose, 245–6
 neonatal air transfers and, 218–19
 septic shock and, 227–9
hypothermia, in cardiac arrest, 151
hypovolaemic shock
 bilious vomiting and, 181–3
 cardiac arrest and, 150

gastro-intestinal bleeding, 172–4
 swallowed foreign body, 171
hypoxia
 in cardiac arrest, 150
 mediastinal mass, 48–50
 tumour lysis syndrome patients, 139
hypoxic ischaemic brain injury
 drowning victims, 197–201
 neurological diagnostic criteria, 201

infection, diabetic ketoacidosis and, 254
inhalational induction, airway security for transfer and, 32–3
inhalation injuries, 191–6
inhaled foreign body, removal guidelines, 44–5
inhaled nitric oxide, pulmonary hypertension, 75–6
inodilators, cardiogenic shock patients, 97–8
inotropic support
 abdominal sepsis and, 181–2
 chemotherapeutic septic shock, 265–6
 in critically ill infants, 281–3
 diabetic ketoacidosis, 254
 multidrug overdose, 246
 septic shock and, 227–9
intra abdominal trauma, as PEG insertion complication, 202–6
intracranial pressure (ICP)
 aetiology, 168–9
 blocked or infected ventriculo-peritoneal shunt, 155–6
 in collapsed neonate, 259–61
 encephalitis and, 210–15
 encephalopathy diagnosis and management, 102–3, 165–70, 208–9
intra-tracheal DNase, asthma management, 73
intravenous immunoglobulin (IVIG)
 autoimmune encephalopathy, 212–13
 COVID-19 complications, 230
 septic shock and, 125

intravenous therapy,
    pneumonia/empyema,
    53–7
intubation. *See also* ETT
    (endotracheal tube)
    abdominal sepsis, 182, 188–9
    airway security for transfer
        and, 32–3
    anesthestisation guidelines,
        19–28
    apnoeic episodes, 35–40
    assessment, 24
    asthma management, 70–1
    blades, 20–1
    bradycardia and risks of,
        105–6
    cardiogenic shock, 113
    congenital heart disease
        patients, 81–2, 86–7, 92
    in critically ill infants,
        283–4
    in croup patients, 66–9
    difficulties, 21–2, 24
    drugs, 22–3
    equipment, 19–20
    foreign body aspiration, 44–5
    gastro-intestinal bleeding,
        175
    indications for, 19
    inhalation injuries, 191–2
    IV access, 24
    location, 25–7
    mediastinal mass patients,
        50–1
    monitoring, 22
    optimisation, 24
    oxygenation, 20
    parental presence, 27–8
    patient positioning, 24
    pertussis patients, 62–3
    pneumonia/empyema
        patients, 56–7
    post-intubation sedation and
        instability, 23, 27–8
    pre-procedural checklist, 25–7
    pulmonary hypertension,
        76–8
    role assignments for, 25–7
    safety protocols, 27–8
    seizure management, 165–70
    suction, 21–2
    tube size and length, 20–1
intussusception, small bowel
    obstruction risk and, 187
invasive ventilation, transfer
    procedures and, 224

irreversible shock, differential
    diagnosis, 111–13
IV access, intubation and, 24

Kawasaki Disease, COVID-19
    syndromes and, 229–30
ketamine
    acute liver failure, 279–80
    asthma management, 73
    chemotherapeutic septic
        shock, 265–6
    intubation, 23
King, Rumi, 19–28
kit bag components, retrieval
    procedures and, 13–14
knee to chest position, spelling
    episodes, 89–93
Knight, Dawn, 248–52

Laddie, Jo, 231–6
language interpreters, parental
    communication and,
    183–4
laryngoscope blades, 20–1
laryngoscopy, inhaled foreign
    body, 44–5
laryngotracheal reconstruction
    (LTR), 31
lethargic patients
    assessment and
        management, 109–15
    differential diagnosis,
        111–13
leucocytosis, bronchiolitis and,
    59–62
leucodepletion, pertussis
    patients, 59–62
Lillie, Jon, 141–6, 148–53
lipid emulsion therapy,
    multidrug overdose, 246
lobar collapse, airway clearance
    protocols and, 301–2
lobar pneumonia, acute
    abdomen and, 179–81
local referring team
    guidelines fo, 17–18
    resource management using,
        289–90
low dose aspirin, COVID-19
    complications, 230
Lund and Browder chart, burn
    injury assessment,
    193–5
lung collapse, airway clearance
    protocols and, 301–2
lung ultrasound, 303–4

lymphocytosis, pertussis and,
    59–62
lymphopenia, septic shock, 229

MacGruer, Kenneth, 74–8
macrolide antibiotics, pertussis
    patients, 63
magnetic extractors, foreign
    body aspiration, 45
manual hyperinflation (MHI)
    central airway secretion
        clearance, 300–1
    lung or lobar collapse, 301–2
maternal health and wellbeing,
    neonatal flight transfers
    and, 9, 82–3, 87–8, 219–20
Max and Kiera's Law, 200–1,
    231–2
maxillofacial fractures,
    diagnosis and
    management, 160–1
McCaffery staging system, 22,
    29–31
McDougall, Marilyn, 53–8,
    122–33, 210–15, 227–30,
    277–80, 293–8
mean airway pressure (MAP),
    calculation of, 141–3
mechanical decompression,
    asthma management, 72
mediastinal mass
    asthma differential diagnosis
        and, 70–1
    facial swelling and, 48
    respiratory or cardiovascular
        emergencies with, 48–50
    transfer and management of
        children with, 50–1
Medical Certificate of
    Certification of Death
    (MCCD), palliative care
    patients, 233–4
medical equipment, HFNC
    apparatus, 221–4
medications
    for palliative care patients, 234
    retrieval and transfer,
        guidelines for, 15–16
meningitis, encephalitis and, 212
metabolic disorders
    in collapsed neonate, 217–18,
        259–62
    renal failure and, 269
    sickle cell crisis and, 273
methylxanthine, asthma
    management, 72–3

milrinone
  in cardiogenic shock
    patients, 114
  guidelines for using, 308
Minen, Federico, 141–6
Minnesota intubation, gastro-
    intestinal bleeding, 175
mucus plugging, asthma and,
    70–3
Multisystem Inflammatory
    Syndrome in Children,
    229–30
myocarditis, acute abdomen
    and, 179–81

nasogastric intubation, in
    ventilated child, 17–18
necrotizing enterocolitis, small
    bowel obstruction risk
    and, 187
necrotizing fasciitis, chicken
    pox and, 126
neuromuscular disorders,
    disease progression,
    224–6
neuroprotective measures
  drowning victims, 197–9
  neonatal air transfers and,
    219
neurosurgical emergency,
    154–8
  physiological target
    identification in, 168–9
  time-critical neurosurgical
    transfer, 166–8
neutropenic sepsis, childhood
    cancer and, 263–5
non-accidental injuries,
    examination for, 241–2
non-Hodgkin lymphoma,
    mediastinal mass with, 48
non-invasive ventilation (NIV)
  contraindications, 223–4
  methods, 223–4
non-pharmacological
    treatment, congenital
    heart block, 107
non-steroidal anti-
    inflammatory drugs
    (NAIDS), chicken pox
    and, 124
noradrenaline
  in cardiogenic shock
    patients, 114
  guidelines for using, 308
  septic shock, 227–9

notifiable disease status,
    pertussis, 63
Nyman, Andrew, 29–33, 41–6,
    70–3

oesophageal obstruction,
    foreign body aspiration,
    41–3
open lung ventilation strategy,
    paediatric ARDS, 141–3
optiflow oxygenation,
    laryngoscopy, 20
optimisation
  congenital heart disease
    patient transfers, 86–7
  intubation, 24
organ donation
  clinical and logistic
    considerations, 200–1
  drowning victims, 197–201
  ethical issues, 201
  life-limiting conditions,
    infants with, 201
  parental communication
    about, 231–2
osmotherapy, diabetic
    ketoacidosis, 254–5
osmotic oedema, diabetic
    ketoacidosis, 254–5
ovarian teratoma, autoimmune
    encephalitis, 212–14
oxygenation
  fetal bradycardia and, 105–6
  intubation and, 20
  pulmonary hypertension,
    75–6
  Tetralogy of Fallot
    management, 91–2
oxygen index (OI) formula,
    141–3
oxygen saturation index (OSI)
    formula, 141–3

pacemaker implantation,
    congenital heart block,
    108
Paediatric Acute Lung Injury
    and Sepsis Investigators
    (PALISI), 128–32
Paediatric Critical Care
    Retrieval
  checklists of processes and
    tasks, 4–5
  data quality and audit
    procedures, 5–6
  growth of, 1–2

integrated vs. independent
    models, 1
  logistics and organisation,
    3–6
  model criteria for, 1–2
  team performance, 13–18
Paediatric Multisystem
    Inflammatory Syndrome -
    Temporally Associated
    with SARS-CoV-2 (PIM-
    TS), 229–30
pain management, in
    functional decline, 95–6
palliative care
  community support for,
    233–4
  handover of drugs and
    documentation following,
    234–5
  memory making strategies
    for, 235–6
  organ donation
    communications during,
    231–2
  paperwork for, 233
  team communication and
    management, 232–3
  transfer home for, 231–6
para-pneumonic effusion,
    pneumonia/empyema,
    55–5
Parecho virus, tachycardia and
    encephalopathy, 103–4
parent accompaniment
  acute liver failure transfer,
    279–80
  congenital heart disease
    patients, 82–3, 87–8
  neonatal flight transfers, 9,
    219–20
  options for, 226
parental communication
  acute liver failure, 279–80
  chemotherapeutic septic
    shock, 266
  congenital heart disease
    patients, 82–3, 87–8
  diabetic ketoacidosis and
    septic shock, 257–8
  distressed mother, 226
  encephalopathy diagnosis
    and management, 209
  fall injuries, 163–4
  hospice care procedures and
    home transfer, 231–6
  language barriers, 183–4

neonatal flight transfers,
219–20
neuromuscular disorder
progression, 224–6
organ donation discussions,
231–2
pertussis patients, 63–4
ventilation emergencies and,
40
parenting issues, foreign body
aspiration and, 45–6
Parkland fluid replacement
formula, 193–5
patient positioning, intubation
and, 24
patient safety and security
equipment
air retrievals, 9–11
in-flight patient
complications, 12
Pavcnik, Maja, 59–64, 259–66
pCO₂, management in diabetic
ketoacidosis, 255–6
peak pressure measurements,
asthma patient ventilation
and, 72
percutaneous endoscopic
gastrostomy (PEG),
insertion/change
complications, 202–6
perindopril, 244–5
Perkins, Joanne, 19–28,
197–201, 243–7
pertussis
diagnosis and management,
59–62
infant mortality rates for,
63–4
morbidity and mortality
factors, 59
pharmacological treatment,
congenital heart block, 107
phenylephrine, Tetralogy of
Fallot management, 91–2
phosphodiesterase type-5
inhibitors, pulmonary
hypertension, 75–6
physiotherapy, asthma and, 72
Pienaar, Alison, 74–8, 154–8,
178–90
Pinto, Catia, 89–93
pneumo/haemothorax, fall
injuries, 162–3
pneumonia/empyema
acute abdomen and, 179–81
complications, 55–6

epidemiology and treatment,
53–5
physiologic observations and
blood tests, 53
point of care ultrasound
(POCUS), retrieval using,
303–4
positive end-expiratory pressure
(PEEP) procedures
in cardiogenic shock
patients, 113
in pneumonia/empyema
shock patients, 57
Tetralogy of Fallot
management, 91–2
post haemorrhagic
hydrocephalus, seizures
and, 154
pre departure checks, air
retrievals, 11–12
prednisolone, COVID-19
complications, 230
pregnancy testing, encephalitis
and, 213–14
pre-load optimisation,
pulmonary hypertension
intubation, 77–8
pre-oxygenation, in
pneumonia/empyema
shock patients, 57
pre-transfer checklist, 27–8
Procopiuc, Livia, 154–8
propofol
intubation, 23
pulmonary hypertension and
avoidance of, 77–8
prostacyclins, pulmonary
hypertension, 75–6
prostaglandin E2/Prostin
congenital heart disease
patients, 81–2, 86–7,
283–4
neonatal air transfers and,
218–19
Prower, Emma, 197–201
psychiatric assessment,
multidrug overdose, 247
psychosis, seizures and, 213
pulmonary disease, cyanosis
and, 79
pulmonary hypertension
aetiology and pathology, 75
assessment, 74
cyanosis and, 80
transfer procedures, 74–8
treatment, 75–6

pulmonary vascular resistance
(PVR), pulmonary
hypertension and,
76–8
pulmonary vein stenosis,
congenital heart disease
patients, 87–8
pulseless electrical activity
(PEA)
cardiac arrest and, 150–2
hypovolaemic shock, 171
septic shock and, 202–6

radiographic findings, chemical
burn, foreign body
aspiration, 43
Rainbow Children's Hospice
Guidelines, 234–5
raised intracranial pressure
(rICP). See intracranial
pressure (ICP)
rashes
cardiogenic shock patients,
94
tachycardia and irritability
and, 99–104
red blood cell replacement,
gastro-intestinal bleeding,
172–4
referral process
advice referrals, 100–2
asthma management,
70–1
cardiac arrest, 148–53
crew resource management,
288–92
croup patients, 65–8
time-critical neurosurgical
transfer, 166–8
refractory shock, intubation
and ventilation, 188–9
religious issues, palliative care,
234–5
renal disease
cardiovascular compromise
and, 268–9
diarrhoea and vomiting and,
267–71
metabolic disorders and, 269
respiratory failure
clinical assessment, 281
DOPES protocol for, 38–40
maximum support protocols
and, 141–6
mediastinal mass and, 48–50
sickle cell crisis and, 273

respiratory support
  abdominal sepsis, 182
  critically ill infant, 281–3
  pulmonary hypertension, 75–6
respiratory syncytial virus
    (RSV)
  bronchiolitis and, 37
  respiratory failure, maximum
    support protocols, 141–6
Resuscitation Council (UK)
    algorithm, foreign body
    aspiration, 41–3
retrieval process
  airway management in acute
    retrieval, 299–302
  apnoeic episodes and, 35–40
  ARDS patients, 132–3
  asthma rescue measures
    during, 72–3
  cardiac arrest, 148–53
  critically ill baby, 285
  delays in, 17–18, 139–40
  pneumonia and empyema,
    53–8
  point of care ultrasound in,
    303–4
  sickle cell crisis, 274
  stridor management during,
    65–6
  tumour lysis patients, 135–40
retrieval team. See also air
    retrieval
  training and monitoring of, 16
return of spontaneous
    circulation (ROSC)
  cardiac arrest patients, 150
  drowning victims, 197–9
Riphagen, Shelley, 1–6, 13–18,
    35–40, 48–52, 65–9,
    79–83, 94–8, 105–8,
    135–40, 159–64, 171–7,
    207–9, 216–26, 237–42,
    248–58, 267–76, 281–7
rocuronium, intubation, 23
Ro/La antibodies, diagnosis of,
    105–8
rotary (helicopter) transfer, 7–8

SAFE triangle, chest drain
    insertion, 295
safety protocols, intubation,
    27–4
salbutamol toxicity, asthma
    management and, 70–1
saline lavage, airway clearance
    with, 299–302

Samasinghe, Nav, 243–7
Satar, Ain, 216–20
sedation
  post-intubation, 23
  Tetralogy of Fallot
    management, 92
seizures
  adolescent psychosis and,
    210–15
  emergency management of,
    154–8, 165–70
  hyperammonaemia and,
    261
  as PEG insertion
    complication, 202–6
Seldinger drain insertion,
    295–6
Sengstaken-Blakemore
    intubation, gastro-
    intestinal bleeding,
    175
Senior Nurses in Organ
    Donation (SNODS) team,
    drowning victim
    assessment by, 199–200
sepsis, pulmonary hypertension
    and, 74
septic shock
  antimicrobial therapy, 125
  bilious vomiting and,
    181–3
  in chemotherapy patients,
    263–5
  collapsed neonate and,
    217–18
  COVID-19 assessment,
    227–9
  diagnosis and management,
    127–33
  differential diagnosis,
    111–13, 203
  percutaneous gastrostomy
    and, 202–6
  sickle cell crisis and, 273
  vasoactive drugs in, 308–9
septic shock, diagnostic criteria
    for, 124
sequential organ failure
    assessment (SOFA) score,
    septic shock assessment,
    128
severe bacterial infection (SBI),
    viral illness concomitant
    with, 126
severe respiratory disease,
    criteria for, 36–7

sevoflurane
  airway security for transfer
    and, 32–3
  asthma management, 73
shock. See also cardiogenic
    shock; hypovolaemic
    shock; refractory shock;
    septic shock
  acute abdomen and, 186–7
  cyanosis and, 84–8
  diabetic ketoacidosis, 253–8
  differential diagnosis,
    111–13
  in pneumonia/empyema
    patients, 56–7
  sickle cell crisis and, 273
  tachycardia management
    and, 118–20
shunt series X-rays, intracranial
    pressure assessment,
    155–6
sickle cell crisis, 272–6
  mortality in, 274
simulated retrievals, team
    training, 18
sinus tachycardia, 116–18
small bowel obstruction
  abdominal sepsis and, 182
  diagnosis and management,
    185–90
  risk factors, 187
Smith, Caroline, 159–64
Smith, Emma, 237–42
social services
  child abuse assessment,
    238–40
  drug abuse assessment,
    213
  fall injuries and, 163–4
  family support for families
    with critically ill children,
    40
  foreign body aspiration, 45–6
source control
  abdominal sepsis, 188–9
  small bowel injury
    management, 182–3
Southampton and Oxford
    Retrieval Service (SORT), 1
South Thames Retrieval Service
    (STRS)
  checklists of processes and
    tasks, 4–5
  establishment of, 1–2
  Evelina PICU integration
    with, 1–2

pharmacy supplies checklist, 15–16
team performance assessment, 13–14
space occupying lesions, encephalitis, 213
Specialist Nurses for Organ Donation (SNODs), 231–2
spelling episodes, cyanosis and CHD with, 89–93
spinal cord injury without radiological abnormality (SCIWORA), fall injuries, 162–3
spinal muscular atrophy, respiratory failure, 221–6
stabilisation procedures, multidrug overdose, 243–7
Starkie, Karen, 3–18
status epilepticus, encephalopathy and, 166–8
steroids, mediastinal mass patients, 50–1
Streptococcal infection, pneumonia/empyema, 53–5
streptococcal toxic shock syndrome (STSS), 125
stridor, management guidelines for, 65–9
stylets, 21–2
subglottic stenosis
  inhalation injury, 191–2
  upper airway obstruction, 29–31
Summers, Rosalie, 299–302
superior vena cava syndrome, mediastinal mass patients, 48–51
supraglottic airway device, rescue ventilation, 20
supraglottic inhalation injury, 191–2
supraventricular tachycardia, 116–18
surgical team, abdominal sepsis and role of, 189–90
Surviving Sepsis Campaign guidelines, 124–5, 128
swallowed foreign body
  assessment and management of, 45
  small bowel obstruction risk and, 187
  vomiting with blood and, 171–7

symptom management plan, palliative care transfers, 233
systemic inflammatory response syndrome (SIRS), 124
systemic toxicity, inhalation injury, 191–2

tachycardia
  abdominal sepsis and, 185
  amiodarone treatment, 120
  DC cardioversion, 120
  differential diagnosis, 116–18
  management priorities, 118–20
  medical management, 119
  observation and test results, 116
  referral structure for assessment of, 102–3
  renal failure and, 268–9
  septic shock and, 227–9
  sickle cell crisis and, 273
  transfer indications, 120
tamponade, in cardiac arrest, 151
Tarres, Anna Canet, 171–7
team communication and management
  air retrievals and transfers, 9, 219
  briefing guidelines, 25–7
  cardiac arrest procedures, 148–53
  cessation of CPR decisions, 152–3
  collapsed neonatal referral, 259–61
  death during transfer and, 248–52
  debriefing, 27–8
  diabetic ketoacidosis and, 257–8
  haemorrhage as PEG insertion complication, 205–6
  intracranial pressure patient transfer, 157–8, 166–8
  intubation preparation, 25–8
  local referring team, 17–18
  non-accidental injury assessment, 242
  paediatric retrieval, 13–14
  palliative care transfers, 232–5

pulmonary hypertension intubation, 76–8
  retrieval team, 13–14, 16
  role assignments, 25–7
  sickle cell crisis, 275–6
  training guidelines, 16–18
  transfer crew resource management, 288–92
temperature regulation, neonatal air transfers and, 219
tension pneumothorax
  in cardiac arrest, 151–2
  chest drain insertion, 294
  ventilation emergencies, 38–40
tertiary care transfers
  complications in, 286
  encephalopathy diagnosis and management, 208–9
  extended resuscitation vs., 132–3
  foreign body aspiration, 41–3
  massive haemorrhage management and, 176
  mediastinal mass patients, 48
  Tetralogy of Fallot patients, 89–93
Tetralogy of Fallot, spelling episodes and, 89–93
The Children's Air Ambulance (TCAA), 7–8
third space fluid loss, abdominal sepsis and, 181–2, 187–8
thoracotomy, foreign body aspiration, 45
thromboprophylaxis, COVID-19 complications, 230
thrombosis, in cardiac arrest, 151–2
thrombotic thrombocytopenic purpura (TTP), 269–70
tidal volumes, asthma patient ventilation and, 72
tonic-clonic seizures, emergency management of, 154–8
Total Anomalous Pulmonary Venous Drainage (TAPVD), 81–4
  diagnosis of, 84–6
Toxbase, medication toxicity, 243–7
toxic shock, mortality from, 248–52

Toxic Shock Syndrome,
COVID-19 syndromes
and, 229–30
toxic shock syndrome (TSS),
chicken pox and, 126
toxins
cardiac arrest and, 152
encephalitis and, 213
in multidrug overdose, 243–7
tracheal obstruction, foreign
body aspiration, 41–3
tracheomalacia, Tetralogy of
Fallot patients and, 91–2
transcutaneous pacing,
congenital heart block,
107
transfer procedures. See also air
retrieval; ambulance road
transfers; ambulance
transfers; flight retrieval
and transfer
anesthestisation for, 32–3
bradycardia patients,
106–7
cardiac arrest, 148–53
cardiogenic shock patients,
97–8, 115
chemotherapeutic septic
shock, 265–6
communication protocols,
169–70
congenital heart disease
patients, 82–3, 86–7, 92–3
crew resource management
and, 288–92
croup patients, 66–8
death during, 248–52
for ECMO patients, 143–5
encephalitis patients, 214
encephalopathy diagnosis
and management, 208–9
fall injuries, 240–1
HFNC during, 221–4
intracranial pressure
patients, 156–7
ischaemic bowel patients,
187–8
medication guidelines, 15–16
metabolic condition in
collapsed neonate, 261–2
multidrug overdose, 247
paedriatic burns centre
transfers, 193–6
palliative home care transfer,
231–6
pertussis patients, 59–63

in pneumonia/empyema
shock patients, 57
pre-transfer checklist, 27–8
pulmonary hypertension,
74–8
tachycardia patients, 120
time-critical neurosurgical
transfer, 166–8
triage protocols for, 290–2
transfusion procedures, sickle
cell crisis and, 274
Transposition of the Great
Arteries (TGA), 81–3
diagnosis of, 84–6
transvenous atrial pacing,
congenital heart block,
107
trauma patients, fall injuries,
159–64, 237–42
triage protocols, transfer
procedures and, 290–2
tricyclic antidepressant
overdose, cardiac arrest
and, 152
tube size and length
intubation and, 20–1
paediatric ARDS
management, 141–3
upper airway obstruction
and, 32–3
tumour lysis, 135–40
pre-retrieval therapy, 135–8
tumour lysis syndrome (TLS),
symptoms and
management, 135–8
two-handed two-person
technique, oxygenation
and, 20

unconscious child
acute liver failure, 277–8
diagnosis and management
of, 253–8
upper airway obstruction
aetiology of, 19–20, 29–31
anesthestisation for
transport, 32–3
blood tests, 29
cannot intubate, cannot
ventilate (CICV) scenario,
33
COMET management
acronym for, 66–8
foreign body aspiration, 41–3
overview, 29–33
predictors, 24

urinary catheter, in ventilated
child, 17–18
urokinase, empyema treatment,
55–6

vaccine schedules, pertussis
and, 63–4
vagal manoeuvres,
tachycardia management
and, 119
Valle Ortiz, Juan Ramon, 272–6
Valsalva method, tachycardia
management and, 119
vancomycin, 125
Van Der Woude, Olga, 105–8
vascular access, management
of, 17–18
vasoactive drugs. See also
specific
drugsadministration
techniques, 309–10
guidelines for,
306–10
vasogenic cerebral ischaemia,
diabetic ketoacidosis,
254–5
vasopressin, guidelines for
using, 308
veno-arterial extracorporeal
membranous oxygenation
(VA-ECMO),
143–5
multidrug overdose, 246
veno-venous extracorporeal
membranous oxygenation
(VV-ECMO), paediatric
ARDS and, 129–33, 141–6
ventilation
abdominal sepsis, 182, 188–9
apnoeic episodes, 35–40
ARDS patients, 132–3
asthma management, 70–2
bradycardia and risks of,
105–6
cardiogenic shock, 113
congenital heart disease
patients, 86–7, 92
inhalation injury,
192–3
invasive ventilation, 224
mediastinal mass patients,
50–1
non-invasive, 223–4
pertussis patients, 62–3
respiratory failure, maximum
support protocols, 141–6

ventilator-induced lung injury
(VILI), mechanisms of,
141–3
ventricular-throacic pressure
gradient, in cardiogenic
shock patients, 113
ventriculo-peritoneal shunt
components of, 155
infected and blocked shunts,
155–6
seizures and, 154
video-assisted thoracostomy
surgery (VATS),
empyema, 55–6
videolaryngoscopes, 21–2
vitamin K, acute liver failure
and, 277–8

volatile anesthetics, asthma
management, 73
volume depletion, asthma
management and, 71
volume resuscitation
gastro-intestinal bleeding,
172–4
septic shock, as PEG
insertion complication,
202–6
vomiting
bilious vomiting, extended
abdomen and,
178–84
bleeding with, 171–7
inguinal hernia patients,
185–90

renal disease and,
267–71
sickle cell crisis,
272–6
V:Q mismatch, asthma patient
ventilation, 72

Waters, Gareth,
29–33
white cell count (WCC),
bronchiolitis patients,
59–64
Whitehouse, Abi,
148–53
Williams, Alex, 191–6

Yankaur suction, 21–2